THE MANAGEMENT OF THE MENOPAUSE

THE MILLENNIUM REVIEW
2000

Dedication

To Robert Benjamin Greenblatt who started it all

THE MANAGEMENT OF THE MENOPAUSE

THE MILLENNIUM REVIEW
2000

Edited by
John Studd

Chelsea & Westminster Hospital, London, UK

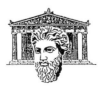

The Parthenon Publishing Group
International Publishers in Medicine, Science & Technology

NEW YORK   LONDON

Published in the USA by
The Parthenon Publishing Group Inc.
One Blue Hill Plaza, PO Box 1564,
Pearl River, New York 10965, USA

Published in the UK and Europe by
The Parthenon Publishing Group Ltd.
Casterton Hall, Carnforth,
Lancs. LA6 2LA, UK

ISSN 1460-1397

Library of Congress Cataloging in Publication Data
Data available on request

British Library Cataloguing-in-Publication Data
The management of the menopause: the millennium review
 1. Menopause   2. Age factors in disease
 I. Studd, John W. W.
 618.1'75

ISBN 1-85070-079-6

Typeset by AMA DataSet Ltd., Preston, UK
Printed and bound by Butler & Tanner Ltd., Frome and London, UK

Contents

List of principal contributors

J. S. Archer
Department of Obstetrics and Gynecology
Medical University of South Carolina
171 Ashley Avenue
Charleston
South Carolina 29425
USA

R. C. Bentley
Department of Pathology
Box 3712
Hospital South, Davidson Bldg.
Room M216a
Duke University Medical Center
Durham
North Carolina 27710
USA

M. L. Brandi
Department of Clinical Physiopathology
University of Florence
Viale Pieraccini, 6
50139 Florence
Italy

A. Cano
Department of Pediatrics, Obstetrics and
   Gynecology
Facultad de Medicina
Av. Blasco Ibéñez 17
46010 Valencia
Spain

J. Compston
Department of Medicine, Level 5
Box 157
Addenbrooke's Hospital
Cambridge CB2 2QQ
UK

C. Di Carlo
Department of Gynecology and Obstetrics
University of Naples 'Federico II'
Via Sergio Pansini, 5
80131 Naples
Italy

L. Dennerstein
Office for Gender & Health
Department of Psychiatry
The University of Melbourne
Royal Melbourne Hospital
Charles Connibere Building
Parkville
Victoria 3050
Australia

C. L. Domoney
Fertility and Research Centre
The Lister Hospital
Chelsea Bridge Road
London SW1W 8RH
UK

J. A. Eden
Royal Hospital for Women
Barker Street
Randwick
New South Wales 2031
Australia

A. R. Genazzani
Department of Reproductive Medicine and
   Child Development
Division of Obstetrics and Gynecology
University of Pisa
Via Roma 35
56100 Pisa
Italy

J. Ginsburg
Department of Medicine
Royal Free Hospital and UCL Medical School
Royal Free Campus
Pond Street
London NW3 2QG
UK

A. Glasier
Family Planning and Well Woman Services
18 Dean Terrace
Edinburgh EH4 1NL
UK

A. Graziottin
Departments of Obstetrics and Gynecology
   and Oncology
4 San Raffaele Resnati
Via San Croce 10/a
Milan
Italy

B. Lunenfeld
7 Harav Ashi Street
69395 Tel Aviv
Israel

N. Manassiev
Menopause Clinic
King's College Hospital
Denmark Hill
London SE5 9RS
UK

M. Neves-e-Castro
Clínica de Feminologia
Av. António Augusto de Aguiar
24, 2°Dto
1050-016 Lisbon
Portugal

A. Paganini-Hill
Department of Preventative Medicine
University of Southern California School of
   Medicine
1721 Griffin Avenue 205E
Los Angeles
California 90089-9680
USA

F. Petraglia
Department of Surgical Sciences
University of Udine
Piazzale Santa Maria della Misericordia
33100 Udine
Italy

A. Pines
Department of Medicine
Tel Aviv Sourasky Medical Center
6 Weizman Street
64239 Tel Aviv
Israel

R. Raz
Infectious Diseases Unit
Haemek Medical Center
18101 Afula
Israel

J.-Y. Reginster
Unité D'Exploration du Métabolisme de L'os
   et du Cartilage
University of Liege
Liege
Belgium

D. Robertson
Department of Psychological Medicine
Institute of Psychiatry
De Crespigny Park
Camberwell SE5 8AF
UK

J. Rymer
Guy's, King's and St. Thomas' Medical School
Guy's Hospital HRT Research Unit
London SE1 9RT
UK

R. H. Sands
Organon Laboratories
Cambridge
UK

H. P. G. Schneider
Department of Obstetrics and Gynecology
University of Münster
Albert-Schweitzer-Str. 33
48129 Münster
Germany

G. Söderqvist
Department of Obstetrics and Gynecology
Karolinska Hospital, Box 140
171 76 Stockholm
Sweden

J. Studd
Department of Obstetrics and Gynecology
The Lister Hospital
Chelsea Bridge Road
London SW1W 8RH
UK

A. Vashisht
Department of Obstetrics and Gynecology
The Lister Hospital
Chelsea Bridge Road
London SW1W 8RH
UK

E. Versi
Brigham & Women's Hospital
Department of Obstetrics & Gynecology
500 Brookline Avenue, Suite E
Boston
Massachusetts 02115
USA

F. Wadsworth
Department of Obstetrics and Gynecology
The Lister Hospital
Chelsea Bridge Road
London SW1W 8RH
UK

C. M. Webb
Imperial College School of Medicine
Dovehouse Street
London SW3 6LY
UK

T. Yasui
Department of Obstetrics and Gynecology
School of Medicine
University of Tokushima
Tokushima 770-8503
Japan

Introduction

For this millennium edition, it is appropriate to remember that the potential role of estrogen in the treatment of depression was first suggested 100 years ago by Easterbrook in the *British Medical Journal*. The classical paper on estrogen replacement therapy by the late and much loved Robert Greenblatt appeared 50 years ago in the *Journal of Clinical Endocrinology*. These events deserve appropriate celebration.

We have now isolated various estrogens and are far more familiar with their potential benefits and problems. We would all accept that estrogens relieve unpleasant menopausal symptoms and prevent, as well as correct, bone demineralization. Most of us will accept that there is cardiovascular protection afforded by long-term estrogen therapy and a beneficial effect upon patients at risk of stroke and Alzheimer's disease. The evidence that estrogens help depression is at last accumulating, although researchers have found it easier to measure lipids and bone density than the complexities of depressive disorders.

In spite of this, the uptake of estrogen therapy remains low, at about 15–20% of women between 50 and 60 years old, with as many as 30% discontinuing therapy within 1 year.

I believe we have all been preoccupied by the benefits of hormone replacement therapy, as well as the potential serious side-effects, such as cancer, and have failed to recognize that many women do not feel better on hormone replacement therapy. With the reappearance of periods, premenstrual syndrome and menstrual headaches, they may even feel worse. This is probably the major problem with compliance and it is a challenge for all of us not only to counsel and communicate with greater skill but to find the correct route and the correct dose of hormone therapy to enable women to feel better as well as reap the long-term benefits of hormone replacement therapy.

The non-bleeding regimens, such as continuous combined preparations, tibolone and SERMs, have to be evaluated and it is also necessary to establish the correct dose of estrogens for specific symptoms, rather than assume that the lowest possible dose is correct for all systems. If there is to be a limit to therapy of approximately 10 years because of an increasing risk of breast cancer, then we must establish whether it is best to start therapy when a woman is in her fifties or start when she is 60 years old to obtain the maximum benefits with the least side-effects. These are all exciting challenges for the future.

I am most grateful to all of the authors, many of whom were recruited with an unreasonable request to contribute within 2 or 3 months. The volume is now more international in its authorship and I hope that it will be a worthwhile text for specialists and family doctors to use in the next millennium.

John Studd, DSc, MD, FRCOG
Chelsea & Westminster Hospital
London, UK

1

Aging for men

B. Lunenfeld

In times when the changes around us are accelerating, but our perceptions of these changes are lagging behind, it becomes of crucial importance to have a vision of the future. I will therefore make an attempt to briefly review in this paper some data from the past and present, and from the lessons learned, attempt to apply these to the most likely projections for the future.

Aging is a triumph, it is a victory of human will, endurance and technology. However, as we near the millennium, new challenges are arising in relation to the lengthening life span. How do we use current and evolving technologies to impart a greater quality of life across that increasing time frame?

A rapidly growing and rapidly aging world population is a new feature in the history of mankind. The human race entered the 19th century with a global population of 978 million, the 20th century with 1650 million and will enter the 21st century with a world-wide population of 6168 million. The estimates and projections of the United Nations (UN) indicate that, between 1900 and 2100, the world population will increase seven-fold, from 1.65 billion to 11.5 billion: an increase of almost 10 billion people. This rapid increase in world population is despite the fact that effective family planning has significantly reduced fertility rates, and that the fertility rates in ten countries, including Italy, France and Germany, are today well below replacement levels (Table 1).

Due to the prolongation of life expectancy and the drastic reduction of fertility rate it is projected that the elderly (over 65 years) will increase within the next 25 years by 82%, whereas the newborn will increase by only 3%. The working age population will increase by only 46%. The UN projects (in its 1998 revision) that, by 2050, the proportion of persons above 60 will exceed, for the first time, the proportion of children below 15, and 13 countries will have more than 10% of the oldest old (> 80 years old), in their population. Italy will be leading, with 14%.

The marked increase in the population of elderly in relation to the working age population will be compounded by a simultaneous decrease in the population of children, who will comprise the working age population of the next generation. Thus a declining labor force

Table 1 Total fertility rate per woman (1990–95) and population (1995) in millions in selected European countries

Country	Total fertility rate	Population
Italy	1.24	57.2
Spain	1.27	39.6
Germany	1.30	81.6
Slovenia	1.36	1.9
Greece	1.38	10.5
Austria	1.47	8.0
Romania	1.50	22.7
Portugal	1.52	9.8
Russian Federation	1.53	148.5
Bulgaria	1.53	8.5
Switzerland	1.53	7.2
Netherlands	1.59	15.5

Reproduced with permission from ref. 17

will have to support an increasing number of elderly.

The 20th century has been marked by the triumph of prolonging life, and we have achieved an increase of life expectancy, which has increased by more than 50% in the last 100 years. The development of antibiotics, vaccines, safer water, better sanitation and better personal hygiene has defeated most infectious diseases.

Life has been prolonged, and acute disease is no longer the major cause of death. Today, one dies from chronic disease, degenerative diseases, metastatic cancer, immunodeficiencies and other diseases which prolong disability, immobility and dependency, and make dying a long, painful and expensive procedure (Figure 1). Therefore, despite the enormous medical progress during the past few decades, 25% of life expectancy after age 65 is spent with some disability, and the last years of life are accompanied by a further increase of incapacity and sickness.

Hence, we must take into account both 'life expectancy' and 'health expectancy' (Table 2). Health authorities should be encouraged to publish both these sets of data, as some already do. Frailty, disability and dependency will increase immensely the demands on the social and health services. The very high cost in relation to these services may strain to the limit the ability of health, social, and even political, infrastructures, not only of developing countries but also of the most developed and industrialized nations.

The ability to maintain independent living, free of disability, for as long as possible is a crucial factor in aging with dignity and would, furthermore, reduce health service costs significantly. The promotion of healthy aging and the prevention, or drastic reduction, of morbidity and disability of the elderly must assume a

Table 2 Life expectancy (LE) versus health expectancy (HE) in selected countries

Country	LE	HE	Difference
United States	70.1	55.5	14.6
Canada	73.0	67.0	6.0
UK	71.8	58.7	13.1
France	70.7	61.9	8.8
Poland	67.0	60.0	7.0
China	66.6	61.6	5.1

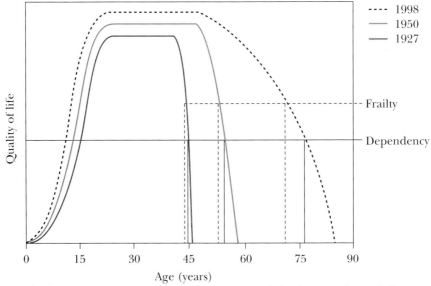

Figure 1 In 1927, the average lifespan was around 45 years and death resulted usually from acute disease. Hospitalization and/or dependency lasted for only days or, at most, weeks. In 1950, the average lifespan was about 58 years and hospitalization or dependency lasted for weeks or months. In 1999, the average lifespan is about 80 years and death results from cancer, degenerative diseases, organ failure, or immune deficiencies. Hospitalization or dependency in 1999 may last months or years

central role in the formulation of the health and social policies of many, if not all, countries in the next century. It must emphasize an all-encompassing lifelong approach to the aging process (Figure 2). If done effectively, it should result in a significant reduction of the health and social costs, reduce pain and suffering, increase the quality of life of the elderly and enable them to remain productive and continue to contribute to the well-being of society.

In contrast to the recent and much needed attention given to the social position and health status in women, the health concerns of men have been relatively neglected. Men continue to have a higher morbidity and higher mortality rate for many of the important causes of mortality, and life expectancy for men is significantly less than that for women in most regions of the world. The course of disease, response to disease and societal response to illness exhibit gender differences and often result in different treatments and different access to health care.

The major causes of morbidity and mortality all take effect over extended periods. Therefore, primary-prevention strategies will be most effective when initiated at the earliest opportunity. Prevention of ischemic heart disease, hypertension and stroke, as well as of lung cancer, needs to be addressed. When problems are more prevalent at older ages, as with prostate and colorectal cancers and osteoporosis, early diagnostic tests, such as appropriate and periodic use of laboratory tests (e.g. prostate-specific antigen) and screening procedures, can

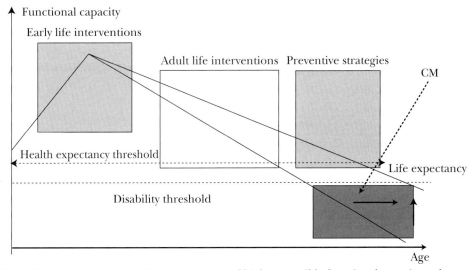

Figure 2   A life-course perspective for maintenance of highest possible functional capacity and compression of morbidity (CM). Early life interventions should be aimed at maximizing functional capacity, bone mass and optimal body composition. They must include effective vaccination, promotion of healthy lifestyle with outdoor activities, healthy nutrition and health and sex education. Adult life interventions should aim at maintaining maximal functional capacity, preventing acute diseases, including sexually transmitted disease. Such intervention must include the promotion of a healthy lifestyle, including physical activity, promotion of healthy dietary habits (preventing alcohol abuse, encouraging low fat consumption and a high-fiber diet, sufficient calcium and anti-oxidant intake, such as vitamins A, C and E). It must encourage the prevention of smoking, since 90% of all lung cancers are attributable to cigarette smoking. Preventive strategies for men over 50 years of age should aim at maintaining functional capacity, delaying 'frailty' (disability threshold) and preventing dependency for as long as possible. These strategies must include the promotion of a healthy lifestyle as described above, avoidance of obesity and control of hypertension. They must also encourage periodic comprehensive clinical screening strategies, including examination of prostate-specific antigen and digital rectal examination for prostate and colo-rectal pathologies. Last, but not least, unsafe living environments should be eliminated or at least modified. Therapeutic interventions must start as soon as a pathological process is diagnosed, and should include: control of hypertension, diabetes, osteoporosis, early interventions for benign prostate hypertrophy and urinary or fecal incontinence, hormone replacement therapy, whenever hormone deficiencies are detected, and should aim at maintaining, restoring, or improving sexual function

THE MANAGEMENT OF THE MENOPAUSE

play an important role in secondary prevention and self-care strategies.

Significant numbers of male-related health problems, such as changes in body constitution, fat distribution, muscle weakness, urinary incontinence, cognitive functioning, reduction in well-being, depression, as well as sexual dysfunction, could be detected and treated in their early stages if both physician and public awareness of these problems were more pervasive. This could effectively decrease morbidity, frailty and dependency, increase quality of life and reduce health-service costs.

When discussing age-related problems, it is often difficult to separate and to distinguish between the natural aging process and an acute or chronic illness or intercurrent diseases. It must not be forgotten that aging is associated with reduced productivity, decreased general vigor ('frailty of the aged') as well as with increased incidence of defined diseases. These include: cardiovascular diseases, malignant neoplasms, chronic obstructive pulmonary diseases, degenerative and metabolic diseases (arthritis, arthrosis, diabetes, osteoporosis, etc.), visual and hearing loss, as well as various dementias (i.e. Alzheimer's disease), anxiety and mood disorders.

Depression is the most common functional mental disorder affecting aging males; it is under-diagnosed and under-treated. It has a high rate of recurrence and is associated with significantly increased mortality. Depression is closely linked in this group with physical illness, and altered presentation can make diagnosis difficult. Thorough holistic assessment and good communication skills are of utmost importance. Nurses and medical professionals can improve the mental health of these patients with therapeutic attitudes and actions. It must be remembered that about 90% of older men who attempt or complete suicide have depression either not diagnosed or inadequately treated.

However, the most important and drastic gender differences in aging are related to the reproductive organs. In contrast to the course of reproductive aging in women, where the rapid decline in sex hormones is expressed by the cessation of menses, men experience a slow and continuous decline of a large number of hormones but do not show an irreversible arrest of reproductive capacity in old age.

In the aging male, endocrine changes and decline in endocrine function involve:

(1) Reduced secretory output from peripheral glands due to sclerosis of blood vessels (in the interstitial tissue of Leydig cells, this process contributes, for example, to a large extent to the decrease of gonadal androgens).

(2) Alterations in the central mechanism controlling the temporal organization of hormonal release. The heterogeneity in basal neuroendocrine function in aging reported in the literature is compounded by the fact that basal hormone levels are far from constant, but fluctuate considerably due to the interaction of circadian rhythmicity, sleep and, for some of the hormones, intermittent pulsatile releases at different intervals. During aging a number of morphological and neurochemical alterations have been found in the suprachiasmatic nuclei (the central circadian pacemaker) and are likely to be responsible for the dampened circadian hormonal and non-hormonal rhythms. These are, in part, responsible for the age-dependent decrease of the peripheral levels of testosterone, dehydroepiandrosterone (DHEA), growth hormone (GH), insulin-like growth factor-1 and melatonin. In addition, the increase in sex hormone binding globulin (SHBG) with age results in a further lowering of the concentrations of free biologically active androgens. Since, however, some Leydig cell function persists during aging, *stricu sensu* the andropause does not exist.

However, a growing body of literature supports the viewpoint that a true decrease in gonadal and adrenal bioavailable androgens[1–4] and in GH[5–7] develops in most aging men and this results in 'partial endocrine deficiencies'. The partial endocrine deficiency syndrome of the aging male (PEDAM) may be associated with a broad spectrum of symptoms:

(1) A decrease of general well-being;

(2) A decrease of sexual pilosity;

(3) A decrease of libido;

(4) A decrease of cognitive function;

(5) A decrease of red blood cell volume;

(6) A decrease in muscle strength;

(7) Osteoporosis;

(8) A decrease of immuno-competence;

(9) An increase of fat mass and change in fat contribution and localization;

(10) An increase in cardiovascular accidents.

Moreover, in aging men, melatonin secretion also decreases and the circadian periodicity of melatonin is gradually disrupted. Sleep in these older men is shallow and fragmented. These alterations influence GH secretion in particular, which occurs with deeper stages of sleep (slow-wave sleep)[5-7]. It has been shown that, in elderly men, the decrease in melatonin secretion and the circadian periodicity of melatonin were correlated with:

(1) Mood disorders;

(2) Decay in cognitive functions;

(3) Increase of sleep disorders;

(4) Regulation of platelet production, probably due to an inhibitory effect of melatonin on macrophage-mediated platelet destruction.

In cases of endocrine deficiencies, traditional endocrinology aims to replace the missing hormone or hormones with substitutes. It has been demonstrated that interventions, such as hormone replacement therapies and use of antioxidant drugs, may favorably influence some of the pathological conditions in aging men, by preventing the preventable and delaying the inevitable.

A comprehensive medical, psychosocial and lifestyle history, a physical examination and laboratory testing are essential for the diagnosis and management of PEDAM. Acute, chronic, or intercurrent diseases must be taken into consideration prior to initiating any hormonal

substitution therapy. Hormone substitution should only be performed by physicians with basic knowledge and clinical experience in diagnosis, treatment and monitoring of endocrine deficiencies. Evidence is available that hormone replacement therapy (HRT) reduces cardiovascular disease and osteoporosis[8-15]. In women, HRT was shown also to delay the onset of Alzheimer's disease. There is an urgent need to obtain such information in men.

Secondary Leydig cell insufficiency in the aging man can often be reversed by stimulation with human chorionic gonadotropin (hCG). But this kind of therapy is only recommended if the testosterone level doubles within 72 hours following the injection of 5000 IU of hCG. In this situation, Leydig cell function can be temporarily restored by weekly injections of 5000 IU hCG. If testosterone levels do not double within 72 hours following injection of hCG, testosterone replacement therapy should be considered (Table 3). Patients with secondary partial androgen deficiency (PADAM) who are older than 40 years of age, receiving supplemental testosterone therapy, should have a clear indication for this therapy (history, physical

Table 3 Testosterone supplementation

(1) Testosterone Depot – 250 mg/2–3 weeks (mixtures of testosterone propionate, isocaproate, decanoate, oroenanthate under development: undecanoate 1000 mg/8–10 weeks bucilate 1000 mg/12–16 weeks MENT 7α-methyl 19-nortestosterone (sustained release subdermal implants)

(2) Testosterone oral – undecanoate (160 mg daily) one tablet morning and noon and two in the evening (lymphatic absorption of this product requires it to be taken with meals) under development: sublingual testosterone cyclodextrin 2.5–5 mg twice daily

(3) Testosterone transdermal – (testosterone in a proprietary, permeation-enhancing vehicle) 2.5 mg or 5 mg patches applied nightly to the back, abdomen, upper arms, or thighs; 5 mg daily is comparable to a normal daily production rate

(4) Testosterone transscrotal – consists of a film containing natural testosterone, 1 mg daily

(5) Testosterone gels – applicable to the skin

examination, and laboratory assessment demonstrating a value of < 13 nm total testosterone, < 0.30 nmol free testosterone/ml). Testosterone therapy is also to be considered for a trial period of 12 months in men with total testosterone < 15 nm/l or where bio-available testosterone is < 10 nm/l if these levels coincide with complaints or physical evidence of androgen deficiency. Furthermore, testosterone replacement may be required in patients with a history of hepatitis, or liver cirrhosis with elevated levels of SHBG and clinical signs of androgen deficiency. Prior to initiation of testosterone therapy all patients should have a digital rectal examination and a serum prostate-specific antigen level taken; this should be repeated within 3 months following initiation of therapy. If clinical history and physical examination show improvement and there is no history of adverse effects, particularly with regard to urinary obstructive symptoms, and no significant increase in prostate-specific antigen is found, they should continue with testosterone therapy and have a digital rectal examination and a prostate-specific antigen determination, lipid profile, hemoglobin and serum calcium at yearly intervals.

Replacement therapies for secondary DHEA, GH, or melatonin deficiencies are currently under development. Within the next few years standardized indications, effective products and treatment protocols will become available.

Hormone replacement therapy will not suffice to increase muscle strength, decrease the fat mass and change the fat contribution and localization of aging men. Proper nutrition and physical exercise targeted at specific muscle groups is mandatory in order to obtain satisfactory results.

It goes without saying that a healthy lifestyle with appropriate nutrition and a healthy and safe environment are critically important in preventing or reducing morbidity and disability. An aging male counselling session will not be complete before detailed information is obtained on nutritional habits and daily food consumption. Individualized supplementation of antioxidants and vitamins will often be required in men over 50 years of age.

Patients can be counselled to start their 'own anti-aging program', to get more active, start to exercise, and lose weight if obese. This will physiologically lead to tiredness, better sleep and, consequently, to higher GH levels. Melatonin secretion will also rise, provided the patient does not sleep in front of the television or with full lights; GH secretion can also be increased by eating only small portions or nothing at all before going to bed (dinner cancelling).

Health professionals, educators and elderly men are becoming increasingly aware that libido, interest, capacity and sexual pleasure can remain throughout a lifetime. It was found that persistent interest in sexual activity results in positive mental and physical healthy benefits. Some men may become less sexually active with age. Reasons for decreased sexual activity include loss of libido (partially due to decreased androgen production), lack of partner, chronic illness and/or various social and environmental factors, as well as to erectile dysfunction. Worldwide, more than 100 million men are estimated to have some degree of erectile dysfunction. The Massachusetts Male Aging Study reported a combined prevalence of 52% for minimal, moderate and complete impotence in non-institutionalized 40–70-year-old men in the Boston area[16]. Erection is a neurovascular phenomenon under hormonal control and includes arterial dilatation, trabecular smooth muscle relaxation and activation of the corporeal veno-occlusive mechanism. Some of the major etiologies in erectile dysfunction are hypertension, diabetes and heart disease (Table 4). Also, genitourinary and colon surgery, as well as many drugs, particularly antihypertensive and psychotropic drugs, may cause

Table 4 Erectile dysfunction: incidence (taken from the Massachusetts Male Aging Study)

Population	New cases/1000 men per year
General	26.0
Hypertension	42.5
Diabetes	50.7
Heart disease	58.3

various degrees of erectile dysfunction. When focusing on the maintenance of quality of life among aging men, efforts to maintain, restore, or improve sexual function should not be neglected. Recent advances of basic and clinical research has led to the development of new treatment options for erectile dysfunction, including new pharmacological agents for intra-cavernosal, intraurethral and oral use (Table 5). The management of erectile dysfunction should only be performed following proper evaluation of the patient and only by physicians with basic knowledge and clinical experience in the diagnosis and treatment of erectile dysfunction.

Men who are educated about the role that preventive health care can play in prolonging their lifespan, and improving their quality of life and their role as productive family members, will be more likely to participate in health screening. To obtain this goal it will be necessary to make available a group of trained medical professionals who can understand, guide, educate and manage the problems of the aging male.

Furthermore, there is a need to obtain the essential epidemiological data to intensify basic and clinical research and to develop new and improved drugs for prevention and treatment of the pathological changes related to aging.

A holistic approach to this new challenge of the 21st century will necessitate a quantum leap

Table 5 Medical management of erectile dysfunction: the revolution!

1982 Virag, the first injection
1986 use of prostaglandin E1
1995 Caverject in the market
1996 MUSE in the market
1998 Sildenafil in the market
Vasomax-

In development:
  Oral phentolamine
  Spontane – oral apomorphine
  Prostaglandin creams
  New phosphodiesterase inhibitors of isoenzymes
  New drug acting on different levels of the
    erectile mechanism
  Topical treatment
  Gene (cell) therapy

in multidisciplinary and internationally co-ordinated research efforts, supported by a new partnership between industry, governments and philanthropic and international organizations.

It is my sincere hope that the next few years will provide us with more facts and clarify the state of our present knowledge, permitting us to recognize some of the missing links and giving us the tools and methodology to design and plan ways to understand the aging of men, allowing us to help to improve the quality of life, prevent the preventable, and postpone and decrease the pain and suffering of the inevitable.

References

1. Gooren LJG. Endocrine aspects of aging in the male. *Mol Cell Endocrinol* 1998;145:153–9
2. Vermeulen A. Some reflections on the endocrinology of the aging male. *Aging Male* 1998; 3:163–9
3. Gooren LJG. Androgen levels and sex functions in testosterone-treated hypogonadal men. *Arch Sex Behav* 1987;16:463–73
4. Martin *et al. Baillier's Clinical Endocrinology and Metabolism, Endocrinology of Aging* 1997;11:223–50
5. Gray A, Feldman HA, McKinlay JB, Longcope C. Age, disease, and changing sex hormone levels in middle-aged men: results of the Massachusetts Male Aging Study. *J Clin Endocrinol Metab* 1991;73: 1016–25
6. Copinschi G, Van Cauter E. Effects of ageing on modulation of hormonal secretion by sleep and circadian rhythmicity. *Horm Res* 1995;43:20–4
7. Holl R, Hartman M, Veldhuis J, Taylor W, Thorner M. Thirty-second sampling of plasma

growth hormone in man. Correlation with sleep stages. *J Clin Endocrinol Metab* 1991;72:854–61

8. Van Cauter E, Kerhofs M, Caufriez A, Van Onderbergen A, Thorner MO, Copinschi G. A quantitative estimation of growth hormone secretion in normal men; reproducibility and relation to sleep and time of day. *J Clin Endocrinol Metab* 1992;74:1441–50

9. Katznelson L, Finkelstein JS, Schoenfield DA, Rosenthal DI, Anderson EJ, Klibanski A. Increase in bone density and lean body mass during testosterone administration in men with acquired hypogonadism. *J Clin Endocrinol Metab* 1996;81: 4358–65

10. Behre HM, Kliesch S, Leifke E, Link TM, Nieschlag E. Long-term effects of testosterone on bone mineral density in hypogonadal men. *J Clin Endocrinol Metab* 1997;82:2386–90

11. Tremblay RR, Morales A. Canadian practice recommendations for screening, monitoring and treating men affected by andropause or partial androgen deficiency. *Aging Male* 1998;1: 213–18

12. Boonen S, Vanderschueren D, Cheng XG, *et al.* Age-related (type II) femoral neck osteoporosis in men: biochemical evidence for both hypovitaminosis D- and androgen deficiency-induced bone resorption. *J Bone Mineral Res* 1997;12: 2119–26

13. Vanderschueren D. Androgens and their role in skeletal homeostasis. *Horm Res* 1996;46:95–8

14. Vanderschueren D, Boonen S. Androgen exposure and the maintenance of skeletal integrity in aging men. *Aging Male* 1998;1:180–7

15. Wu SZ, Weng XZ. Therapeutic effects of an androgenic preparation on myocardial ischemia and cardiac function in 62 elderly male coronary heart disease patients. *Chin Med J* 1998;106: 415–41

16. Feldman HA, Goldstein I, Hatzichristou DG, Krane RJ, McKinlay JB. Impotence and its medical psychological correlates: results of the Massachusetts Male Aging Study. *J Urol* 1994;151:54–61

17. Lunenfeld B. Hormone replacement therapy in the aging male. *Aging Male* 1999;2:1–5

2

Assessing well-being in menopausal women

H. P. G. Schneider, B. Schultz-Zehden, H. P. Rosemeier and H. M. Behre

INTRODUCTION

In recent years, there has been a growing awareness of the aspects of quality of life and aging. By definition, quality of life is a subjective parameter and direct questioning is therefore a simple and appropriate way of accruing information about how patients feel and function. The health-related quality of life measures, whatever their theoretical basis, are generated from subjective responses and open to substantial methodological criticism and are often performed with less quantitative rigor[1]. Using standard questionnaires, however, does ensure that these psychometric properties are well documented. For routine use in clinical practice or in clinical trials, it is essential that the instruments employed are simple and comparatively short. To the medical personnel involved, a critical question has always been whether or not psychological studies upset patients. However, it has been shown that the majority of patients or probands welcome the opportunity to report how symptoms and their subsequent treatment affect daily life[2]. Psychometrically evaluated questionnaires allow uniform administration and unbiased quantification of data, as the response options are pre-determined and thus equal for all respondents[1]. A core set of questionnaires would allow the comparison of study results and patient populations. Increasingly, the emphasis has been on self-administered questionnaires. Certain aspects, e.g. that interviewed individuals, particularly of older age, might have difficulty with reading or writing, or being exposed to interviewers of varying experience, or simply the expenses involved in gathering quality of life data, may act together to produce bias to interpretation. Standardization, compatibility, lack of bias and economy therefore are important aspects of the validity in any type of quality of life assessment.

METHODOLOGICAL CONSIDERATIONS

The administration of health-related quality of life instruments deserves the same scrutiny and attention as the measurement of physiological outcomes. Random and representative samples of the population should be investigated in sufficient numbers and over prolonged periods of time. As far as statistics are concerned, quality of life is, by definition, a multi-state attribute. The use of many measures in the multiple statistical tests reduces the statistical power of the analysis[3]. Health-related quality of life certainly is a multi-dimensional concept; there is a continuing debate on whether or not the aggregation of several dimensions into a summary index is appropriate. A summary score may falsely suggest improvement in one vital area and conceal deterioration in another[3]. Indices however are practical and are a convenient method of information transfer.

HEALTH-RELATED QUALITY OF LIFE IN MENOPAUSE – A DEFINITION

Results obtained from an increasing number of controlled clinical studies indicate that hormone replacement therapy could substantially improve patients' quality of life. Specific questionnaires were recognized as important tools for complete evaluation of treatment effects. Health-related quality of life designates a multi-dimensional psychological construct which includes at least three important components: the physical, emotional and social functioning as main determinants for quality of life. Assessing the impact of a condition on quality of life is particularly relevant in symptomatic conditions such as the menopause. One cause of the growing importance of all aspects of personal well-being and quality of life has been a paradigmatic change in the definition of health. The main reasons for this change can be listed as follows:

(1) The World Health Organisation definition besides somatic aspects also covers the psychological and social components of health;

(2) Demographic variation with a growing population of elderly and the associated incremental chronic illness; a newly defined appropriate goal is to have healthy and independent elders who maintain physical and cognitive function as long as possible;

(3) Rather than looking at classical therapeutic targets, such as reduction of symptoms or extension of life-time, the best health strategies to incremental chronic illness are rather defined as a change of the slope or the rate at which illness develops, thus postponing the clinical illness, and if it is postponed long enough, effectively preventing it.

The methods for postponing illness are obvious to all of us: exercise, elimination of cigarette smoking, discipline over excessive alcohol consumption, elimination of obesity, and – particularly in the elderly – a sense of personal choice in dealing with individual problems. In order to improve the individual sense of controlling health as affected by aging, quality of life assessment becomes more and more important. Monitoring variations in physical, emotional and social life parameters as indicators of improvement of quality of life and general well-being is also important for the discussion of cost-effectiveness of new therapeutic strategies targeted to reduce morbidity in the elderly.

ASSESSMENT OF QUALITY OF LIFE – IN GENERAL AND IN THE CLIMACTERIC

Various instruments have been developed for measuring quality of life. There are two basic types of questionnaire, generic and disease- or treatment-specific. Although quality of life may be defined in different ways, the contents of the different generic scales show many similarities, assessing the ability of patients to cope with their condition physically, emotionally and socially as well as their general performance at work and in daily life[4]. Among the more commonly used instruments are the Sickness Impact Profile[5], the Nottingham Health Profile[6], Quality of Well-being Scale[7], or the Short Form (SF)-36 Health Survey[8]. The generic measures cover the multi-dimensional aspects of quality of life in a wide range of health problems, they might be less responsive to treatment-induced changes, and may be lengthy and time-consuming.

The disease-specific measures are more likely to be responsive and make sense to clinicians as well as to patients. Their specific measures relate to concepts and domains in patient populations, diagnostic groups, or diseases. One of the very first was the Women's Health Questionnaire (WHQ)[9], a menopause-specific instrument. The Women's Health Questionnaire consists of 37 items including nine scales, and it assesses, in addition to vasomotor symptoms, important areas such as other somatic symptoms, mood, sleep problems, cognitive difficulties and sexual functioning.

Other test systems and questionnaires refer to psychiatric problems (e. g. Beck Depression Scale[10]), pain scores, sleep disturbances, sexual dysfunction, mental and cognitive function. A description of the merits and shortcomings of the different tools is presented elsewhere[11].

THE BERLIN STUDIES

Sample

As a first step, we analyzed a group of 230 women living in the city of Berlin, Germany. We contacted the co-operating women via their general practitioners, provided that they had not asked for their consultation because of menopausal complaints. This sample served the purpose of a pilot study on psychosocial aspects of menopausal transition. The age of the subjects ranged from 45 to 55 years. Our second study in 1996 involved 603 participants nationwide and is representative for the Federal Republic of Germany. The age of these women ranged from 47 to 59 years. Their menopausal status was 67% postmenopausal, 31% pre- or perimenopausal; 14% were nulliparous, the parous women had an average of 1.7 children. The marital status showed 61% to be married, 15% divorced, 7% unmarried and 13% already widows. Their level of education was 49% basic, 33% moderate and 16% higher, and professional status 67% in jobs, 10% unemployed and 22% working at home or retired.

Methods

As a basic instrument for quantification of menopausal symptoms in both of our studies we applied the Menopause Rating Scale (see below; ref 12; Schneider and colleagues submitted for publication). For personality identification in our Berlin sample, we used the Freiburg Personality Inventory, widely acknowledged and evaluated in Germany, and a projective sentence-accomplishing technique. The returns were

Table 1 Subscales to the Berlin Menopause Questionnaire

Depressive moods: 'I live in constant worry'
Re-orientation: 'A new life period starts for me'
Sleeping disorders: 'At night, I lie awake'
Irritability: 'When I get frustrated, I cannot control myself'
Problem-free: 'I have no problems with menopause'
Self-esteem: 'I am happy with myself'
Exhaustion: 'I have no energy'
Quality of relationship: 'My partner relationship is trustful'

analyzed as material for the evaluation of well-being in menopausal women. Attitudes of the women towards menopause could be transformed into items and scales of well-defined diagnostic quality. The scales of this Berlin Menopause Questionnaire have been factor-analyzed and evaluated on the nationwide German representative sample of $n = 603$[13].

Results

Our Berlin pilot study in 1994 with 230 women provided psychosocial determinants of menopausal symptoms such as lack of social support, deficit in self-esteem and stressful re-orientation. Based on these results, we developed an item-catalog of psychosocial variables which supposedly influence well-being during menopause. The questionnaire contained 90 items within 13 psychosocial domains. Eight scales were characterized as a result of factor analysis (Table 1).

The first four scales relate to complaints such as depressive mood, sleeping disorders, irritability and exhaustion. Furthermore, the instrument records women's self-confidence, quality of partner relationship, re-orientation initiated by menopause, as well as the absence of menopause-related problems. Based on this information, we developed a validated test instrument consisting of 32 items creating individual profiles of coping and quality of life in menopause conditions.

Perceived positive effects of menopause

According to their own appraisals, menopause occurs subtly in 80% of the women, with no apparent loss in quality of life. Two out of five women emphasized the physical reliefs of menopause with a resultant general improvement in well-being (Figure 1). Rather than interrogating detailed climacteric complaints, the test asked about joy of living and quality of life items. Sixty-two per cent of our probands reported positive attributions to menopause itself. In all, 78% of women looked on the interview experience as a way in which to more consciously handle their life than previously.

Menopause is a critical transition in a woman's life not only because of biological changes, but also because of the co-occurring social and psychological alterations during midlife. Very often, psychosocial reliefs are not remembered as positive aspects during the perimenopause. The fact that children are often leaving home around the mother's menopause is predominantly associated with a loss ('empty nest syndrome'). In the psychoanalytical literature on menopause the 'empty nest syndrome', mental depression and the feeling of no longer being in command of reproductive abilities are generally stressed. In contrast to this general assumption, women in our study pointed to the advantages of greater personal independence. Only 20% of women in our sample complained of empty nest symptoms, pointing to different attitudes in the younger generation; they also felt strong relief from menstrual problems, premenstrual syndrome, contraceptional obligations and the pregnancy complications of older age (Figure 1).

With increasing age, the quality of their sexual life was of growing importance. Tender loving care was a dominant issue for 75% of the women.

Psychosocial factors associated with well-being

In a cluster analysis of the Berlin Study, we found three types of menopausal coping styles.

In a first cluster were the pragmatic women, a more or less problem-free group of 37% with discrete menopausal complaints, but good self-esteem level, regarding themselves as attractive. They neglected to be seriously affected by menopausal changes. It is possible that this pragmatic group has a repressor coping strategy and shield the occurring symptoms with self-discipline.

The majority of the women (75%) stated no loss of their attractiveness. Women who thought themselves to be attractive showed fewer menopausal symptoms. With increasing age, this positive individual body image seemed to modify. The results of a study in 1997[13] with

1000 postmenopausal women (aged 50–70) are depicted in Table 2.

Women with a low self-esteem scored much higher in the Menopause Rating Scale in all of our studies (Figure 2). A very important finding was the high correlation between personal professional activity and a quantified low degree of menopausal complaints.

The positive feedbacks of health-promoting behavior need to be emphasized. Regular exercise correlated significantly with high self-confidence and with fewer menopausal complaints.

In our study, 50% of the women experienced a re-orientation process in their life, initiated by

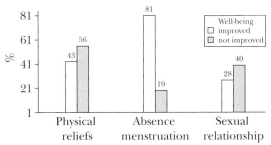

Figure 1 Individual perception of positive effects of menopausal age; $n = 531$

Table 2 Age-related perception of body

Feature	Postmenopausal women aged 50–70 years (%) ($n = 1038$)
Drop in efficiency	49
Figure changes	39
Gain in weight	35
Skin slackness	35
Get wrinkles	30
Decrease in attraction	13

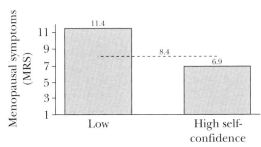

Figure 2 Self-confidence and well-being in menopausal women; $n = 531$, ***$p < 0.001$, m = 8.4

the menopause and with the consequence of arranging a change of life-style.

A trend towards a creative form of re-orientation dominated. Those subjects presenting with a high level of positive re-orientational motives in the questionnaire were the ones with a lower level of psychological complaints (Menopause Rating Scale). This group of women looked forward to new perspectives in their individual lives. Another group considered themselves forced towards a form of re-orientation which was not dominated by their own intentions. Here we found a correlation with high levels of psychological complaints (Figure 3).

A further predictor for a relatively problem-free menopause was a satisfactory partner relationship. The importance of a stable relationship and of a secure social net was clearly evident. The personal relationship and its quality were of increasing impact during midlife. Women without partners scored both low and high levels of menopausal complaints on the Menopause Rating Scale. When the group with partners was asked about the quality of their partnerships, those who were dissatisfied were

also those who suffered more complaints (Figure 4).

In summing up the Berlin experience, important sequelae for the understanding of well-being in menopausal women are the women's self-confidence, the quality of their partner relationship and the re-orientation process initiated by the menopause or by their psychosocial condition. Good self-confidence is a predictor for successful coping. A satisfying relationship and social network improve quality of life. Employment is confirmed as a protective factor. Furthermore, there are several physical and psychosocial reliefs which have to be considered in the assessment of well-being in menopausal women. Introducing these variables into the interaction between a woman and her counseling doctor would allow us to predict a better co-operation and a higher degree of compliance.

MENOPAUSE RATING SCALE

In 1996, a questionnaire was completed by a representative random sample of 683 German women aged 40–60 years in order to evaluate the newly established Menopause Rating Scale[12,14]. A follow-up investigation was organized one and a half years later including the same women who had participated in 1996. The purpose was to identify those conditions relevant to the individual rating (Schneider and co-workers, submitted for publication). The Menopause Rating Scale is a self-administered standardized questionnaire for complaints in menopausal women (Table 3). The majority

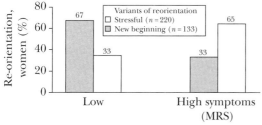

Figure 3 Re-orientation and well-being in menopausal women

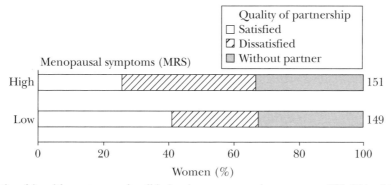

Figure 4 Relationship with partner and well-being in menopausal women; $n = 536$, $**p < 0.01$

Table 3 Menopause Rating Scale (MRS)

| | Degree of severity | | | |
| | None (no point) | Mild (1 point) | Moderate (2 points) | Severe (3 points) |
Items				
Hot flushes, sweating				
Anxiety				
Sleep disorders				
Irritability				
Depressive mood				
Heart symptoms				
Exhaustion				
Muscle and joint pain				
Sexual complaints				
Urinary symptoms				
Vaginal dryness				
Score $\Sigma \leq 33$ points				

of women demonstrated a stable level of complaints over the period of observation. The mean change of the Menopause Rating Scale scores was 2 points at follow-up. Differences occurred with changes in health status. The Menopause Rating Scale scores varied mainly with co-morbidity such as cardiac failure, chest pain, chronic gastrointestinal problems, rheumatoid/muscle complaints or others and produced differences up to 5 Menopause Rating Scale scoring points on average. The variation over time was similar across various degrees of severity and menopausal complaints. The Menopause Rating Scales scores also varied with medications such as hormone replacement therapy, phyto-hormones and psychotropic drugs.

Menopause complaints and quality of life

As of their fifth decade, women will experience a loss of quality of life. One of the most widely accepted measurement systems is the Short Form-36 Health Survey which depicts generic health concepts relevant across age, disease and treatment groups. It provides a comprehensive, psychometrically sound, and efficient way to measure health from the patient's point of view by scoring standardized responses to standardized questions. The SF-36 was constructed to represent eight of the most important health concepts. These are listed in Table 4.

The SF-36 includes eight multi-item scales containing two to ten items each, and a single-item measure of reported health transition that is not used to score any of the eight multi-item scales. Within our Menopause Rating Scale follow-up survey, quality of life was measured over age groups (Schneider and colleagues, submitted for publication). Figure 5 depicts physical functioning and psychological well-being as typical examples. The segment of physical functioning, at younger age, starts from a very high level and from 40 years and older will drop considerably. This loss of quality is not continuous over all age groups. A loss of psychological well-being with progressing age is much less pronounced. The complete eight multi-item scales of the Short Form-36 have been analyzed across age groups in the same cohort of Menopause Rating Scale-investigated women (Figure 6). The age groups comprise all women aged 40–49 years and 50–59 years. This graph demonstrates the eight Short Form-36 scales on the horizontal axis. The dimensions of the Short Form-36 profile are arranged in such a way that physical scales are shown to the left and psychological scales to the right side of the horizontal axis. Higher scores on the vertical axis relate to better quality of life. The course of the two profiles is characteristic for many studies in the literature. There is a trend for lower quality of life profiles in the older age group, which is more pronounced in the segment of physical

Table 4 Health concepts, number of items and levels, summary of content for eight Short Form-36 scales and the health transition item

Concepts	Number of items	Number of levels	Summary of content
Physical functioning (PF)	10	21	Extent to which health limits physical activities such as self-care, walking, climbing stairs, bending, lifting and moderate and vigorous exercises
Role functioning – physical (RP)	4	5	Extent to which physical health interferes with work or other daily activities, including accomplishment less than wanted, limitations in the kind of activities, or difficulty in performing activities
Bodily pain (BP)	2	11	Intensity of pain and effects of pain on normal work, both inside and outside the home
General health (GH)	5	21	Personal evaluation of health, including current health, health outlook and resistance to illness
Vitality (VT)	4	21	Feeling energetic and full of pep versus feeling tired and worn out
Social functioning (SF)	2	9	Extent to which physical health or emotional problems interfere with normal social activities
Role functioning – emotional (RE)	3	4	Extent to which emotional problems interfere with work or other daily activities, including decreased time spent on activities, accomplishing less, and not working as carefully as usual
Mental health (MH)	5	26	General mental health, including depression, anxiety, behavioral–emotional control, general positive affect
Reported health transition (HT)	1	5	Evaluation of current health compared to 1 year ago

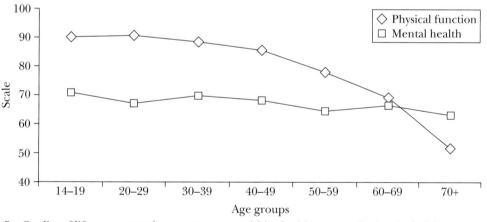

Figure 5 Quality of life as measured over age groups within the Menopause Rating Scale follow-up survey

functioning. The biggest differences are seen with the concepts of physical functioning (PF) and role functioning – physical (RP). On the other hand, vitality (VT), social functioning (SF), role functioning – emotional (RE) and mental health (MH) differ only slightly between age groups.

In order to depict the relation of menopausal complaints with quality of life more clearly, we looked at the Short Form-36 scores in the three, Menopausal Rating Scale degrees of severity, slight, moderate and severe (Figure 7). There was a striking difference in quality of life between groups of women with different degrees of menopausal complaints as compared to the variation seen between age groups. Moreover, loss of quality of life was maximal in women with severe menopausal symptoms, less

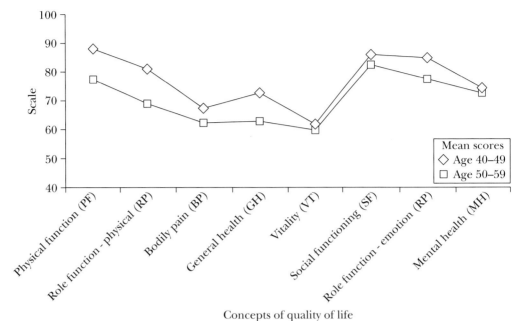

Figure 6   Analysis of the complete eight multi-item scales of the Short Form-36 across age groups in the cohort of Menopause Rating Scale investigated women

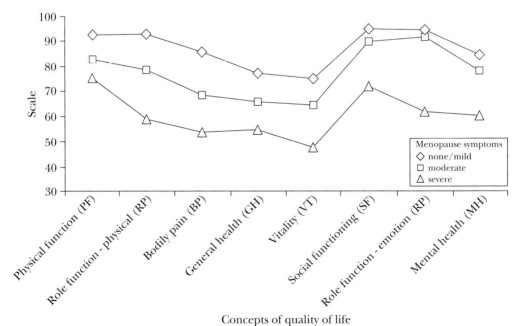

Figure 7   Short Form-36 scores in relation to the three Menopause Rating Scale degrees of severity

pronounced in those with moderate symptoms and just subtly apparent in the slight Menopause Rating Scale scorers. These differences are most evident in the Short Form-36 concepts role functioning – physical (RP), bodily pain (BP), vitality (VT) and role functioning – emotional (RE).

DISCUSSION

Our data clearly demonstrate a striking dependence of the Menopause Rating Scale classification of menopausal symptoms on the quality of life. Aging, on the other hand, has a much smaller impact on menopausal symptoms. However, the interpretation of these phenomena should be done with caution as women with a low quality of life might sense their menopausal symptoms more profoundly than would women with high levels of quality of life. In other words, a good quality of life may be protective against the clinical manifestation of menopausal symptoms. However, such causal interpretations of close correlations on the basis of population studies need further periods of longitudinal observation.

Hormone replacement therapy leads to a major improvement in quality of life for women with menopausal symptoms. A well-defined menopausal complaint rating scale may serve as a less troublesome, practical and less time-consuming instrument with which to investigate the impact of treatment on various aspects of quality of life and at the same time avoid wide-range batteries of questionnaires with their draw-backs in practicability.

References

1. Wiklund, I. Methods of assessing the impact of climacteric complaints on quality of life. *Maturitas* 1998;29:41–50
2. Fallowfield L, Baum M, Maguire GP. Do psychological studies upset patients? *J R Soc Med* 1987; 80:59
3. Fletcher AE, Gore S, Jones D, *et al.* Quality of life measures in health care. II: Design, analysis and interpretation. *Br Med J* 1992;305:1145–8
4. Fitzpatrick R, Fletcher A, Gose S, *et al.* Quality of life measures in health care. I: applications and issues in assessment. *Br Med J* 1992;305: 1074–7
5. Bergner M. Development, use and testing of the Sickness Impact Profile. In Walker S, Rosser M, eds. *Quality of Life Assessment: Key Issues in the 1990s.* Dordrecht: Kluwer Academic Press, 1993; 201–9
6. Hunt SM, McKenna SP, McEwen J, *et al.* The Nottingham Health Profile: Subjective health and medical consultations. *Soc Sci Med* 1981;15A: 221–9
7. Kaplan RM, Anderson JP, Ganiats T. The Quality of Wellbeing Scale: rationale for a single quality of life index. In Walker S, Rosser M, eds. *Quality of Life Assessment: Key Issues in the 1990's.* Dordrecht: Kluwer Academic Press, 1993;65
8. McHorney CA, Ware JE, Raczek AE. The MOS 36-item Short-Form health status survey (SF-36): II. Psychometric and clinical tests of validity in measuring physical and mental health constructs. *Med Care* 1993;31:247–63
9. Hunter M. The Women's Health Questionnaire (WHQ): a measure of mid-aged women's perceptions of their emotional and physical health. *Psychology and Health* 1992;7:45–54
10. Beck AP. *Depression: Clinical, Experimental and Therapeutic Aspects.* New York: Harper and Row, 1967
11. Wiklund I, Dimenäs E, Wahl M. Factors of importance when evaluating quality of life in clinical trials. *Control Clin Trials* 1990;11:169–79
12. Hauser GA, Huber JC, Keller PJ, Lauritzen C, Schneider HPG. Evaluation der klimakterischen Beschwerden (Menopause Rating Scale [MRS]). *Zentralbl Gynakol* 1994;116:16–23
13. Schultz-Zehden B. *FrauenGesundheit in und nach den Wechseljahren. Die 1000 Frauenstudie.* Gladenbach: Verlag Kempkes, 1998
14. Schneider HPG, Dören M. Traits for long-term acceptance of hormone replacement therapy – results of a representative German survey. *Eur Menopause J* 1996;3:94–8

3

Relative and absolute contraindications to hormone replacement therapy

J. Rymer

INTRODUCTION

Despite the proven long-term benefits of hormone replacement therapy (HRT), adherence remains poor. Why are women not taking HRT? Is it because we are not succeeding with the initial consultation, or is it because the contraindications preclude the majority of women? One approach to improve adherence may be to concentrate more on the first consultation covering benefits of long-term therapy, and be quite clear as to which women have contraindications to HRT.

ADHERENCE

Whether or not women take HRT and continue to take it depends on many factors, and these relate to the patient, the doctor, the medication itself, and other factors, e.g. media, friends.

Women who consult are a different population from those who do not. They are therefore a self-chosen group and their motivation for consultation is influenced by their health beliefs and many may perceive menopause as a natural process and not one requiring medication. Their previous experience of medication is influential as are their concerns about possible side-effects or risks of medication.

With regard to the doctor, the direction of the consultation will depend on his knowledge of the subject, his confidence and competence, and his ability to negotiate and agree a management strategy with the patient. The doctor–patient interaction can be described as the push–pull effect. The physician's willingness to prescribe hormones (the push effect) and the woman's desire to use them (the pull effect).

With regard to the medication itself, adherence would be dependent on the perceived benefits, tolerability and convenience of the medication, the side-effects that it may produce and the cost.

Other factors include what the woman has heard or read in the media, and what her relatives and friends have experienced and advised. Therefore, if we are to improve adherence, in the initial consultation we need to clearly state the long-term benefits of HRT, discuss possible side-effects and talk about possible long-term risks. With regard to the latter, we need to be clear as to which patients are at risk.

CONTRAINDICATIONS TO HRT

Hartmann and Huber in 1997 published an article *The Mythology of Hormone Replacement Therapy*[1]. In this article they evaluated the literature on contraindications to HRT contained in the pharmaceutical data-sheets of five currently available estrogen replacement preparations. These contraindications included cardiovascular disease, diabetes, liver diseases, otosclerosis, endometriosis, melanoma and hormone-dependent tumors. They showed that the contraindications had been taken from the data-sheets of oral contraceptives, despite the fact that oral contraceptives use alkylestrogens, which are very different from the esterized or micronized estrogens used in HRT. They concluded that the information in the pharmaceutical data-sheets of HRT regimens should be modified as it influences how these medications are prescribed by doctors, as well as affecting patient adherence. This brings us to one of the major influences on why adherence with HRT is so poor. Once a woman is prescribed HRT, one of the first things she does is read the data-sheet contained in the drug packaging. The result is shocking to any lay person as the side-effects listed are endless and the list of contraindications is enormous. Therefore, women become frightened and are reluctant to commence the medication. If they do commence HRT, as soon as they experience anything that may be interpreted as a side-effect, e.g. headache, then they discontinue the drug. This incorrectly frightens women (not to mention their litigation-sensitive physicians) and we must be clear that the pharmaceutical data-sheets are wrong. It is important to remember that the data-sheets are mainly describing the side-effects of the alkylestrogens rather than the esterized and micronized estrogens, which have quite different pharmacological characteristics. We must therefore distinguish between oral contraceptives and HRT preparations.

ABSOLUTE CONTRAINDICATIONS

The list of absolute contraindications is small and is listed in Table 1.

Pregnancy

It would be inappropriate to give exogenous hormones after conception unless ovum donation had occurred.

Active venous thromboembolism

Until the acute episode is over and the appropriate investigations have been performed then HRT would be inappropriate.

Severe active liver disease

Assuming that this was an acute event it would be prudent to wait until liver function had normalized before prescribing HRT.

Endometrial and breast carcinoma with recurrence

Strictly speaking these both should be absolute contraindications, although quality of life must be taken into account and each case should be dealt with on an individual basis.

RELATIVE CONTRAINDICATIONS

Relative contraindications are listed in Table 2.

Abnormal vaginal bleeding

This must be fully investigated prior to commencing HRT.

Breast lump

It would be unwise to commence HRT without completing full investigation of a breast lump.

Table 1   Absolute contraindications to hormone replacement therapy

Pregnancy
Active venous thromboembolism
Severe active liver disease
Endometrial carcinoma with recurrence
Breast carcinoma with recurrence
Patient does not want it

Table 2   Relative contraindications to hormone replacement therapy

Abnormal vaginal bleeding
Breast lump (prior to investigation)
Previous endometrial cancer
Previous breast cancer
Strong family history breast cancer
Previous venous thromboembolism
Family history of thromboembolism

Previous endometrial carcinoma

If the original disease was early stage and there was complete surgical resection then there is no contraindication to HRT. If there was incomplete resection or evidence of recurrence then this would, strictly speaking, be an absolute contraindication and the risks would have to be weighed up against quality of life.

Previous breast cancer

If there was early Stage I disease, presumably cured by the initial treatment, or in women who were hormone-receptor-negative, then the benefits outweigh the risks. The remaining cases are controversial because of the high incidence of late recurrence. In each case one needs to individualize treatment and ensure that the patient is aware of the benefits and risks so that she is able to make the ultimate decision for herself.

Breast cancer patients may be at particular risk of developing estrogen-deficient symptoms because, not only may they undergo a natural menopause, but they may have hot flushes secondary to tamoxifen or have ovarian castration either surgically induced or by radiotherapy or chemotherapy. This means that they may have an acute onset of severe flushes, significantly affecting their quality of life.

Strong family history of breast cancer

If a woman has two or more first-degree relatives with breast cancer under the age of 45, then she should be referred for genetic counselling to test for *BRCA1* and *BRCA2* genes. Depending on the outcome of the genetic testing, the decision for HRT would be much easier.

Previous venous thromboembolism

Previously, HRT was not considered to be associated with venous thromboembolism (VTE)[2]. However, recent case–control studies have shown an increase in the relative risk of VTE in women on HRT. One study from the United States, which was a population-based, nested, case–control study, showed that women with idiopathic VTE had a matched relative risk estimate for VTE of 3.6 (95% CI 1.6–7.8) for current users of estrogen compared to non-users. The absolute risk was estimated at 9 per 100 000 women per year in non-users compared to 32 per 100 000 per year in users[3]. A UK study, which was a hospital-based, case–control study, looked at women in the 45–64-year-old age group with idiopathic VTE and they found the adjusted odds ratio for current users of HRT compared to non-users to be 3.5 (95% CI 1.8–7.0). Furthermore, the risk appeared to be highest among short-term current users. The estimate of absolute risk was 11 per 100 000 women per year for non-users and 27 per 100 000 women per year for current users[4]. The general practice research database in the UK performed a population-based, case–control study and found an adjusted odds ratio of VTE for current users of 2.1 (95% CI 1.4–3.2) relative to non-users. This study also showed the increase in risk was restricted to the first year of use with odds ratio of 4.6 (95% CI 2.5–8.4) during the first 6 months[5].

An analysis of the nurses cohort study estimated the adjusted relative risk of primary pulmonary embolism to be 2.1 (95% CI 1.2–3.8) for current users[6]. All these studies seem to agree that there is an increased relative risk of VTE with HRT in the order of three times, although the absolute risk is low.

At the time of ovarian failure there are marked changes in the coagulation system, and these include an increase in factor VII and fibrinogen which are known risk factors for vascular disease. If exogenous estrogen is given there are changes in the coagulation system, including a reduction in fibrinogen, factor VII, antithrombin and enhanced fibrinolysis. This produces a mixed profile as some factors are associated with a reduction and others with an increase in thrombotic risk. Therefore it seems unlikely that these changes on their own are responsible for the increased risk of VTE. These studies also suggested that the increase in risk was restricted to the first year of use and this suggests that HRT may be unmasking a congenital thrombophilia. It appears that more genetic defects are associated with thrombotic problems and affect a significant proportion of the population. These genetic defects include antithrombin deficiency, protein C deficiency, protein S deficiency, factor V Leiden, pro-thrombin gene variant and hyperhomo-cysteinemia. The prevalence of antithrombin, protein C and protein S deficiencies in European populations is low, in the order of 2 to 5.5 per 1000. However, they comprise 10% of women who have a past history of VTE. Factor V Leiden is more common. The heterozygote gene frequency in the population is 2–15% in Western countries and an investigation of patients with VTE has found an underlying frequency of 20–60%. This thrombophilic defect manifests itself as a resistance to activated protein C which is the endogenous anticoagulant directed against factor VA and factor VIIIA. Interestingly, there has been an association with pregnancy and the pill, with 59% of women with VTE in pregnancy and over 30% of women with VTE on the pill being found to be resistant to activated protein C.

In practice, what could the management be? In a woman who has a past history of a venous thromboembolic event one needs to assess the history and clarify the evidence and subsequent management. It would be prudent to do a thrombophilia screen and further management may depend on these results. One should avoid HRT if ongoing risk factors apply, for example obesity and immobilization. One should then discuss the risk of HRT with the woman (assuming the thrombophilia screen is negative) and if HRT is to be prescribed then a low-dose trans-dermal preparation would be recommended. If the thrombophilia screen was positive, one may consider low-dose aspirin or low-dose warfarin. If HRT is given in conjunction with coumarins, care must be taken to avoid potentiation of the anticoagulation effect and more frequent monitoring of the International Normalized Ratio of the prothrombin time would be required.

The Royal College of Obstetricians and Gynaecologists have issued recommendations regarding HRT and venous thromboembolism and they are as follows:

(1) There is no indication for routine screening for thrombophilia in women starting HRT.

(2) Women starting HRT should have a personal and family history taken of thrombo-embolic events.

(3) Women on, or starting, HRT should have an assessment made of additional risk factors for thromboembolic disease.

(4) Women with a personal or family history of venous thromboembolic disease should undergo thrombophilia screening.

NOT CONTRAINDICATIONS BUT CONDITIONS OF WHICH TO BE AWARE

Diabetes

When ovarian failure occurs there is a decrease in insulin secretion, an increase in insulin resistance and an increase in the metabolism of insulin, and this results in an overall increase in the levels of circulating insulin. Oral contraceptives will increase insulin resistance but 17β-estradiol will decrease insulin resistance by improving insulin sensitivity and elimination. Elevated insulin concentrations are associated with an atherogenic profile and may also have a direct effect on increasing atherogenesis. Therefore diabetic women should be encouraged to take HRT, although an alteration in their diabetic management may result due to the effect of HRT.

Gallstones

If there are pre-existing gallstones then trans-dermal therapy would be preferable, and in women who are not known to have gallstones, oral therapy may unmask pre-existing gallstones.

Past history of liver disease

It would be wise to check liver function tests first and recheck after 3 months of treatment. Avoidance of the liver is advised, so a non-oral route would be preferable.

Endometriosis

There is a theoretical risk that giving HRT may stimulate previous endometriosis; even if a pelvic clearance has been performed endometrial deposits may have been left. In reality this does not appear to be a significant problem, but if at all concerned it would be advisable to give continuous combined HRT or tibolone.

Fibroids

As these are known to shrink after ovarian failure, HRT may stimulate regrowth. Practically this does not seem to be a major problem, but it would be worthwhile monitoring the size of the fibroids and discontinuing therapy if there was a significant increase.

Endometrial hyperplasia

Endometrial monitoring needs to be performed and progestogens must be given either 12 days of each 4-week cycle or continuously.

Varicose veins

These are associated with a doubling of the risk of postoperative deep vein thrombosis; therefore, the use of HRT in women with varicose veins who are undergoing surgery must be reviewed in the light of other risks factors. The non-oral route would be advised.

Superficial phlebitis

There is an association with deficiency of proteins S and C, and one should consider whether to do a thrombophilia screen. The non-oral route is preferred to avoid the liver, and if the disease is still active one should defer HRT.

Migraine

Some women improve on HRT and some get worse. The pattern needs to be observed and medication should be adjusted accordingly.

Epilepsy

Some anti-epileptic drugs induce hepatic enzymes and reduce estrogen levels, so it is advisable to use a non-oral route or to change the anti-epileptic drug to one that does not induce hepatic enzymes.

Systemic lupus erythematosis

This sometimes deteriorates on HRT.

Multiple sclerosis

HRT will not cause deterioration of the disease, but other risk factors, for example immobilization and obesity, should be considered.

Hypertriglyceridemia

Oral estrogens elevate triglycerides, so a transdermal route is advised.

Recent myocardial infarction or stroke

HRT should be avoided during acute episodes when the patient is immobilized in bed. Most observational studies have suggested a significant effect for secondary prevention, but the more recent HERS study, which was a prospective randomized study, did not confirm this[7]. This area remains controversial.

CONDITIONS QUOTED AS CONTRAINDICATIONS BUT NOT SUBSTANTIATED

Otosclerosis

This condition is inherited as a Mendelian dominant trait and may be activated by viral infection. It involves premature hearing loss due to ossification of the inner ear. There have been case reports showing that, in pregnancy or on the oral contraceptive pill, otosclerosis may deteriorate. There are no substantial reports confirming deterioration of otosclerosis with HRT.

Melanoma

It has been suggested that melanocytes are responsive to estrogen, hence the rationale behind quoting melanomas as contraindications. There are estrogen and androgen receptors in about 50% of melanomas; however, survival is better in women compared to men with melanomas, especially in cases of estrogen-positive lesions. Animal work, both *in vivo* and *in vitro*, has shown that melanoma cells exposed to estradiol underwent inhibition of growth[8]; therefore, melanoma does not appear to be a contraindication, apart from the very aggressive melanotic adenocarcinoma of the uterus which is highly sensitive to estrogen stimulation.

Cardiovascular disease

This area is controversial, although it is worth remembering that, although stated in the datasheets as a contraindication, the studies to back this up are based either on estrogens being given to men for prostate cancer or oral contraceptive studies which used alkylestrogens. This emphasizes the fact that there is a significant difference between the alkylestrogens and the estrogens used in HRT.

Current evidence suggests that HRT provides protection against cardiovascular disease, although the magnitude of this is not clear.

CONCLUSION

It is time to recognize that there are very few contraindications to HRT. There are many conditions where we must observe caution before prescribing HRT, but we must be confident in understanding the pharmacological differences between oral contraceptives and HRT. With each patient we must individualize management and be clear in weighing up the long-term benefits against the possible side-effects and long-term risks. However, progress will be retarded for as long as the pharmaceutical datasheets remain incorrect.

References

1. Hartmann BW, Huber C. The mythology of hormone replacement therapy. *Br J Obstet Gynaecol* 1997;104:163–8
2. Carter C. Pathogenesis of thrombosis. In Greer IA, Turpie AGG, Forbes CD, eds. *Haemostasis and Thrombosis in Obstetrics and Gynaecology*. London: Chapman and Hall, 1992:229–56
3. Jick H, Derby LE, Myers MW, Vasilakis C, Newton KM. Risk of hospital admission for idiopathic venous thromboembolism among users of postmenopausal oestrogens. *Lancet* 1996;348:981–3
4. Daly E, Vessey MP, Hawkins MM, Carson JL, Gough P, Marsh S. Case control study of venous thromboembolism risk in users of hormone replacement therapy. *Lancet* 1996;348:977–80
5. Gutthann SP, Garcia Rodrigues LA, Castallsague J, Oliart AD. Hormone replacement therapy and risk of venous thromboembolism: population based case control study. *Br Med J* 1997;314:796–800.
6. Grodstein F, Stampfer MJ, Goldhaber SZ, *et al.* Prospective study of exogenous hormones and risk of pulmonary embolism in women. *Lancet* 1996;348:983–7
7. Hully S, Grady D, Bush T, *et al.* Randomized trial of estrogen plus progestin for secondary prevention of coronary heart disease in postmenopausal women. *J Am Med Assoc* 1998;280:605–13
8. Schleicher RL, Hitselberger MH, Beatt CW. Inhibition of hamster melanoma growth by oestrogen. *Cancer Res* 1987;47:453–9

4

Effects of oral and transdermal hormone replacement therapy in relation to serum estrogen levels

T. Yasui, M. Irahara and T. Aono

INTRODUCTION

Postmenopausal hormone replacement therapy (HRT) can benefit women in the short term by reducing the frequency of hot flushes or improving vulvovaginal atrophy, and in the long term by reducing the risk of osteoporosis and cardiovascular disease. Despite this evidence, HRT is not widely used because of adverse effects, such as unscheduled bleeding or breast tenderness, with the continuous combined regimen. HRT also increases the risk of breast cancer after long-term treatment in postmenopausal women[1].

An estrogen threshold hypothesis has also been reported which states that each tissue has a different sensitivity to estradiol. A significant decrease in urinary calcium excretion was very sensitive to estradiol level as low as 20 pg/ml and effective estradiol levels for vasomotor symptoms are between 35 and 70 pg/ml, whereas for a change in the serum lipid profile an estradiol level over 70 pg/ml is needed[2,3]. Furthermore, breast cancer can be very sensitive to the growth-promoting effects of estradiol concentrations as low as 10–20 pg/ml, and estradiol levels in the range of 30 pg/ml produce regression in the endometriotic lesions[2]. Therefore, it is necessary to know the association of serum estrogen levels with the effects of estrogenic preparations in postmenopausal women treated with HRT. In the present study,

we measured the serum levels of estrone and 17β-estradiol precisely in postmenopausal Japanese women receiving HRT, and clarified the relationship between the effects on vasomotor symptoms, bone mineral density and lipid metabolism, and estrogen levels.

PATIENTS AND METHODS

Eighty-four postmenopausal or bilaterally ovariectomized women aged 30–64 years who suffered from vasomotor symptoms, such as hot flush or atrophy of the vagina, were divided into three groups and treated with HRT as follows. Group A (33 patients) received oral administration of 0.625 mg conjugated equine estrogen (CEE, Premarin, Wyeth) and 2.5 mg medroxyprogesterone acetate (MPA, Provera, Upjohn) every other day. Group B (37 patients) received oral administration of 0.625 mg CEE and 2.5 mg MPA every day. Group C (14 patients) received 25 µg/day transdermal estradiol (Estraderm TTS, Novartis) percutaneously and daily oral 2.5 mg MPA. All women were in good health, as shown by medical history, physical examination, blood chemistry profile, and had not received any hormonal therapy before. As shown in Table 1, age, years since menopause, body mass index (BMI) and bone mineral density (BMD) of lumbar spine (L2–4) were not

Table 1 Group characteristics at the initial examination

	Group A	Group B	Group C
Number of patients	33	37	14
Age (years)	50.7 ± 1.2	52.0 ± 0.8	51.1 ± 2.1
Years since menopause	4.4 ± 0.9	3.8 ± 0.6	6.2 ± 1.5
Body mass index	22.9 ± 0.5	22.8 ± 0.5	21.6 ± 0.5
Spine BMD (g/cm^2)	0.929 ± 0.023	0.894 ± 0.021	0.882 ± 0.043
Estrone (pg/ml)	14.7 ± 1.7	19.1 ± 1.7	16.6 ± 3.7
17β-estradiol (pg/ml)	3.7 ± 0.5	4.4 ± 0.7	5.2 ± 0.9

Mean ± SEM; BMD, bone mineral density

significantly different among the three groups. The mean levels of estrone and 17β-estradiol before treatment with HRT were 14.7 and 3.7 pg/ml in group A, 19.1 and 4.4 pg/ml in group B, 16.6 and 5.2 pg/ml in group C, respectively. We measured the serum levels of estrone and 17β-estradiol, BMD of lumbar spine, total cholesterol, triglyceride, high-density lipoprotein (HDL) cholesterol, apolipoproteins A1, B, E before and 12 months after treatment. The Kupperman index was determined every 3 months for the study of vasomotor symptoms. Incidence of breakthrough bleeding between oral HRT daily and every other day was compared every month.

Measurement of bone mineral density

BMD of the L2–4 vertebral bodies was measured by dual energy X-ray absorptiometry (Hologic QDR 2000, Hologic Corp, MA, USA) before the initiation of therapy and 12 months later. The coefficients of variation of these measurements were less than 1.0% for lumbar BMD. Data were expressed as bone mineral density in g/cm^2.

Measurements of lipids and lipoproteins

Serum total cholesterol, triglyceride and HDL cholesterol were analyzed by using an enzymatic calorimetric method. The low-density lipoprotein (LDL) cholesterol level was calculated according to the Friedewald formula. Apolipoprotein Al, B and E levels were estimated by an immunoturbidimetric method.

Measurements of estrone and estradiol

We have developed a highly sensitive assay for estrone and 17β-estradiol in serum. Estrone and estradiol, obtained by solid-phase extraction using a Sep pak tC18 cartridge, were purified by high-performance liquid chromatography. Quantification of estrone and 17β-estradiol were carried out by radioimmunoassay. The minimum detectable doses for estrone and 17β-estradiol were 1.05 pg/ml and 0.65 pg/ml, respectively. The serum levels of 17β-estradiol using this method strongly correlated with those from gas chromatography mass spectrometry. In our preliminary work, serum levels of estrone and 17β-estradiol after a single oral administration of CEE reached peaks of 125.9 and 13.7 pg/ml, respectively, 12 hours after administration. Based on the result that levels of estrone and 17β-estradiol reached a plateau and were not significantly different between 12 and 18 hours, blood samples were drawn at 12–18 hours after the ingestion of CEE during HRT. The blood was centrifuged at 4 °C and the serum samples obtained were frozen until analysis.

Statistical analysis

Results were expressed as mean ± SE. Statistical differences between baseline and treatment values within the groups were determined by the two-sided paired t test, and the difference between the groups by analysis of variance assessed by Student's t test. Values of p less than 0.05 were considered to be statistically significant.

RESULTS

As shown in Figure 1, the Kupperman index in all groups reduced significantly ($p < 0.01$) after 3 and 6 months' treatment. Incidence of breakthrough bleeding during treatment in group A was less than that in group B. During 1 year of treatment, the incidence of breakthrough

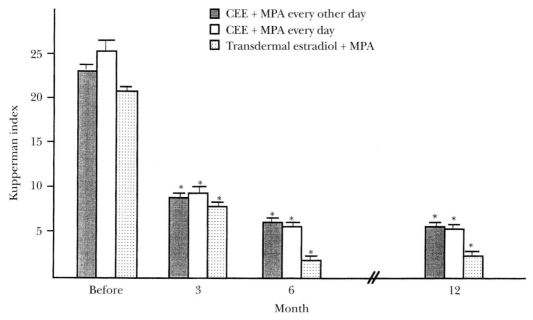

Figure 1 Changes of the Kupperman index in postmenopausal women before and during HRT. Each value represents the mean ± SE. *$p < 0.01$ versus before treatment

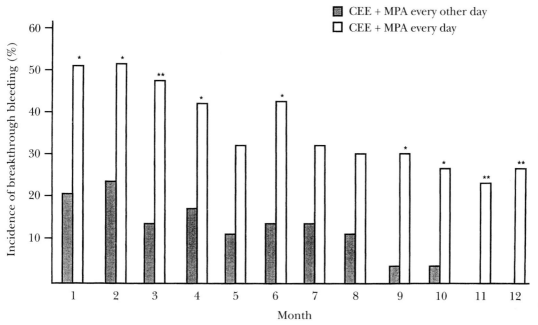

Figure 2 Incidence of breakthrough bleeding in oral HRT daily and every other day. *$p < 0.05$ versus CEE + MPA every other day; **$p < 0.01$ versus CEE + MPA every other day

bleeding in both groups reduced, and that in group A (0%) was significantly ($p < 0.01$) less than in group B (25.8%) at 12 months (Figure 2).

The mean levels of estrone and 17β-estradiol at 12–18 hours after treatment in group A were 71.7 and 14.9 pg/ml at 12 months, respectively, whereas those levels in group B were 139.8 and 22.8 pg/ml, respectively. On the other hand, the mean levels of estrone and 17β-estradiol in group C were 51.7 and 40.5 pg/ml, respectively (Figure 3).

The percentage changes in spine BMD in the three groups are shown in Figure 4. The HRT in group B significantly increased BMD over baseline at the lumbar spine (3.4%, $p < 0.0001$), and HRT in groups A and C increased significantly (1.8% ($p < 0.05$), 2.6% ($p < 0.01$), respectively).

Table 2 shows changes in total cholesterol, triglyceride, HDL cholesterol, LDL cholesterol and apolipoprotein Al, B and E levels before and after 12 months of treatment. Levels of total cholesterol decreased significantly in group B ($p < 0.01$) and group C ($p < 0.05$) (–8.1% and –7.5%, respectively), whereas group A had a mean decrease of 1.6%, which was less than the response in groups B and C. Changes in the levels of LDL cholesterol were similar to those of total cholesterol: group A, –3.5%; group B, –18.1% ($p < 0.01$); group C, –10.5% ($p < 0.05$), respectively. HDL cholesterol levels rose significantly in groups B ($p < 0.01$) and C ($p < 0.05$) (14.2% and 10.3%, respectively), but increased only slightly in group A. Relative to the baseline value, serum triglyceride levels decreased slightly in groups B and C, whereas those in group A showed a 10.5% decrease. The treatment in all groups caused a significant increase in the levels of apolipoprotein Al (A, 5.1%; B, 9.8%; C, 7.2%). The levels of apolipoprotein B decreased significantly ($p < 0.05$) in group B (–9.1%), but no significant changes were found in the other two groups. The level of apolipoprotein E decreased significantly ($p < 0.01$) in group B (–23.6%), whereas those in groups A and C showed no significant changes.

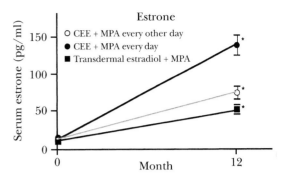

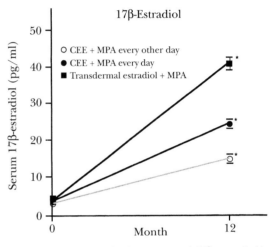

Figure 3 Mean levels of estrone and 17β-estradiol in the serum of postmenopausal women before and during HRT. *$p < 0.01$ versus before treatment. Each value represents the mean ± SE

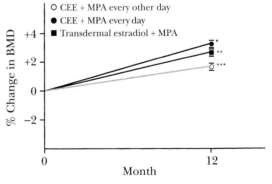

Figure 4 Mean percentage change from baseline in bone mineral density (BMD) of lumbar spine after 12 months of treatment. *$p < 0.01$ versus baseline values; **$p < 0.05$ versus baseline values. Each value represents the mean ± SE

Table 2 Changes in lipid profile after 12 months of treatment

	Group A	Change (%)	Group B	Change (%)	Group C	Change (%)
Total cholesterol (mg/dl)						
0	214.9 ± 5.7	−1.6	213.1 ± 5.7	−8.1*	210.9 ± 7.9	−7.5**
12 months	211.5 ± 4.8		195.9 ± 4.0		195.1 ± 9.4	
Triglyceride (mg/dl)						
0	120.5 ± 11.7	−10.5	114.7 ± 9.6	−4.0	99.9 ± 10.5	−0.8
12 months	107.9 ± 8.8		110.1 ± 9.7		99.1 ± 8.5	
HDL cholesterol (mg/dl)						
0	62.7 ± 3.0	+3.7	60.4 ± 2.5	+14.2*	56.4 ± 3.7	+10.3**
12 months	65.7 ± 3.2		69.0 ± 2.5		62.2 ± 3.9	
LDL cholesterol (mg/dl)						
0	129.4 ± 5.2	−3.5	129.7 ± 5.1	−18.1*	131.0 ± 7.8	−10.5**
12 months	124.9 ± 5.1		106.2 ± 4.2		117.2 ± 8.5	
Apolipoprotein A1 (mg/dl)						
0	148.6 ± 4.5	+5.1**	145.2 ± 3.9	+9.8*	131.7 ± 6.0	+7.2**
12 months	156.2 ± 4.1		159.5 ± 3.6		141.2 ± 6.3	
Apolipoprotein B (mg/dl)						
0	107.0 ± 4.9	−1.1	103.1 ± 4.8	−9.1**	99.8 ± 5.4	−4.6
12 months	105.8 ± 4.2		93.7 ± 4.3		95.2 ± 4.8	
Apolipoprotein E (mg/dl)						
0	4.7 ± 0.2	0	5.5 ± 0.3	−23.6*	4.8 ± 0.3	−2.0
12 months	4.7 ± 0.2		4.2 ± 0.2		4.7 ± 0.4	

Mean ± SE; *$p < 0.01$ versus baseline value; **$p < 0.05$ versus baseline value

DISCUSSION

Hormone replacement therapy is well established as an effective treatment for vasomotor symptoms, and for preventing the postmenopausal bone loss that underlies the development of osteoporotic fractures[4]. There is a body of opinion that states that a minimum of 0.625 mg of conjugated equine estrogen or 0.05 mg transdermal estrogen is required to relieve vasomotor symptoms and prevent bone loss, at least in the perimenopausal period[5–7]. In postmenopausal women with hypercholesterolemia, CEE at a dose of 0.625 mg and transdermal estradiol at a dose of 0.05 mg are also effective for lowering the levels of total cholesterol and LDL cholesterol, and for increasing the level of HDL cholesterol[8].

However, side-effects are particularly important in elderly women[9]. There is a low level of compliance because of unscheduled bleeding, breast tenderness, or fear of cancer[10]. Thus, a demonstration that low doses of HRT are successful in preventing bone loss is very important to this group of users. The groups of Ettinger[11] and Webber[12] demonstrated that a daily dose of 0.31 mg of CEE was effective in preventing postmenopausal bone loss if administered with calcium. Mizunuma and colleagues[13] also reported that HRT using 0.31 mg of CEE can increase lumbar BMD and be an appropriate option for prevention of postmenopausal bone loss in women wishing to minimize genital bleeding and to reduce hormonal side-effects as well as vasomotor symptoms. In the present study, we also reveal that HRT with CEE and MPA every other day as a low-dose therapy is effective for relieving vasomotor symptoms and preventing bone loss and is associated with fewer side-effects, such as unscheduled bleeding or breast tenderness, while it has no beneficial effects on lipid profile.

On the other hand, it is important for women taking HRT to monitor the serum level of estrogen because the level is strongly related to the estrogenic effects on various tissues. However, it has been very difficult to measure the precise serum level of estrogen in women receiving oral conjugated equine estrogen, which is widely used for the treatment of postmenopausal estrogen deficiency symptoms. This preparation, derived from pregnant mares' urine, is a mixture of estrogens, estrone sulfate being the major component, and the other estrogens, such as sodium equilin sulfate, probably contribute as much to the biological potency of the drug as estrone sulfate, which, after absorption, is converted to unconjugated estrone and estradiol. Therefore, there are some difficulties in clinical assay techniques. Lobo and colleagues[14] reported that serum levels of estrone and estradiol after 25 days of treatment with 0.625 mg CEE increased to 153 and 39.4 pg/ml, respectively. Jurgens and co-workers[15] have also demonstrated that serum levels of estrone and estradiol after 1 month's administration of 0.625 mg CEE increased to 100 and 20.0 pg/ml, respectively. Furthermore, serum levels of estrone and estradiol after 72 hours of treatment with 50 µg transdermal estradiol have been reported to be 45 and 41.1 pg/ml, respectively[16]. We developed a highly sensitive assay using high-performance liquid chromatography for serum estrone and 17β-estradiol in Japanese women, and could detect the precise levels of estrone and 17β-estradiol after 12 months of treatment. The mean serum levels of 17β-estradiol after treatment with CEE and MPA every other day (Group A), every day (Group B) and 25 µg transdermal estradiol (Group C) were 14.9, 22.5 and 40.5 pg/ml, respectively.

Based on our results of the association of 17β-estradiol levels with the effects of estrogenic preparations, those levels required to relieve vasomotor symptoms and increase bone mineral density are at least 15 pg/ml, which gives less breakthrough bleeding. Furthermore, the level to decrease total cholesterol and LDL cholesterol, and increase HDL cholesterol, is more than 30 pg/ml. Excessive levels of estradiol may result in marked side-effects and complications[17]. Therefore, HRT given every other day as a low-dose therapy can be chosen as a candidate treatment for avoiding side-effects, such as unscheduled bleeding and breast tenderness, but retaining a normal lipid profile. Transdermal estradiol is also recommended to avoid hepatic first-pass effects, because hypertension, thromboembolism, cholelithiasis and increased hepatic protein formation may relate to high oral doses of non-physiological estrogens. We advise that the precise levels of estradiol be monitored and maintained in the suitable range individually for postmenopausal women receiving HRT, in order to have beneficial effects and to avoid adverse effects due to overdose of estradiol levels.

ACKNOWLEDGEMENTS

The authors wish to thank Dr Hirokazu Uemura, Dr Naoto Yoneda, Dr Masayo Yamada, Dr Michiko Okada for preparing the manuscript, and Mitsubishi Kagaku Bio-Clinical Laboratories for measuring the serum levels of estrone and 17β-estradiol.

References

1. Colditz GA, Hankinson SE, Hunter DJ, *et al.* The use of estrogens and progestins and the risk of breast cancer in postmenopausal women. *N Engl J Med* 1995;332:1589–93
2. Barbieri RL. Hormone treatment of endometriosis: the estrogen threshold hypothesis. *Am J Obstet Gynecol* 1992;166:740–5
3. Nichols KC, Schenkel L, Benson H. 17β-estradiol for postmenopausal estrogen replacement therapy. *Obstet Gynecol Surv* 1984;39:230–45
4. Lindsay R, Hart DM, Aitken JM, *et al.* Long-term prevention of postmenopausal osteoporosis by estrogen. *Lancet* 1976;1:1038–41
5. Lindsay R, Hart DM, Clark HD. The minimum effective dose of estrogen for the prevention of post-menopausal bone loss. *Obstet Gynecol* 1984; 63:759–63
6. Haas S, Walsh B, Evans S, *et al.* The effect of transdermal estradiol on hormone and metabolic dynamics over a six-week period. *Obstet Gynecol* 1988;71:671–6

7. Stevenson J, Cust MP, Gangar KF, *et al.* Effect of transdermal versus oral hormone replacement therapy on bone density in spine and proximal femur in post-menopausal women. *Lancet* 1990; 335:265–9

8. Zichella L, Perrone G, Steefanutti C, *et al.* Hormonal replacement therapy in hypercholesterolemic women. In Nencioni T, Ognissanti F, Polvani F, eds. *Menopause Update '92* Italy: Monduzzi Editore, 1992:219–22

9. Grey AB, Cundy TF, Reid IR. Continuous combined estrogen/progestin therapy is well tolerated and increases bone density at the hip and spine in post-menopausal osteoporosis. *Clin Endocrinol* 1994;40:671–7

10. Ravnikar VA. Compliance with hormone therapy. *Am J Obstet Gynecol* 1987;156:1332–4

11. Ettinger B, Genant HK, Cann CE. Postmenopausal bone loss is prevented by treatment with low-dosage estrogen with calcium. *Ann Int Med* 1987;106:40–5

12. Webber CE, Blake JM, Chambers LF, *et al.* Effects of 2 years of hormone replacement upon bone mass, serum lipids and lipoproteins. *Maturitas* 1994;19:13–23

13. Mizunuma H, Okano H, Soda M, *et al.* Prevention of postmenopausal bone loss with minimal uterine bleeding using low dose continuous estrogen/progestin therapy: a 2-year prospective study. *Maturitas* 1997;27:69–76

14. Lobo RA, Brenner P, Mishell DR. Metabolic parameters and steroid levels in postmenopausal women receiving lower doses of natural estrogen replacement. *Obstet Gynecol* 1983;62:94–8

15. Jurgens RW, Downey LJ, Abernethy WD, *et al.* A comparison of circulating hormone levels in postmenopausal women receiving hormone replacement therapy. *Am J Obstet Gynecol* 1992;167:459–60

16. Scott RT, Ross B, Anderson C, *et al.* Pharmacokinetics of percutaneous estradiol: a crossover study using a gel and a transdermal system in comparison with oral micronized estradiol. *Obstet Gynecol* 1991;77:758–64

17. Steingold KA, Laufer L, Chetkowski RJ, *et al.* Treatment of hot flushes with transdermal estradiol administration. *J Clin Endocrinol Metab* 1985; 61:627–32

5

Continuation with hormone replacement therapy

C. L. Domoney and J. Studd

INTRODUCTION

Compliance, concordance, adherence, or whatever terminology is appropriate to describe the therapeutic alliance between doctor and patient in the 1990s, is a major problem in prescribing. Many studies have examined the dismal adherence rate of patients to their medication. Up to 30% of patients may not even pick up their prescription from the pharmacy[1]. Compliance with hormone replacement therapy (HRT) reflects the more generalized problem of differing perceptions of patients and doctors regarding the benefits of a particular medication for an individual.

Since 1975, public knowledge regarding the use of HRT has been fuelled by the great media interest in women's health. Some of the major improvements in women's quality of life in the 20th century have been due to medical advances, HRT being arguably one of the most important. When doctors consider the prescription of HRT, it will often be prompted by enquiry from the woman herself. Yet misunderstandings regarding the short- and long-term use of HRT are rife amongst medical practitioners and women as consumers of health care.

WOMEN'S PERSPECTIVE

Women have generally incurred a significant number of consultations with physicians during their reproductive lifetime. An increasingly health-conscious female population has become conversant with the medicalization of many aspects of women's health. Although a substantial proportion of health-seeking behavior will occur informally, the initiation of medical consultations for menopause-related issues is commonly accepted by a significant proportion of Western women. It is no longer considered necessary for women to suffer the consequences of hormonal deprivation, just as it is accepted that choice with respect to family planning or antenatal care should be available for all women. It is increasingly understood, by the lay population and the medical profession, that the menopausal transition causes significantly more problems than vasomotor symptoms alone. The balance of risks and benefits of HRT versus the polypharmacy that may be necessary for the potential multitude of short- and long-term consequences of the menopause must be deliberated.

However, it is not clear that the health-care professions fully understand women's perceptions of the need for HRT. A recent qualitative analysis of decision-making and HRT suggested that women consider different criteria from health professionals when determining use of medication at the menopause[2]. Interestingly, there appears to be a discrepancy between media discourse and women's own attitudes to menopause, health and medication. The poor continuation rate of HRT can only be challenged by a greater understanding of these issues.

Ethnographic investigation of a North American population[3] indicated women's HRT anticipations could be divided into six broad categories ('trusting in nature', 'fixing', 'sceptical experimenting', 'restabilizing', 'life enhancement', or 'trusting in science'.) Yet sociological investigation of the characteristics of women with express attitudes to HRT suggested that lack of knowledge caused rejection and poor compliance with treatment[4]. This study also indicated that familiarity with the health-care system promoted HRT use. Several studies have confirmed that prior use of oral contraceptives increases the likelihood of HRT experimentation[5,6].

Rates of HRT usage

Studies indicate that women are not unwilling to try HRT in the younger age groups[7], but significant numbers have stopped within 1 year (20–60% depending on country and study). In the United States, it has been estimated that less than 20% of postmenopausal women will have ever used HRT and of those that are prescribed HRT, less than 40% will continue for longer than 1 year[8]. A British study with data from 1400 general practices, contributing to the Oral Contraception Study of the Royal College of General Practitioners, determined that, between 1981 and 1990, there had been a three-fold increase in the use of HRT. By 1990, 16% of non-hysterectomized and 36% of hysterectomized women were ever users of HRT[9]. However, only 9% were classified as current users. A Spanish study revealed 9% of a group of 331 postmenopausal women being seen at a tertiary referral center did not pick up their prescription, 15% discontinued during the first year and 14% followed treatment intermittently[10]. The two factors associated with poor compliance in this study were addition of progestogens and oral route of administration. Many others have confirmed this poor adherence, but with varying causes ascertained (Table 1).

More recent papers have suggested that a supportive and interested group of health

Table 1 Factors associated with non-use of HRT

Safety concerns
Not medically recommended
Lack of awareness
Weight gain
Fear of cancer
Bleeding
'Unnatural'

professionals, whether general practitioners, specialist nurses, or special interest hospital clinics, can achieve much higher levels of compliance. Coope and Marsh reported compliance with long-term therapy (assessed by repeat prescription audit) of between 84% and 92% over a 5-year period in a general practice population, although only 20% of the eligible population were current users[11]. A cohort of patients ever prescribed HRT from a single physician over a 10-year period revealed an 85% current usage from a 65% questionnaire response rate[12]. This study, perhaps not surprisingly, also suggested the most important factor for continuation was physician recommendation. A population in Hong Kong has been studied retrospectively and the results reported recently[13]. A concordance rate of 68.3% was determined 2 years after commencement of therapy. Yet 9% of women who stopped did so because other physicians had told them there was no need for treatment. The lack of consensus amongst the medical profession promotes misunderstanding in the lay population.

THE WOMAN OVER 60

This special group are not so well targeted for health-care input as the younger age groups. At present, few women over 65 use HRT[14,15], although there are some more encouraging reports of increasing uptake and continuation (see Figure 1)[16]. Menopausal symptoms may no longer be present (or they feel unable to complain about them) yet the long-term consequences of estrogen deficiency become more apparent. The generalized connective tissue deterioration can alter urinary function, sexual function, skin appearance and the underlying bone strength. The exposure to a more adverse

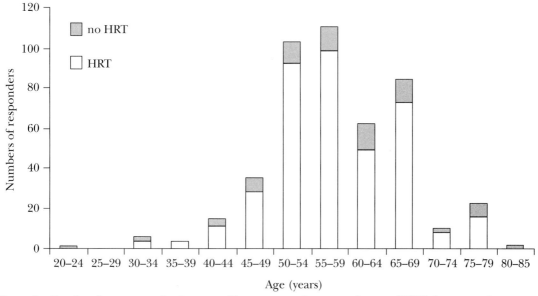

Figure 1 Results of survey monitoring use of hormone replacement therapy (HRT) in women hysterectomized between 1986 and 1997 in our unit

lipoprotein profile may enhance the atherosclerotic process. Deteriorating cognitive function may be accepted as a normal consequence of aging.

The findings of the Collaborative Group on Hormonal Factors in Breast Cancer[17], however, suggest that our rationale for advising women on their HRT use should perhaps swing more towards increasing the uptake of the older woman as she will benefit most from the increase in bone mass. The reduction in risk of fracture appears to be more substantial in those taking HRT later than an equivalent exposure time during the climacteric[18]. If 10 years is the maximum period a woman is prepared to take or a physician is willing to prescribe estrogen replacement, then cost–benefit analyses would suggest that there may be two 'ages' when HRT should be considered: the perimenopausal and the late postmenopausal[19].

If an older woman agrees to initiate estrogen replacement, the key to continuation is careful counselling and choice of preparation. The longer the period of estrogen deficiency, the greater the incidence of side-effects. There are now several low-dose continuous combined products available developed in response to the needs of these women.

DOCTORS' PERSPECTIVE

General practitioners are the ideal personnel to encourage HRT uptake and continuation. Yet experts in the field must support them to minimize the damage that conflicting opinion propagates amongst women. A British epidemiological study[9] suggests that women with a history of fracture or vascular problems were not more likely to be offered HRT by general practitioners. Non-hysterectomized women with ischemic heart disease, diabetes mellitus, or hypertension were less likely to be receiving HRT, although this did not concur with prescribing practice for hysterectomized women. Doctors may be more aware of the hormonal contribution to these common diseases when alerted by a history of surgical intervention. General practitioners may be aided by the reinforcement of hospital specialists, including orthopedic surgeons, geriatricians and general physicians, who themselves may not feel confident enough to initiate therapy. However, there is continuing misinformation amongst medical practitioners regarding the risks and benefits of HRT. Data sheets have been directly transferred from the guidelines given with the oral contraceptive pill (i.e. synthetic estrogens), which promotes this confusion[20]. Many contraindications stipulated on the data sheets would in fact be considered as relative indications for use in expert opinion. Professional concerns are readily transmitted to women who are unsure of the safety, and therefore the practical long-term preventive role, of estrogen replacement. The majority of HRT prescribing is now performed by general practitioners, who may have few misgivings with respect to short-term prescribing for acute estrogen deficiency, yet are sometimes reluctant to prescribe long-term treatment. Our unit's survey of hysterectomized long-term HRT users revealed a significant proportion had been advised not to continue by their general practitioners[21]. Unfortunately, conflicting and contradictory data are exemplified by the recent HERS trial[22], which will only serve to confuse the emerging future role of HRT.

For primary-care providers, access to investigations that may serve to improve both patient and physician compliance is restricted in many areas of the country. Bone-density scans have been demonstrated to be the only reliable means of identifying those at highest risk of fracture[23]. Reinforcement of health issues with the use of medical technology has occurred with other groups of patients, perhaps most notably in antenatal patients with the use of ultrasound scanning. Yet Ryan and co-workers[24] revealed in 1992 that 40% of women with low bone density were not taking HRT 8 months after diagnosis. Women in the 50–60-year age group were most likely to accept HRT. This group is frequently targeted by GPs for attendance at 'well woman clinics' and it should be possible, in a motivated general practice, to discuss the problems and consequences of the menopause with a majority of the relevant age group. Different methods for educating women need further investigation, but it appears that informal information is an important source of initial interest in HRT. A paper investigating the impact of videos on HRT compliance, however, did not suggest a significant improvement in compliance[25]. More research is required to elicit the benefits derived from the pharmaceutical companies' literature.

A survey of views of general practitioners and consultant gynecologists on HRT published in 1994 revealed that, although 97% and 98% of general practitioners and gynecologists, respectively, believed that HRT decreased subsequent risk of osteoporosis, only 17% and 33%, respectively, would prescribe it for over 10 years[26]. Wallace and co-workers[27] found that only 23% of osteoporotic women over 69 agreed to have estrogen replacement. Until a higher rate of HRT uptake and long-term prescribing is achieved, a national bone density screening program is unlikely to be cost-effective. Alternative treatments for osteoporosis are relatively expensive, do not have as wide a range of beneficial effects and in this age of financial caution may not be so willingly prescribed.

Women doctors as health-care consumers and providers

Female doctors' uptake of HRT in Britain was investigated, revealing that 55% of women doctors aged 45–65 years without regular menstruation were ever uses of HRT and, of these, 70% were still taking HRT 5 years after starting therapy and 48% 10 years after beginning HRT[28]. When asked about their future intentions in 1995, over half anticipated continuing for over 10 years. A Swedish study reported current HRT use amongst 88% of postmenopausal female gynecologists and 72% of female general practitioners[29]. Women doctors may be expected to have a higher HRT usage linked to socioeconomic status, but will also be less influenced by their caregivers, particularly regarding duration of use. In 1989, doctors in the MRC general practice research framework prescribed HRT to approximately 9% of their patients aged between 40 and 64, an average of 24.6 women each (range 0–150) but with female doctors treating five times more women than male doctors[30]. More recently it has been suggested from an American epidemiological study that women who see a male physician are more likely to be non-compliant[31], although this does not appear to be the case in Europe.

Side-effects

The possibility of side-effects should be discussed with all women initiating therapy to encourage a crucial alliance between doctor and patient. The transient nature of the more minor effects, such as nausea, breast tenderness, mild headaches and bloating, can be compared to those of the 'pill' and it can be suggested that generally there will be some amelioration over a few cycles.

FACTORS AFFECTING HRT UPTAKE AND CONTINUATION

Bleeding

It is commonly believed that initiation of HRT for prophylactic reasons heralds the return of regular bleeding, and 'non-bleed' preparations are probably still underused. Studies suggest that bleeding is the main reason for non-continuation of short- as well as long-term treatment. In a group of previous hormone users, 44.8% stated that bleeding was the significant factor in their decision to discontinue HRT[32]. Ulrich and co-workers[33] have reported patient preference for a continuous combined preparation in a group comprised of two-thirds previous sequential preparation users and one-third previous non-users. Of those who completed the study, 91% suggested a preference for the particular brand of non-bleeding preparation. This has significant implications for the long-term usage of HRT and therefore the long-term health benefits. Higher rates of continuation have been achieved with continuous combined preparations when used appropriately, i.e. in women more than 1 year from their last menstrual period when low levels of endogenous estradiol are present, therefore resulting in less erratic bleeding during the first 3–6 months[34]. There is a suggestion that regular bleeding rather than flow or duration is most important to women.

Breast cancer

It is not clear what effect the well-publicized, but not well-portrayed, breast cancer data from the Collaborative Group on Hormonal Factors in Breast Cancer will have on future HRT usage[17]. The medical profession's interpretation of the 1 in 12 lifetime risk of breast cancer and excess risk with long-term usage of HRT is likely to be different from that of the lay population. It is our opinion that conveying the absolute risk in numbers and reinforcing the unaltered mortality rate of tumors associated with HRT, allows women to make an informed choice without the sensationalism of the media publicity. We must, however, acknowledge the very real fear that women have of 'cancer'[35], even if the probability of death is higher by a disease process that may be ameliorated by estrogen.

Osteoporosis

In a Scottish study[36], 96% of women had heard of HRT and 84% understood the concept of osteoporosis. This information was generally gathered from friends and women's magazines. Although 79% of the group aged 45–49 years had never taken HRT, and half had concerns regarding its use, 96% would consider HRT if their bone density suggested an increased risk of osteoporosis. However, Torgerson and colleagues[37] reported a 48% uptake of HRT within 1 year of bone densitometry in non-hysterectomized women compared with 59% in those with a simple hysterectomy. It is not clear whether bone density screening will greatly reduce fracture incidence given the poor continuation rates, even in screen-positive women[38,39].

Weight gain

This problem that is perceived by menopausal women as one of the consequences of HRT, but not corroborated by any studies, must be addressed[40]. A general discussion regarding change in energy requirements and distribution of body fat at the menopause is likely to increase patient confidence.

Breast pain

Although some women welcome the changes in breast shape secondary to estrogen administration, the pain encountered on commencement of treatment can be a major deterrent. Tailoring the dose of estrogen is usually all that is required, but occasionally the addition of evening primrose oil may alleviate the initial symptoms.

Progestogen intolerance

It is now widely accepted that the progestogen component of HRT can be most problematic[41,42] with respect to both progestogenic adverse effects and bleeding patterns. The necessity of progestogens in non-hysterectomized women to induce secretory transformation or atrophy of the endometrium and therefore prevent hyperplasia is well documented[43]. Withdrawal bleeds with sequential preparations should prevent endometrial hyperplasia and reduce the risk of endometrial carcinoma[44]. Unopposed estrogen increases the risk of endometrial carcinoma and this risk remains elevated for some years after cessation of therapy[45]. This should be reinforced at the time of counselling, particularly if women are not taking pre-packaged medications.

There is evidence to suggest that women with a previous history of premenstrual syndrome are more likely to suffer side-effects with the combined oral contraceptive pill[46] and therefore also with HRT preparations. It is our understanding that this is frequently caused by progestogen intolerance causing symptoms which are premenstrual in nature: bloating, irritability, depression, headaches, lethargy. Re-creation of this phenomenon has been reported in a group of estrogen-using hysterectomized women with two doses of norethisterone as compared to placebo[47]. These symptoms are readily identifiable by women who have experienced them during their fertile years and a proportion of them will neglect to regularly take the progestogen component of their HRT. Progestogen intolerance should be approached with an understanding of the derivation of these products. This will be discussed further later.

INDICATIONS AND TIMING

Symptomatic improvement

Both general practitioners and gynecologists are agreed on the use of HRT for menopausal symptoms[26], but the categorization of these symptoms may vary. Estrogen replacement for treatment of depression was only considered by approximately 55–60% of doctors in this survey of medical practitioners' views. A Dutch study assessing determinants of first prescription of HRT, however, did associate use of HRT without 'typical' (vasomotor) complaints with a lower level of well-being[48]. Vasomotor symptoms are generally relieved by standard doses of estrogens compared to the higher doses frequently required for relief of psychological complaints. This effect may be, in part, due to the mood-elevating effects of high-dose estrogens and the additional consequences of ovulation suppression in a perimenopausal woman suffering hormonal fluctuations. Young women undergoing hysterectomy and oophorectomy may need higher-dose estrogen initially or the addition of androgen to achieve total relief of hormone deficiency symptoms.

Urogenital symptoms are susceptible to alleviation by most modes of delivery, including local delivery systems, therefore benefiting even the most estrogen-intolerant women.

Long-term prevention

Bone

The prevention of osteoporosis has been the mainstay of long-term benefits of HRT, as the case for its use is clear and unequivocal. Whether newer agents, such as bisphosphonates and selective estrogen receptor modulators (SERMS), have a major role to play in this market remains to be seen. Their expense, lack of multiorgan benefit and less significant improvement in bone density may limit their use. Yet in 1994, only 50% of practitioners would use HRT to treat established osteoporosis in women over 60[26]. A French study indicated that the strongest determinant of HRT use was an expectation that it would prevent osteoporosis[49]. Bone density may be declining in Western populations[50] due to an increasingly sedentary lifestyle, greater exposure to environmental pollutants and poorer nutritional intake. The attainment of maximal bone density at the menopause may encourage a less traditional timing of HRT use, i.e. perimenopause, in the light of the increased incidence of breast cancer with prolonged HRT use. Breast cancer concerns may rationalize the use of estrogen for population benefits to the older age group for a 5- or 10-year period. As the lowest bone density shows most improvement and bone benefits of HRT may be lost after 5 years, the cost–benefit analysis may fall in favor of delayed HRT prescribing in asymptomatic women[19].

Vascular disease

The benefits of HRT for cardiovascular and cerebrovascular disease continue to be poorly estimated by physicians. Stampfer and Colditz[51] and Paganini-Hill and colleagues[52] demonstrated the reduction in risk of ischemic heart disease and stroke, respectively, in epidemiological studies. Surrogate markers for these diseases can be measured and changes in cholesterol and lipoproteins can be reported to the woman to enhance compliance. The difference between synthetic and naturally occurring estrogens needs reinforcing to both physicians and women. The disappointing results of the HERS study have confused the picture for secondary cardiovascular disease prevention.

Brain

Studies examining the cognitive effects of estrogen in healthy women are inconsistent, but there appears to be a general trend towards improved verbal memory. Women with Alzheimer's disease have demonstrable improvements in cognition, often within a remarkably short timespan, suggesting a direct estrogenic effect[53]. Although poor memory may be a frequently reported perimenopausal symptom amenable to estrogen therapy, it is also worth discussing the evidence in favor of long-term protection of cognitive function to those women deliberating the pros and cons of prophylactic HRT.

Hysterectomized women

Hysterectomized women are a subgroup of women that comprise approximately 20% of the perimenopausal female population. This group are acknowledged to be at high risk for estrogen deficiency diseases, yet the National Osteoporosis Society reported in 1995 that only 37% were receiving HRT advice at the time of hysterectomy. Targeting of HRT recommendations should include those without oophorectomy as there is much evidence to suggest that these women's earlier menopause is often overlooked. It has been demonstrated that bone mass begins to decline at a younger age than in their non-hysterectomized contemporaries[54]. In 1989, Spector[55] reported that only 25% of women who had undergone a bilateral oophorectomy before the age of 40 were taking HRT. More optimistically, a well-motivated practice in Middlesborough found that 71% of their hysterectomized women under the age of 52 were users[56]. The risk–benefit analysis of prophylactic oophorectomy by Speroff and colleagues[57] suggests that compliance with replacement therapy in perimenopausal women is such that survival may be longer with ovarian conservation. All women undergoing oophorectomy premenopausally should be aware of the necessity to replace their endogenous estrogens until at least the age they would have been expected to undergo a 'natural' menopause. In our practice, a substantial number of women will endure hysterectomy and oophorectomy as definitive treatment of their premenstrual syndrome[58]. This would not be suitable management if long-term replacement therapy was not agreed.

DURATION OF USE

Duration of use is an issue poorly discussed by both patient and doctor. For this reason it is often not addressed directly. Many women will stop their HRT without any further consultation with their doctor, therefore not allowing time for adequate counselling. Until recently, there was little evidence to suggest to a woman who was stable on an HRT product that suited her (and if undergoing therapeutic monitoring, was demonstrated to have measurable beneficial effects) that she should not take lifelong HRT. Regular, but not necessarily frequent, checks offer an opportunity to discuss the risks and benefits to an individual at any particular time in her postmenopausal life. Yet the widely publicized data from the Collaborative Group on Hormonal Factors in Breast Cancer now gives us some guidance for counselling women considering long-term use of HRT. Those women wanting short-term symptom relief can be reassured of no additional risk of breast cancer. It has been suggested that 'the clock' should be started from the age of 50, i.e. approximately the average age of a 'natural' menopause. This must be reinforced to women with premature ovarian failure or premenopausal oophorectomized women. The increased risk of breast cancer appears to be equivalent to the additional risk incurred with a later menopause, i.e. 2.3% per year.

The purpose of HRT prescribing should be put into the context of the gain by the individual and society. As discussed previously, the benefits to bone mass from estrogen are maintained for a limited period; therefore, the rationale for short-term use in an asymptomatic, perimenopausal woman should be questioned. The population benefits of HRT as a preventive intervention may be far greater at the age of 70. This is not the current approach to prescribing. Reluctance on the part of both physicians and women to cause unnecessary side-effects in older women is coupled with ignorance of the wide range of estrogen products. Products such as bisphosphonates and SERMS can fill this area of the market that may be neglected by ignorance and fear but may have much less far reaching health benefits in comparison. It could be suggested that this is a natural treatment for an evolutionarily unnatural lifespan. Women now spend on average a third of their lifespan in a postmenopausal state. The decision to use endogenously occurring steroids should be suggested in addition to normal lifestyle advice,

Table 2 Reasons why women continue with HRT

Minimal side-effects, well tolerated
Improvement in symptoms
Improved sense of well-being
Osteoporosis prevention
Medical encouragement
Cardiovascular protection
Satisfaction with advice given

rather than the alternative they are promoted as by opponents[59]. However, women will themselves decide how long to continue HRT based on initial motivations for starting therapy, their experience of the treatment and their knowledge of the long-term risks and benefits[60] (Table 2).

REGIMENS

The plethora of products on the market should make it possible to find a suitable HRT preparation for most women. There is certainly an element of 'fashion' for different preparations, but an important factor for compliance is patient satisfaction with mode of delivery. Unless there is a definite contraindication to a particular delivery form (of which there are few, generally favoring a non-oral route to avoid the hepatic first-pass effects), patient choice should be the main determinant[61].

In the USA, conjugated equine estrogens still remain the most commonly prescribed; in France, 80% of women using HRT will be prescribed transdermal estradiol gel. In Britain, the majority of hormone users are taking oral regimens, but many more are now experimenting with transdermal regimens. Tolerability and convenience must be sufficient to warrant change. The acceptability of these preparations has been reported frequently, particularly since the development of single-membrane matrix patches, causing less frequent skin reactions. Once-weekly patches are now available and may be more convenient than those lasting 3–4 days, but occasional replacement before 7 days for hygiene, skin irritation, or lack of effect makes them potentially more expensive. More recently, several transdermal estrogen and progestogen patches have been introduced onto the HRT formulary that appear to be well tolerated with sufficient progestogenic effect.

Estrogen gels are becoming more popular due to convenience and lack of skin reactions. It becomes easier for physician and patient to titrate estrogen dose according to symptoms and it can enhance the doctor–patient relationship when the responsibility of finding an individualized regimen is shared. Many women appreciate informed control of their estrogen intake, although care must be taken to ensure this is not abused. One case report had documented evidence of 17β-estradiol levels of 21 000 pmol/l in a woman previously using implants but supplementing with an estrogen gel[62].

Topical estrogen therapy for vaginal and/or urinary symptoms with or without progestogenic opposition may be a useful therapy in the few women who cannot tolerate higher estrogen doses or are unwilling to do so. In the near future, estrogen may be delivered transnasally, which is well tolerated and less intrusive than transdermal methods, but may induce very high estradiol levels immediately after intake then subside to lower steady-state levels.

Percutaneous implants have a unique role in the hormone replacement armamentarium due to the significant convenience of a biannual consultation. We have reported compliance rates in hysterectomized women in excess of most other surveys (97% at 5 years in 200 consecutive hysterectomized women[63]), the majority of long-term users receiving hormone implants (Figure 2). The efficacy of subcutaneous implants is remarkable: hot flushes were reduced in all patients and there was an improvement in depression and libido in 99% and 92%, respectively[64]. It is assumed by many that hormone implants are synonymous with high-dose estrogens, as reported by Garnett and colleagues[65] (mean levels of 760 pmol/l in 1388 long-term users of 50–75 mg), but 25-mg doses at 6-month intervals have demonstrably beneficial skeletal and cardiovascular effects[66].

Testosterone replacement can be considered for continuing lethargy, tiredness and loss of libido in spite of adequate estrogen replacement, as demonstrated by Burger in non-hysterectomized women[67]. The ovary significantly contributes to androgen levels in both premenopausal and postmenopausal women. A 30% fall in testosterone is seen postoophorectomized premenopausal women to levels below that of a postmenopausal state. The postmenopausal woman produces 50% of circulating testosterone and 30% of androstenedione from her 'quiescent' ovaries. The lack of efficacy of estrogen therapy alone in oophorectomized or perimenopausal women may lead to disillusionment with HRT and consequent poor adherence. Testosterone replacement should therefore be discussed with all oophorectomized women, although at present this commits her to subcutaneous implants as this is the only androgen therapy currently licensed for women in Britain. Gonadomimetics, such as tibolone, may

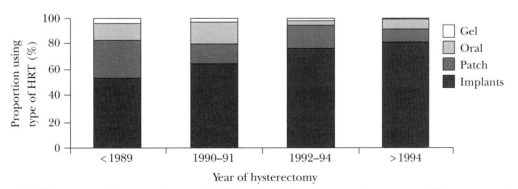

Figure 2 Hormone replacement therapy (HRT) preparation use according to year of hysterectomy in a follow-up survey of 545 women

have a role for those not suitable or reluctant for hormone implants, as they display estrogenic, progestogenic and androgenic properties. An improvement in libido greater than that experienced with estrogen replacement alone has been reported[68].

Progestogens

Progesterone is the most physiological compound in its psychological, physical and metabolic effects. Its use in the treatment of premenstrual syndrome for many years has elicited few side-effects[69]. Unfortunately, it is rapidly metabolized in the gut and it was not until the creation of oral micronized progesterone that a suitable product for endometrial transformation was available. However, at this time it is still underused due to the efficacy of synthetic progestogens. Progesterone pessaries/suppositories are licensed for endometrial opposition, but are unacceptable to many women due to the inconvenience of copious waxy discharge. A new progesterone-containing vaginal biogel may be more acceptable due to its smaller amount of carrier medium and a possible moisturizing effect on the vagina. Reversal of endometrial hyperplasia has also been demonstrated[70]. There is some evidence that a 'uterine first-pass' effect occurs, which would account for the efficacy of low serum levels of progesterone with this product[71] and the good side-effect profile.

Recent interest has been generated in transdermal progesterone cream, synthesized from diosgenin derived from a plant source. Although it is promoted as a product to be substituted for estrogen replacement, its lack of therapeutic effect in current doses on menopausal symptoms as compared to estrogen has led to some women adding estrogen therapy to their progesterone cream or exchanging the progestogen component of their HRT for the cream. The safety of this will soon be ascertained in controlled clinical trials, but, at present, all women presenting to doctors on these regimens should be discouraged or carefully monitored. The risks of unopposed or inadequately opposed estrogen therapy must be reinforced and the persistence of this increased risk for some years after cessation of therapy must be explained[72]. Those women wishing to use 'natural' products should be reassured of the molecular structure and origin of estradiol and a suitable product should be prescribed. The vast array of preparations on the market in the Western world makes it possible to create a regimen suitable for the majority of women wanting or needing to take HRT. The element of consumer choice must enhance the likelihood of concordance.

The C-19 nortestosterone-derived progestogens tend to have a more detrimental profile with respect to psychological outcomes, androgenic-type physical effects and less advantageous metabolic effects[73]. The progesterone-derived C-21 progestogens may have a more modified mood response in some women, although, as with the majority of hormonal prescribing, there is wide interindividual variation. It is difficult to predict the symptoms of bloating, edema, weight gain and migraine, which may be due to the mineralocorticoid activity of progestogens[74]. Androgenic symptoms are more likely in the C-19 progestogens, which have a relatively strong binding affinity for androgen receptors compared with pregnane progestogens such as medroxyprogesterone acetate[75]. Progesterone, dydrogesterone and norpregnane derivatives do not appear to have androgenic effects.

Duration of progestogen rather than dose is the most important factor for endometrial control. It may be necessary to respond to problems encountered with any regimen by varying type, duration, or, occasionally, dose of progestogen according to each individual woman.

The long-term safety of continuous combined preparations is still under review, but it appears from histological data that atrophic endometrium can be maintained in the majority of users[76].

An alternative mode of progestogen delivery being investigated intensively is the intrauterine system. The levonorgestrel intrauterine system (LNG IUS) releases levonorgestrel at a rate of 20 µg per day, which is sufficient to cause endometrial suppression[77] and is adequate to prevent endometrial proliferation in women using oral, transdermal, or subcutaneous estrogen[78]. The adverse metabolic, psychological and physical effects of progestogens are generally ameliorated by the significantly lower, stable plasma levels induced[79,80].

Starting HRT after a period of estrogen deprivation

Those women who are starting estrogen therapy after a long period of estrogen deprivation should have a gradual increase in dose even if hormone replacement has been suggested for treatment of osteoporosis or depression (i.e. relatively higher doses required) to minimize initial unacceptable effects and therefore maximize compliance. Non-bleed preparations may be a good option for the older woman some time from her menopause. High drop-out rates have been encountered due to the initial irregular bleeding in 40% of women. A trial of continuous combined HRT should be undertaken at the correct time with respect to the menopause, i.e. 1 year since last menstrual period, at least 1 year of sequential HRT or age over 54. All patients must be informed of initial bleeding problems, but be reassured that 60–75% should achieve a bleed-free regimen. The smaller dose of progestogen may alleviate the progestogenic side-effects and cause minimal alteration of the estrogenic effect on the high-density to low-density lipoprotein ratio, but occasionally persistent low-grade premenstrual-like symptoms can be incurred by the most progestogen-intolerant women.

REVIEW

A review appointment with the initial prescriber within 3–4 months of starting therapy should improve the willingness of the patient to try alternative regimens if the first choice is not suitable. A Danish study[81] evaluating the effect of introducing treatment alternatives on compliance revealed approximately 50% concordance in non-hysterectomized women compared with 65% in hysterectomized, but no statistical difference after introduction of an alternative regimen. A flexible approach to the search for the optimum HRT formulation for an individual with frequent review, in a manner well-rehearsed by general practitioners and family planning doctors with regard to contraceptive prescribing, should be encouraged. Once stabilized, follow-up can be reduced to annual check-ups (Table 3).

CONCLUSION

Although the majority of HRT prescribing can, and should, occur in the community by general practitioners, specialist menopause clinics can support the work of other clinicians by the suggestion of alternative regimens, regular update sessions and rapid review of related problems. Experts involved in women's health care should be counteracting the misinformation and misunderstandings delivered daily in the media. Written, up-to-date information that is readily available for patients would improve the situation that at present may set the primary health carers at odds with the specialists. Nachtigall[82] suggests that preparing women for potential problems, offering a solution and putting them into perspective, in addition to written information, will enhance continuation. Cost–benefit analysis with all factors considered will still, in our opinion, justify the prescription of HRT in the majority of women, but adherence may be largely determined by society's attitudes.

Table 3 Issues to be addressed at follow-up visits

Breast cancer (particularly at 5- and 10-year continuation)
Bleeding pattern
Mastalgia
Weight gain
Sexuality
Possible progestogenic side-effects
Concerns regarding the use of HRT arising from previous months (including addressing possible media messages)
General health advice (including diet, exercise and smoking)

References

1. Ravnikar VA. Compliance with HRT. *Am J Obstet Gynecol* 1987;156:1332–4

2. Hunter MS, O'Dea I, Britten N. Decision making and hormone replacement therapy: a qualitative analysis. *Soc Sci Med* 1997;45:1541–8

3. Wardell DW, Engebretson JC. Women's anticipations of hormone replacement therapy. *Maturitas* 1995;22:177–83

4. Jensen LB, Hilden J. Sociological and behavioral characteristics of perimenopausal women with an express attitude to hormone substitution therapy. *Maturitas* 1996;23:73–83

5. Sinclair HK, Bond CM, Taylor RJ. Hormone replacement therapy: a study of women's knowledge and attitudes. *Br J Gen Pract* 1993;43:365–70

6. Stampfer MJ, Willett WC, Colditz GA, *et al.* A prospective study of postmenopausal estrogen therapy and coronary heart disease. *N Engl J Med* 1985;313:1044–9

7. Draper J, Roland M. Perimenopausal women's views on taking hormone replacement therapy to prevent osteoporosis. *Br Med J* 1990;300:786

8. Hammond CB. Women's concerns with hormone replacement therapy – compliance issues. *Fertil Steril* 1994;62(Suppl 2):157s–160s

9. Moorhead T, Hannaford P, Warskyj M. Prevalence and characteristics associated with use of hormone replacement therapy in Britain. *Br J Obstet Gynaecol* 1997;104:290–7

10. Cano A. Compliance to hormone replacement therapy in menopausal women in a third level academic centre. *Maturitas* 1994;20:91–9

11. Coope J, Marsh J. Can we improve compliance with long term HRT? *Maturitas* 1992;15:151–8

12. Halbert DR, Lloyd T, Rollings N, *et al.* Hormone replacement therapy usage: a 10 year experience of a solo practitioner. *Maturitas* 1998; 29:67–73

13. Chung TH, Lau TK, Cheung LP, *et al.* Compliance with hormone replacement therapy in Chinese women in Hong Kong. *Maturitas* 1998; 28:213–19

14. Rozenberg S, Kroll M, Vandromme J, *et al.* Factors influencing the prescription of hormone replacement therapy. *Obstet Gynecol* 1997;90:387–91

15. Cauley JA, Cummings SR, Black DM, Mascioli SR, Seeley DG. Prevalence and determinants of estrogen replacement therapy in elderly women. *Am J Obstet Gynecol* 1990;163:1438–44

16. Leveille SG, LaCroix AZ, Newton KM, Keenan NL. Older women and hormone replacement therapy: factors influencing late life initiation. *J Am Geriatr Soc* 1997;45:1496–500

17. Collaborative group on hormonal factors in breast cancer. *Lancet* 1997;359:1047–59

18. Ettinger B, Grady D. Maximising the benefit of estrogen therapy for the prevention of osteoporosis. *Menopause* 1994;1:19–24

19. Barrett-Connor E. Hormone replacement therapy. Clinical review. *Br Med J* 1998;17:457–61

20. Hartmann BW, Huber JC. The mythology of hormone replacement therapy. *Br J Obstet Gynaecol* 1997;104:163–8

21. Domoney CL, Studd JWW. Long term continuation of hormone replacement therapy in hysterectomised women. Presented at *British Menopause Society Meeting*, Manchester, June 1999

22. Hulley S, Grady D, Bush T, *et al.* Randomised trial of estrogen plus progestin for the secondary prevention of coronary heart disease in postmenopausal women. Heart and estrogen/ progestin replacement study (HERS) research group. *J Am Med Assoc* 1998;280:605–13

23. Stevenson JC, Bees B, Devenport M, *et al.* Determinants of bone mineral density in normal women: risk factors for osteoporosis. *Br Med J* 1989;298:924–8

24. Ryan PJ, Harrison R, Blake GM, *et al.* Compliance with hormone replacement therapy (HRT) after screening for post menopausal osteoporosis. *Br J Obstet Gynaecol* 1992;99:325–8

25. Powell KM, Edgren B. Failure of educational videotapes to improve medication compliance in a health maintenance organization. *Am J Health Syst Pharm* 1995;52:2196–9

26. Norman SG, Studd JWW. A survey of views on hormone replacement therapy. *Br J Obstet Gynaecol* 1994;101:879–87

27. Wallace WA, Price VH, Elliot CA, *et al.* Hormone replacement therapy acceptability to Nottingham postmenopausal women with a risk factor for osteoporosis. *J R Soc Med* 1990;83:699–701

28. Isaacs AJ, Britton AR, McPherson K. Utilisation of hormone replacement therapy by women doctors. *Br Med J* 1995;311:1399–401

29. Andersson K, Pedersen AT, Mattsson LA, Milsom I. Swedish gynecologists' and general practitioners' views on the climacteric period: knowledge, attitudes and management strategies. *Acta Obstet Gynecol Scand* 1998;77:909–16

30. Wilkes HC, Meade TW. Hormone replacement therapy in general practice: a survey of doctors in the MRC's general practice research framework. *Br Med J* 1991;302:1317–20

31. Berman RS, Epstein RS, Lydick E. Risk factors associated with women's compliance with estrogen therapy. *J Wom Health* 1997;6:219–26

32. Karakoc B, Erenus M. Compliance considerations with hormone replacement therapy. *Menopause* 1998;5:102–6

33. Ulrich LG, Barlow DH, Sturdee DW, *et al.* Quality of life and patient preference for sequential versus continuous combined HRT: the UK Kliofem multicenter study experience. *Int J Gynecol Obstet* 1997;59(Suppl 1):S11–17

34. Rymer JM. The effects of tibolone. *Gynecol Endocrinol* 1998;12:213–20

35. Griffiths F. Women's health concerns: is the promotion of hormone replacement therapy for prevention important to women? *Fam Pract* 1995; 12:54–9

36. Garton M, Reid D, Rennie E. The climacteric, osteoporosis and hormone replacement; views of women aged 45–49. *Maturitas* 1995;21:7–15

37. Torgerson DJ, Donaldson C, Russell IT, *et al.* Hormone replacement therapy: compliance and cost after screening for osteoporosis. *Eur J Obstet Gynecol Reprod Biol* 1995;59:57–60

38. Torgerson DJ, Donaldson C, Reid DM. Bone mineral density measurements: are they worthwhile? *J R Soc Med* 1996;89:457–61

39. Kanis JA. Estrogens, the menopause and osteoporosis. *Bone* 1996;19(Suppl 5):185S–190S

40. Kritz-Silverstein D, Barrett-Connor E. Long-term postmenopausal hormone use, obesity and fat distribution in older women. *J Am Med Assoc* 1996;275: 46–9

41. Studd JWW. Complications of hormone replacement therapy in post menopausal women. *J R Soc Med* 1992;85:376–8

42. Ferguson KJ, Hoegh C, Johnson S. Estrogen replacement therapy: a survey of women's knowledge and attitudes. *Arch Int Med* 1989;149:133

43. Thom M, Studd JWW, *et al.* Prevention and treatment of endometrial disease in climacteric women receiving oestrogen therapy. *Lancet* 1979; 2:455–7

44. Gambrell RD. The prevention of endometrial cancer in postmenopausal women with progestagens. *Maturitas* 1986;8:159–68

45. Grady D, Gebretsadik T, Ernster V, *et al.* Hormone replacement and endometrial cancer risk: a meta-analysis. *Obstet Gynecol* 1995;85:304–11

46. Cullberg J. Mood changes and menstrual symptoms with different gestagen/estrogen combinations. A double blind comparison with placebo. *Acta Psychiatr Scand* 1972;236(Suppl):1–46

47. Magos AL, Brewster E, Singh R, O'Dowd T, Brincat M, Studd JWW. The effects of norethisterone in postmenopausal women on oestrogen replacement therapy: a model for premenstrual syndrome. *Br J Obstet Gynaecol* 1986;93:1290–6

48. Groeneveld FP, Bareman FP, Barentsen R, *et al.* Determinants of first prescription of hormone replacement therapy. A followup study among women aged 45–60 years. *Maturitas* 1994;20:81–9

49. Ringa V, Ledesert B, Breart G. Determinants of hormone replacement therapy among postmenopausal women enrolled in the French GAZEL cohort. *Osteo Int* 1994;4:16–20

50. Carey A, Carey B. Nutritional support for osteoporosis. In Studd JWW, ed. *The Management of the Menopause: Annual Review 1998.* Carnforth: Parthenon Publishing, 1998:159–68

51. Stampfer MJ, Colditz GA. Estrogen replacement and coronary heart disease: a quantitative assessment of the epidemiological evidence. *Prev Med* 1991;20:47–63

52. Paganini-Hill A, Ross RK, Henderson BE. Postmenopausal oestrogen treatment and stroke – a prospective study. *Br Med J* 1988;297: 519–22

53. Henderson VW, Paganini-Hill A, Emanuel CK, *et al.* Estrogen replacement therapy in older women: comparisons between Alzheimer's disease cases and nondemented control subjects. *Arch Neurol* 1994;51:896–900

54. Watson NR, Studd JWW, Garnett T, *et al.* Bone loss after hysterectomy with ovarian conservation. *Obstet Gynecol* 1995;86:72–7

55. Spector TD. Use of oestrogen replacement therapy in high risk groups in the United Kingdom. *Br Med J* 1989;299:1434–5

56. Griffiths F, Convery B. Women's use of hormone replacement therapy for relief of menopausal symptoms, for prevention of osteoporosis and after hysterectomy. *Br J Gen Pract* 1995;45: 355–8

57. Speroff T, Dawson NV, Speroff L, *et al.* A risk–benefit analysis of elective bilateral oophorectomy: effect of changes in compliance with estrogen therapy on outcome. *Am J Obstet Gynecol* 1991;164:165–73

58. Leather AT, Holland EFN, Andrews GD, Studd JWW. A study of the referral patterns and therapeutic experiences of 100 women attending a specialist premenstrual syndrome clinic. *J R Soc Med* 1993;86:199–201

59. Price EH, Little HK. Women need to be fully informed about the risks of hormone replacement therapy. *Br Med J* 1996;312:1301

60. Garnett T, Studd JWW. For how long should women take hormone replacement therapy? *Mat Ch Health* 1990;16:274–8

61. Stevenson JC. Handling hormone replacement therapy: key issues for the prescriber. *Eur J Obstet Gynecol Reprod Biol* 1996;64S:S25–7

62. Panay N, Studd JWW. Excessive supraphysiological levels of estradiol due to self medication and overdosage with estradiol gel. *Menopause* 1996;4:120–2

63. Studd JWW. Continuation rates with cyclical and continuous regimen of oral oestrogen and progestogens. *Menopause* 1996;3:181–2

64. Cardozo L, Gibb DMF, Studd JWW, *et al.* The use of hormone implants for climacteric symptoms. *Am J Obstet Gynecol* 1984;148:336–7

65. Garnett T, Studd JWW, Henderson A, *et al.* Hormone implants and tachyphylaxis. *Br J Obstet Gynaecol* 1990;97:917–21

66. Holland EFN, Leather AT, Studd JWW. The effect of 25 mg percutaneous estradiol implants on the bone mass of postmenopausal women. *Obstet Gynecol* 1994;83:43–6

67. Burger H, Hailes J, Nelson J. Effect of combined implants of oestradiol and testosterone on libido in postmenopausal women. *Br Med J* 1987;1:936–7

68. Nathorst-Boos J, Hammar M. Effect on sexual life – a comparison between tibolone and a continuous estradiol–norethisterone acetate regimen. *Maturitas* 1997;26:15–20

69. Dalton K. *Premenstrual Syndrome and Progesterone Therapy.* London: Heinemann Press, 1977

70. Affinito P, Di Carlo C, Di Mauro P, *et al.* Endometrial hyperplasia: efficacy of a new treatment with a vaginal cream containing natural micronised progesterone. *Maturitas* 1995;20:191–8

71. Casanas-Roux F, Nisolle M, Marbaix E, *et al.* Morphometric, immunohistological and three dimensional evaluation of the endometrium of menopausal women treated by oestrogen and Crinone, a new slow-release vaginal progesterone. *Hum Reprod* 1996;11:357–63

72. Whitehead MI, Hillard TC, Crook D. The role and use of progestogens. *Obstet Gynecol* 1990;75(Suppl):59S–76S

73. Panay N, Studd JWW. Progestogen intolerance and compliance with hormone replacement therapy in menopausal women. *Hum Reprod* 1997;3:159–71

74. Oelkers W, Schoneshofer M, Blumet A. Effects of progesterone and four synthetic progestogens on sodium balance and the renin–aldosterone system in man. *J Clin Endocrinol Metab* 1974;39:882–90

75. Rozenbaum H. How to choose the correct progestogen. In Birkhauser MH, Rozenbaum H, eds. *Menopause.* European Consensus Development Conference, Montreux, Switzerland. Paris: Editions ESKA, 1996:211–17

76. Leather A, Savvas M, Studd JWW. Endometrial histology and bleeding patterns after 8 years of continuous combined estrogen and progestogen therapy in postmenopausal women. *Obstet Gynecol* 1991;78:1008–10

77. Silverberg SG, Haukkamaa M, Arko H, *et al.* Endometrial morphology during long term use of levonorgestrel-releasing intrauterine systems. *Int J Gynaecol Pathol* 1986;5:235–41

78. Suhonen SP, Holmstrom T, Allonen HO, *et al.* Intrauterine and subdermal progestin administration in postmenopausal hormone replacement therapy. *Fertil Steril* 1995;63:336–42

79. Raudaskoski TH, Tomas EI, Paakkari IA, *et al.* Serum lipids and lipoproteins in postmenopausal women receiving transdermal oestrogen in combination with a levonorgestrel intrauterine device. *Maturitas* 1995;22:47–53

80. Panay N, Studd JWW, Thomas A, *et al.* The levonorgestrel intrauterine system as progestogenic opposition for oestrogen replacement therapy. Presentation at *Annual Meeting of the British Menopause Society,* Exeter, July 1996

81. Vestergaard P, Harmann AP, Gram J, *et al.* Improving compliance with hormone replacement therapy in primary osteoporosis prevention. *Maturitas* 1997;28:137–45

82. Nachtigall LE. Enhancing patient compliance with hormone replacement therapy at menopause. *Obstet Gynecol* 1990;75(Suppl 4):77S–80S

6

Monitoring of women on hormone replacement therapy: what should we be doing?

C. Page and A. Glasier

Hormone replacement therapy (HRT) improves quality of life for menopausal women by relieving vasomotor symptoms, and improving other menopausal symptoms such as vaginal dryness, loss of libido, poor memory and mood disturbance. Long-term treatment is thought to improve overall survival by decreasing the risks of both osteoporotic fracture and coronary heart disease. To obtain the long-term benefits it is recommended that women remain on HRT for at least 10 years, but the information available regarding monitoring of treatment for these women is vague and often confusing.

Special surveillance is recommended for patients with medical conditions such as diabetes, liver disease, heart disease, or hepatic disorders. However, in the case of diabetic women on HRT, there is little scientific justification at present to routinely recommend more intensive monitoring[1].

This review will look at what we should be doing for healthy women taking HRT. There are no clear guidelines on how women on HRT should be monitored. Different pharmaceutical companies recommend various levels of follow-up, and often their guidelines are unclear and non-specific. Analysis of the ABPI Compendium of Data Sheets[2] for the 15 top selling preparations of HRT in Lothian region from August 1998 to October 1998 confirmed this.

The following recommendations were made for assessment prior to starting treatment. All manufacturers recommended a full physical and gynecological examination, and for eight products it was advised that there should be special emphasis on examination of blood pressure, breasts, abdomen and pelvic organs. In the case of six preparations it was specifically stated that an endometrial assessment should be carried out if indicated.

None of the manufacturers advised a routine pre-treatment mammogram but for eight products it was recommended that patients be instructed in the technique of breast self-examination.

The makers of five preparations advised that body weight should be recorded at the initial examination. Although this may be a useful baseline, repeated measurements are unnecessary, as there is no evidence to suggest that HRT is associated with weight gain. Although HRT is frequently blamed for weight gain, it has been demonstrated that women who do not take HRT actually gain more weight than those on treatment. The Postmenopausal Estrogen/Progestin Investigation (PEPI) study showed that estrogen alone, or in combination with a progestogen, had little or no effect on weight or fat distribution[3].

In summary, the manufacturer's recommendations for assessment before starting a woman on HRT seem reasonably consistent. All women should have a thorough physical examination with special emphasis on examination of blood pressure, breasts, abdomen and pelvic organs. A mammogram should be performed only if clinically indicated. Women with abnormal bleeding should be investigated and may require an endometrial biopsy[4]. Those with a significant past or family history of venous thrombo-embolism should have a thrombophilia screen prior to commencing HRT.

However, for women established on HRT, the recommendations for subsequent monitoring become much less consistent. Follow-up examinations were recommended 'at least' 6-monthly for Nuvelle and Cycloprogynova, 6–12-monthly for seven other preparations, 'within one year' for Femoston and Tridestra, and 'periodically' for the four remaining preparations.

For ten products, specific advice was given that follow-up should include a full physical and gynecological examination, but for the remaining five, there was no indication of what the follow-up examination should include.

Breast examination was recommended 6-monthly for patients on Trisequens, and yearly for those on Femoston. For eight products, a 'regular' breast examination was advised, but this is unhelpful as the term 'regular' is open to a wide range of interpretation. For five products there was no specific mention of breast examination at follow-up.

'Regular' mammograms were recommended for all patients on Estraderm and Estracombi. The manufacturers of six preparations advised a regular mammogram if considered appropriate, and the data sheets stated that this should specifically include women with breast nodules or fibrocystic disease. For women on Evorel preparations the advice was that 'changes noticed during breast examination require further evaluation'. The remaining six products made no mention of indications for mammography.

The data sheets for eight products recommended 'regular monitoring of blood pressure in hypertensive patients'. Those for Climesse and Climagest stated that an idiosyncratic rise in blood pressure may occur, and for patients on Elleste it was recommended that treatment should be stopped at once if there was a significant rise in blood pressure. Data sheets for seven products made no mention of blood

pressure monitoring in hypertensive women, and for the eight that did, there was no mention of specific time intervals for rechecking blood pressure.

All data sheets stated that an endometrial biopsy should be performed if there was persistent breakthrough bleeding.

When considering the recommendations above, it is important to bear in mind that the data sheets are produced by the pharmaceutical companies. Although, in the UK, The Medicines Control Agency and Committee of Safety of Medicines review the data sheets before granting a licence, the recommendations are not evidence-based and are certainly driven to some degree by a desire to avoid successful litigation.

SO WHAT SHOULD WE BE DOING?

Research indicates that monitoring varies between different health professionals. This was highlighted by a study carried out in Sweden which showed that significantly more general practitioners than gynecologists measured blood pressure, weight and lipoproteins, and palpated the breasts before starting treatment and at the follow-up visits. On the other hand, significantly more gynecologists performed pelvic examination, transvaginal ultrasound scan, endometrial biopsy and mammography[5]. So what should we be doing?

In view of the fact that many women discontinue HRT because of minor side-effects, it seems sensible to arrange a follow-up visit after a short interval. Women on HRT should be reviewed 3 months after starting therapy to ensure that it is providing effective relief of menopausal symptoms and to assess bleeding patterns and side-effects. This is also an opportunity for women to clarify any areas of uncertainty they have about their treatment.

To determine the frequency and content of subsequent monitoring, the evidence for specific aspects of the follow-up examination will be considered in greater detail. These will include breast examination, mammography, blood pressure measurement, endometrial assessment and pelvic examination. It is important to bear in mind that monitoring which is too invasive may discourage women from starting or continuing HRT. On the other hand, sensible monitoring may enhance compliance by conferring confidence in the treatment.

BREAST EXAMINATION AND MAMMOGRAPHY

In 1997, the Collaborative Group on Hormonal Factors in Breast Cancer published data on analysis of 52 705 women with breast cancer, and 108 411 women without breast cancer, from 51 studies in 21 countries. The outcome of this analysis showed that the risk of breast cancer increases slightly in women using HRT and that the risk increases the longer the treatment is used[6].

The risk of breast cancer in non-users of HRT is calculated at 45 cases per 1000 women aged 50–70 years[6]. Extrapolating from the findings of the meta-analysis above, the use of HRT for 5 years would be expected to result in the diagnosis of two extra breast cancers by the age of 70 years. Use of HRT for 10 years would mean an extra six cases per 1000 women, and for 15 years an extra 12 cases[7]. As a consequence of this, doctors have an ethical responsibility to advise women of the increased risk of breast cancer associated with the use of HRT. However, if general practitioners were to perform an annual breast examination on all women on HRT, then in the case of 1000 women on treatment for 10 years we can calculate that general practitioners would have to perform 10 000 breast examinations. Despite this there is no guarantee that they would identify any of the six extra cases of breast cancer predicted, and indeed, the vast majority of breast cancers are identified by women themselves[8].

Mammography

In view of the prevalence of breast cancer in the UK, it would probably be desirable for all women to undergo mammography prior to starting treatment with HRT, however this is not economically feasible at present.

In 1993, The Royal College of Radiologists (RCR) recommended that; 'Commencement of HRT is not an indication for baseline mammographs. There is no evidence to suggest that mammography is cost effective in this situation and routine mammography outside the National Breast Screening Programme is not justified'[9]. This recommendation appeared unchanged in the RCR Guidelines for Doctors published in 1998[10].

Prior to starting HRT, women under the age of 50 years should only be offered mammography if they have significant risk factors for breast cancer, such as a history of benign breast disease with atypia, or a first-degree relative with premenopausal breast cancer. In the UK, women between 50 and 65 years of age should be encouraged to participate in the National Health Service Breast Screening Programme, which involves a routine 3-yearly mammogram. Beyond this age the national policy states that women can elect to continue with mammographic surveillance at their own request.

Breast self-examination

The role of breast self-examination is controversial. Self-examination is a systematic method of self-inspection and palpation of the breast, performed by a woman at the same time each month (preferably following the menstrual period). There has never been any consistent evidence that it reduces mortality from breast cancer and moreover it produces a high number of false positives leading to unnecessary investigation and anxiety.

Two large prospective trials have looked at the effect of self-examination on breast cancer stage and survival. In one study, women between the ages of 40 and 64 years were randomized either to perform or not perform breast self-examination. Follow-up at 5 years on a total study population of 120 310 women showed no significant differences in tumor size, axillary node involvement and stage between the groups[11]. In the second study women aged 45–64 years were invited to attend self-examination instruction[12]. Results at 7 years compared subsequent cancers in 89 010 women invited for education with a group of age-matched historical controls. Of the women with identified tumors, 47% had tumors less than 2 cm in diameter in the breast self-examination group compared with 37% in the controls. More of the self-examination group were node-negative (42% versus 33%), but they were also more likely to have advanced disease (18% versus 13%). The results at 7 years showed no survival advantage between breast cancer patients who attended the self-examination program and the control group.

The findings of these studies were backed up by an English language literature review of 45 papers on breast self-examination, which concluded that the procedure should not be promoted for mass screening[13]. The author did however go on to suggest that breast self-examination should be selectively applied, and that education about self-examination should be offered to all women 'at risk'. Women with a positive family history, or personal past history of breast cancer, and all women on HRT were included in the author's examples of those 'at risk'. The recommendation that women on HRT should perform breast self-examination must be challenged however, as there are no scientific data looking specifically at self-examination in women on HRT. Data from the general female population suggest that it does not reduce mortality from breast cancer and may actually increase anxiety[14].

Breast awareness

In 1989, the Government's Advisory Committee on breast cancer screening recommended that breast self-examination should not be promoted as a screening procedure. The Advisory Committee issued a further statement in 1991 promoting breast awareness[15]. This involves a woman being aware of what is normal for her regarding the look and feel of her breasts throughout the menstrual cycle. The committee recommended that women, particularly those over the age of 40 years, should be conscious of their breasts in everyday activities such as bathing, showering and dressing.

Breast palpation

The Department of Health in 1998 recommended that doctors and nurses should no longer perform routine breast palpation[16]. The Chief Medical Officer, Sir Kenneth Calman, stated that such examinations were likely to give false reassurance to patients and that it was more important to promote breast awareness, as over 90% of breast cancers are found by women themselves. The five-point code of 'Breast awareness'[17] states that women should:

(1) Know what is normal for them,

(2) Become familiar with the look and feel of their own breasts,

(3) Know what changes to look for,

(4) Report any changes without delay,

(5) Attend for breast screening if aged 50 or over.

The emphasis is on checking for normality and seeing the doctor only if something in the breast changes.

BLOOD PRESSURE MONITORING

A large body of epidemiological evidence suggests that estrogen use after the menopause may reduce the incidence of cardiovascular disease by over 40%[18]. It is thought that estrogens may act on vascular endothelial cells to enhance the synthesis and release of nitrous oxide and other vasodilators, and may also inhibit the synthesis and release of vasoconstricting agents, thus favoring vasodilatation[19]. These findings are backed up by evidence from the PEPI Trial, which failed to demonstrate any major effect of HRT on blood pressure. This was a randomized, double-blind, placebo-controlled trial with 3 years of follow-up, conducted to assess the influence of estrogen, with or without progestogen, on heart disease risk factors. The PEPI study concluded that estrogen alone, or in combination with a progestogen, improved lipoprotein patterns, lowered fibrinogen levels, and had no detectable effect on insulin levels or blood pressure[3].

Despite these findings, some doctors remain anxious about prescribing HRT to women with hypertension or other risk factors for cardiovascular disease. This was highlighted by a study from Birmingham which involved a postal survey of HRT prescribing habits among 285 general practitioners, physicians and gynecologists[20]. The results showed that 20% of general practitioners, 21% of physicians and 9% of gynecologists thought that HRT increased blood pressure. A minority in each group considered that HRT increased the risk of stroke, myocardial infarction and thrombosis, and 21% of all the doctors reported that they would not prescribe HRT to women whose hypertension was difficult to control. On the other hand, the same study showed that 9% of physicians did not routinely measure blood pressure before starting HRT, and 24% did not monitor blood pressure at follow-up. The figures for gynecologists were 13% and 10% respectively. All general practitioners stated that they routinely measured blood pressure before starting HRT, and at follow-up, 40% of them measured blood pressure 3-monthly, and 43% measured every 6 months.

A large prospective study carried out in 1991 demonstrated that HRT had no adverse effect on blood pressure in hypertensive women[21]. The authors of this study concluded that menopausal women with hypertension should not be denied HRT.

Considering the evidence presented above, the following guidelines are suggested for the monitoring of blood pressure in women on HRT (adapted from ref. 20).

All clinicians should measure a baseline blood pressure before starting HRT.

In normotensive women, HRT does not appear to raise the blood pressure and may even lower it[22,23]. A small number of women however, respond idiosyncratically to HRT with an acute rise in blood pressure. This effect was first reported in 1971 in association with conjugated estrogens[24]. The blood pressure should therefore be checked at the first follow-up visit at 3 months. Thereafter, there is no scientific justification for repeated blood pressure measurement in women on HRT. It is however a simple and quick procedure to perform. As many women taking HRT are in the age range where they may develop essential hypertension, or raised blood pressure due to some other cause, it would seem worthwhile to perform an annual blood pressure measurement as part of general well-woman screening.

In hypertensive women, blood pressure should be measured 6-monthly if well controlled, and 3-monthly if labile or difficult to control. If there is a rise in blood pressure, anti-hypertensive therapy should be adjusted as considered necessary.

ENDOMETRIAL ASSESSMENT

The use of estrogen monotherapy is known to promote growth of the endometrium, leading to hyperplasia and eventually to malignant transformation. Unopposed estrogen was first linked to endometrial cancer in the 1970s, when studies demonstrated a four- to sevenfold increased risk among women on estrogen monotherapy[25]. The addition of cyclical or continuous progestogen has been shown to protect the endometrium from hyperplastic change, a finding which was confirmed by the PEPI trial[26]. Although this trial was conducted to assess the influence of HRT on heart disease risk factors, it offered a unique opportunity to study the effect of HRT on the endometrium. The authors concluded that non-hysterectomized, postmenopausal women on estrogen replacement therapy should also receive a progestogen, administered either cyclically or continuously, for endometrial protection. In women unable to tolerate a progestogen, estrogen monotherapy could be considered, but follow-up of these women should include an annual endometrial assessment with discontinuation of the regimen following the diagnosis of endometrial hyperplasia.

Many women stop taking HRT after just a few months of use. The main reasons for this are bleeding problems and fear of cancer[27]. Unfortunately, bleeding problems such as spotting, and irregular or heavy bleeding remain major obstacles to the widespread and long-term use of HRT. The questions to be answered are, which women should we investigate, and which methods should we be using?

As endometrial cancer presents with abnormal uterine bleeding early in its clinical course, routine screening of asymptomatic women offers no advantage over evaluating women when they present with symptoms[28]. Vigilant surveillance leads to early discovery and improved chances for cure, therefore, all women with unexplained bleeding should undergo endometrial sampling[29]. In women who are taking cyclical progestogen, withdrawal bleeding is expected, and endometrial assessment is unnecessary if bleeding occurs exclusively at this time. It is well recognized that women on continuous-combined therapy have a high rate of breakthrough bleeding during the first 6 months of therapy.

In summary, postmenopausal women on HRT should undergo endometrial assessment if they continue to have breakthrough or irregular bleeding after the first 6 months of therapy (cyclical or continuous-combined), or if they develop new or irregular bleeding once stabilized on HRT[30].

METHODS OF ENDOMETRIAL ASSESSMENT

Endometrial biopsy

Endometrial biopsy can be performed by a variety of methods including the Pipelle sampler or the Z-sampler, and does not require anesthesia. It gives comparable results to dilatation and curettage (D&C) for specimen adequacy and diagnostic accuracy. One study showed a 97% sensitivity when specimens obtained with the Pipelle sampler were compared with those obtained at hysterectomy in patients with known endometrial cancer[31]. Other studies confirm these findings, showing a detection rate for endometrial hyperplasia and cancer which exceeds 95%[32,33]. In one of these studies[32], follow-up biopsies were performed at least 2 years after the initial biopsy. Two per cent of patients had endometrial cancer detected on the repeat biopsy, of which half were in the group that had a 'benign tissue' diagnosis and half were from the group that had 'insufficient tissue' obtained at the initial biopsy. Therefore, a repeat sample, or resampling by another method should be considered if bleeding continues after a normal biopsy. Compared with D&C, endometrial biopsy has fewer complications, including a lower rate of hemorrhage, infection and uterine perforation. It is also considerably less costly and is more convenient for patients, and should therefore be considered the first-line diagnostic procedure for abnormal uterine bleeding. This was the conclusion of the Gynaecology Audit Project in Scotland (GAPS 2) feedback report on endometrial sampling and D&C[34]. The authors went on to state that hysteroscopy should be regarded as a second-line procedure and that D&C should only be considered if the cervical canal cannot be cannulated, or if insufficient tissue for histological examination is obtained from initial endometrial biopsy and symptoms persist.

Hysteroscopy

Hysteroscopy allows direct visualization of the endometrium and it is possible to biopsy or excise identified abnormalities. It is superior to D&C and endometrial biopsy for its ability to detect endometrial polyps and submucous myomas, however, it cannot be used in patients with cervical stenosis or in patients who are actively bleeding, as this impairs the ability to visualize the cavity. Compared to endometrial biopsy it is relatively expensive and therefore should be considered a second-line measure for endometrial sampling.

Transvaginal sonography

Transvaginal sonography can be used to demonstrate the thickness and echogenicity of the endometrium, and it is also useful for imaging the ovaries. The importance of this was highlighted by a study from Dundee in which five out of 76 women presenting with postmenopausal bleeding were found to have ovarian tumors, which were detected by ultrasound[35]. This clearly shows that adnexal pathology should be excluded in women with postmenopausal bleeding.

With transvaginal scanning the ability to identify endometrial polyps and submucous myomas can be enhanced by instilling isotonic saline into the endometrial cavity prior to imaging, a process known as saline infusion sonography[30].

Multiple studies suggest that an endometrial thickness of less than 4 mm is associated with a low risk of endometrial pathology including adenocarcinoma. In women who are receiving cyclical HRT however, the endometrial thickness varies between 4 and 8 mm, and is about 5 mm in women on continuous-combined therapy[29]. Transvaginal sonography therefore cannot be relied upon as the sole diagnostic test for women on HRT with uterine bleeding. In these women, significant pathology must be ruled out with endometrial sampling[30]. The presence of fluid in the endometrial cavity has been associated with carcinoma of the endometrium and therefore requires investigation with endometrial biopsy.

In summary, endometrial biopsy is the first-line choice of investigation because of its diagnostic accuracy, convenience and lower cost. Pelvic ultrasonography is a non-invasive outpatient procedure, which has the advantage of not only predicting endometrial pathology, but also excluding ovarian pathology. Transvaginal ultrasound and endometrial biopsy can be performed in the clinic as a 'one-stop' assessment. In this situation it is advisable to do the ultrasound scan first, as changes induced by the biopsy make the ultrasound difficult to interpret. If endometrial biopsy and transvaginal sonography do not provide a satisfactory diagnosis then hysteroscopy is a reasonable next step. D&C should be reserved for patients in whom none of the other methods are possible.

PELVIC EXAMINATION

It is widely stated in the ABPI data sheets that bimanual pelvic examination should form part of the routine follow-up of women on HRT; but what evidence is there in favor of this procedure which many women find unpleasant?

Obviously a pelvic examination is mandatory in any woman on HRT who has symptoms such as irregular bleeding or pelvic pain. However, what do we hope to achieve by examining asymptomatic women?

Researchers in Melbourne attempted to answer this question by performing a pelvic examination on 2623 healthy, asymptomatic volunteers with a mean age of 51 years[36]. A bulky or fibroid uterus was detected in 12.9% of women and the prevalence of abnormal adnexal findings was 1.5%, with a positive predictive value of 22% for a subsequent diagnosis of benign adnexal abnormality. No ovarian malignancies were identified from further investigation of the group with abnormal adnexal findings. The authors concluded that there was no clear benefit to asymptomatic women of detecting a fibroid uterus, or bulky uterus due to adenomyosis, as progression to malignancy is rare. They went on to question the value of bimanual pelvic examination as a screening procedure for ovarian malignancy. This was in view of the low incidence of ovarian cancer in the population (1 in 2500 women per year after age 45 years)[37], and the fact that the number found at a potentially curable stage would be even lower still.

These findings were backed up by a study of 18 753 women, in which only one of six asymptomatic women with ovarian carcinoma detected by pelvic examination was cured of her disease[38]. In another study, in which 6470 women underwent screening with transvaginal sonography, six patients were found to have primary ovarian cancers. Of these patients, only one had a palpable abnormality on pelvic examination[39]. These studies confirm that pelvic examination as a screening test for ovarian cancer is ineffective in changing the likelihood of a favorable outcome. The risks of pelvic examination include unnecessary investigation, anxiety and surgery after a false-positive screening result.

From review of the literature, there appears to be little to be gained from performing pelvic examinations in asymptomatic women, and therefore this should not form part of the routine follow-up of women on HRT.

Cervical smears

HRT is not associated with an increased risk of cervical cancer and therefore smears should be taken in accordance with the national screening programs.

CONCLUSIONS

After considering all the evidence, the following recommendations can be made for the follow-up of women on HRT.

(1) The initial review should take place 3 months after starting therapy. This is an opportunity to ensure symptom control, assess side-effects and clarify any areas of uncertainty the woman may have about her treatment. The blood pressure should be checked at this visit and thereafter can be measured once a year as part of opportunistic well woman screening.

(2) The next review should take place 3–6 months later in order to assess the bleeding pattern. Women who continue to have irregular or breakthrough bleeding after the first 6 months of therapy should undergo endometrial assessment.

(3) Once established on HRT, women should be reviewed once a year. At each annual review, the doctor should assess symptom control and side-effects, enquire about the bleeding pattern, and consider how much longer the patient should remain on therapy. The blood pressure can be measured, and women reminded that if they develop new or irregular bleeding they should seek a medical opinion, as they will require endometrial assessment. The concept of breast awareness should be discussed, and women over the age of 50 years should be encouraged to attend the National Breast Screening Programme for mammography.

(4) In asymptomatic women there is no need to perform a breast or pelvic examination.

(5) Finally, women should be encouraged to attend their doctor at any time if new problems arise during treatment.

References

1. Studd J. ed. *The Management of the Menopause. Annual Review 1998.* Carnforth: Parthenon Publishing, 1998:273
2. *ABPI Compendium of Data Sheets and Summaries of Product Characteristics 1998–1999.* London: Datapharm Publications Limited, 1999
3. Writing Group for the PEPI Trial. Effects of estrogen or estrogen/progestin regimens on heart disease risk factors in postmenopausal women. The Postmenopausal Estrogen/Progestin Interventions (PEPI) Trial. *JAMA* 1995;273:199–208
4. Speroff L. Treating the perimenopausal patient. *Contemp Obstet Gynaecol* 1993;27:124–41
5. Andersson K, Pedersen AT, Mattsson L, Milsom I. Swedish gynaecologists' and general practitioners' views on the climacteric period: knowledge, attitudes and management strategies. *Acta Obstet Gynecol Scand* 1998;77:909–16
6. The Collaborative Group on Hormonal Factors in Breast Cancer. Breast Cancer and HRT: collaborative reanalysis of data from 51 epidemiological studies of 52 705 women with breast cancer and 10 8411 women without breast cancer. *Lancet* 1997;350:1047–59
7. Wise J. HRT increases risk of breast cancer. *Br Med J* 1997;315:969
8. DOH 1998. *Clinical Examination of the Breast.* PL/CMO/98/1
9. Royal College of Radiologists. Hormone Replacement Therapy and Mammography. *Reference List for Royal College of Radiologists Guidelines* 1993: FCR/5/93
10. Royal College of Radiologists Working Party. *Making the Best Use of Clinical Radiology: Guidelines for Doctors*, 4th edn. London: RCR, 1998.
11. Semiglazov VF, Bavli JL, *et al.* The role of breast self examination in early breast cancer detection

(results of the 5 years USSR/WHO randomised study in Leningrad). *Eur J Epidemiol* 1992;8: 498–502

12. Locker AP, Caseldine J, Mitchell AK, Blarney RW, Roebuck EJ, Elston CW. Results from a seven year program of breast self examination in 89 010 women. *Br J Cancer* 1989;60:401–5

13. Vafiadis P. Breast self-examination: should general practitioners bother? *Aust Fam Physician* 1997;26(suppl 1):S41–6

14. Brain K, Norman P, Gray J, Mansel R. Anxiety and adherence to breast self-examination in women with a family history of breast cancer. *Psychosom Med* 1999;61:181–7

15. DOH. *Breast Awareness*. London: DOH, 1991 (Professional Letter: PL/CMO (91) 15, PL/CNO (92) 12)

16. DOH. *Clinical Examination of the Breast*. London: DOH, 1998 (Professional Letter: PL/CMO/98/1, PL/CNO/98/1)

17. DOH. *Be Breast Aware*. London: DOH, 1998 K64/ 006 14343 PDD 50K 2P Nov. 98 SA (CLO)

18. Stampfer MJ, Colditz GA. Estrogen replacement therapy and coronary heart disease: a quantitative assessment of the epidemiological evidence. *Prev Med* 1991;20:47–63

19. Pines A, Mijatovic V, van der Mooren MJ, Kenemans P. HRT and cardioprotection: basic concepts and clinical considerations (Review). *Eur J Obstet Gynecol, Reprod Biol* 1997;71:193–7

20. Lip G, Beevers M, Churchill D, Beevers DG. Do clinicians prescribe HRT for hypertensive post-menopausal women? *Br J Clin Pract* 1995;49:61–4

21. Peck K, Perry IJ, Leusley DM, *et al.* The effect of HRT on blood pressure in hypertensive women (Abstract). *J Hypertens* 1991;9:1087

22. Von Eiff AW, Plotz EJ, Beck KJ, Czernik A. The effects of oestrogens and progestogens on blood pressure regulation of normotensive women. *Am J Obstet Gynecol* 1971;4:31–47

23. Perry I, Beevers M, Beevers DG, Leusley D. Oestrogens and cardiovascular disease. *Br Med J* 1998;297:1127

24. Crane MG, Harris JJ, Winsor W. Hypertension, oral contraceptive agents and conjugated oestrogens. *Ann Intern Med* 1971;74:13–21

25. Smith DC, Prentice R, Thompson DJ, *et al.* Association of exogenous estrogens and endometrial carcinoma. *N Engl J Med* 1975;293:1164

26. The Writing Group of the PEPI Trial. Effects of hormone replacement therapy on endometrial histology in postmenopausal women. The postmenopausal estrogen/progestin interventions (PEPI) trial. *JAMA* 1996;275:370–5

27. Ravnikar VA. Compliance with hormone replacement therapy. *Am J Obstet Gynecol* 1987; 156:1332–4

28. Archer DF, McIntyre-Seltman K, Wilborn WW, *et al.* Endometrial morphology in asymptomatic postmenopausal women. *Am J Obstet Gynecol* 1991;165:317

29. Good AE. Diagnostic options for assessment of postmenopausal bleeding. Concise review for primary care physicians. *Mayo Clin Proc* 1997;72: 345–9

30. Fontaine P. Endometrial cancer, cervical cancer, and the adnexal mass. *Primary Care* 1998;25: 433–57

31. Stovall TG, Photopulos GJ, Poston WM, Ling FW, Sandles LG. Pipelle endometrial sampling in patients with known endometrial carcinoma. *Obstet Gynecol* 1991;77:954–6

32. Chambers JT, Chambers SK. Endometrial sampling: When? Where? Why? With what? *Clin Obstet Gynecol* 1992;35:28

33. Grimes DA. Diagnostic dilatation and curettage: A reappraisal. *Am J Obstet Gynecol* 1982;142:1

34. *Gynaecology Audit Project in Scotland 2. Endometrial sampling and D&C. Feedback Report.* Scottish Executive Committee of the RCOG, June 1996

35. Gupta JK, Wilson S, Desai P, Hau C. How should we investigate women with postmenopausal bleeding? *Acta Obstet Gynecol Scand* 1996;75:475–9

36. Grover S, Quinn M. Is there any value in bimanual pelvic examination as a screening test? *Med J Aust* 1995;162:408–10

37. Cutler SJ, Young JL. Third national cancer survey: incidence data. *Natl Cancer Inst Monogr* 1075;41:1–25

38. MacFarlane C, Sturgis MC, Fetterman FS. Results of an experiment in the control of cancer of the female pelvic organs and report of a fifteen-year research. *Am J Obstet Gynecol* 1955;69:294

39. DePriest PD, Gallion HH, Pavlik EJ, Kryscio RJ, van Nagell JR Jr. Transvaginal sonography as a screening method for the detection of early ovarian cancer. *Gynecol Oncol* 1997;65: 408–14

7

The place of tibolone in menopausal therapy

J. Ginsburg and G. M. Prelevic

WHAT IS TIBOLONE?

Tibolone is a synthetic steroid, an analog of norethynodrel (Figure 1), which relieves hot flushes, maintains urogenital and skeletal integrity and improves mood and libido. In laboratory animals the drug has been found, on the basis of conventional pharmacological testing, to have weak estrogenic, progestogenic and androgenic activity. From the clinical point of view, tibolone cannot however be considered either a classical estrogen, progestogen, or androgen, in particular since it does not stimulate the growth of endometrial or breast tissue. A welcome consequence of the lack of stimulant activity of the drug on the uterus is that no concurrent progestogen therapy is required and vaginal bleeding is thereby obviated.

METABOLISM AND MECHANISM OF ACTION OF TIBOLONE

That the alleviation of vasomotor symptoms by tibolone and its beneficial effects on bone strength, mood and libido – classical estrogen effects – are achieved without endometrial or breast stimulation, can now be explained in terms of the varying proportions of the different metabolites (Figure 1) of the drug produced in specific tissues. The three main metabolites – $\Delta 4$-tibolone, 3α-hydroxytibolone and 3β-hydroxytibolone – have different binding affinities for estrogen, progesterone and androgen receptors (Table 1). Thus the $\delta 4$ metabolite has a higher affinity for progesterone and

androgen receptors than the parent drug and does not bind to estrogen receptors.

In the endometrium, tibolone is metabolized virtually exclusively to the $\Delta 4$ metabolite by the enzyme 3β-hydroxysteroid dehydrogenase and since the $\Delta 4$ metabolite has no estrogenic affinity, there is no endometrial stimulation – indeed the endometrium atrophies. In the breast, the reduced stimulation of breast tissue – an effect

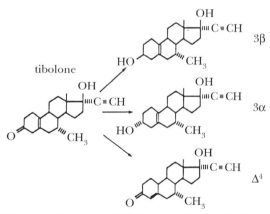

Figure 1 Structure of tibolone and its metabolites

Table 1 Binding affinities of tibolone and metabolites

	Steroid receptor		
	Estrogen	*Progesterone*	*Androgen*
Tibolone	+	+	+
$\Delta 4$ tibolone	0	++	++
3α hydroxytibolone	+	0	0
3β hydroxytibolone	+	0	0

that is manifest clinically and also in tissue culture of normal and malignant breast cells – relates to the fact that tibolone and its metabolites inhibit sulfatase and thereby formation of estrone and estradiol[1,2]. This is another example of the differential pattern of metabolism of tibolone in different tissues.

As far as the skeleton is concerned, although the precise mechanism of the action of tibolone on bone metabolism has not been defined, the fact that the effects of the drug on bone are blocked by a synthetic anti-estrogen (ICI 164.384) but not by an anti-androgen (flutamide) or an anti-progestogen (Org 31710)[3] suggests that the maintenance of skeletal integrity by tibolone depends on a mechanism akin to that of the action of estrogens on bone.

Similarly, whilst the mechanism of the effects of tibolone on central nervous system activity, manifest clinically by the alleviation of hot flushes and improvement in mood and libido, is not yet known, this must likewise relate to an influence of the drug and/or its metabolites on central nervous system activity. Indeed, some data suggest that tibolone may stimulate endorphin release[4].

The foregoing unique combination of an estrogenic effect in the skeleton and central nervous system, with a simultaneous absence of stimulatory effects on the endometrium and breast, has led to the description of tibolone as a 'tissue-specific' drug, which can exert estrogenic or progestogenic effects in different tissues depending on the amount and relative distribution of the main metabolites of tibolone produced in that particular tissue.

Tibolone itself binds, albeit weakly, to all three receptors – estrogen, progesterone and androgen. The 3α and 3β metabolites bind weakly to estrogen receptors but not to progesterone or androgen receptors (Table 1).

EFFECTS OF TIBOLONE ON MENOPAUSAL SYMPTOMS

Hot flushes

Numerous studies have documented the effectiveness of tibolone in alleviating climacteric symptoms[5–8]. In a randomized double-blind, placebo-controlled study in 60 postmenopausal women, tibolone was significantly more effective than placebo in reducing hot flushes, sweats, sleeplessness, fatigue, irritability and psychic instability[7]. A study comparing tibolone with estradiol valerate and with placebo showed that tibolone was as effective as estradiol valerate with regard to symptoms and mood ratings[9].

In our own experience[8] climacteric symptoms were relieved in the majority of women within 3–5 weeks. Classical vasomotor symptoms (hot flushes, night sweats and sleep disturbance) were present initially in 38.2% but only 2.63% had symptoms at the first follow-up visit 6–8 weeks after starting tibolone. A very high proportion of our patients presented with 'psychological' problems, such as mood change, loss of libido or depression, but only 2.25% reported any 'psychological' problem a few weeks after starting tibolone. The overwhelming majority of patients taking tibolone felt much better than before therapy and wanted to continue on the drug.

Mood

Changes in mood are difficult to measure, particularly since they are often associated with alleviation of other menopausal symptoms. Most studies assessing the effect of tibolone on menopausal symptoms indicate, however, that it has a beneficial influence on mood.

Vaginal dryness and libido

Tibolone also produces significant improvement in libido and in sexual enjoyment. It has been claimed that women with major sexual problems show the greatest improvement[10]. Tibolone seems to be more effective with regard to sexual enjoyment and frequency than an estrogen–norethisterone combination. The fact that tibolone appears to be superior to conventional menopausal therapy for sexual well-being may be attributable to its androgenic effects.

Vaginal dryness and dyspareunia are relieved by tibolone[11]. An increased karyopyknotic index and maturation index of the vagina[11] after tibolone are clearly an estrogenic effect.

But despite this estrogenic effect on the vagina, tibolone does not stimulate the endometrium, another example of its 'tissue specificity'.

In a recent open, but randomized, parallel group study of postmenopausal women who had atrophic vaginitis, tibolone was highly effective in reducing vaginal dryness, dyspareunia and signs of atrophic vaginitis[12].

PREVENTION AND TREATMENT OF OSTEOPOROSIS WITH TIBOLONE

Tibolone reduces bone resorption as indicated by decreases in urinary hydroxyproline to creatinine and calcium to creatinine ratios in a short-term study[13] and prevents cortical bone loss in experimental animals[14].

Tibolone has been shown to increase bone mineral density at both the spine and the hip in postmenopausal women to a similar extent to estrogens[15–18]. Both prevention of bone loss[19] and increased spine bone mineral density were also demonstrated with tibolone in women with established osteoporosis, with or without previ-

ous fractures, treated with tibolone[16,20,21]. Concurrent treatment with tibolone also prevents the adverse effects on bone mineral density and on cancellous bone microstructure induced by gonadotropin releasing hormone agonists given to women with endometriosis[22,23].

We reviewed the comparative effects on bone mineral density of 3 years tibolone or estrogen (either unopposed or combined with cyclical progestogen) in postmenopausal women who had not previously received estrogen or other menopausal therapy[18]. The increase in spine bone mineral density we observed after tibolone was greater than that recorded with either transdermal estradiol or conjugated equine estrogens (Figure 2) and also than that reported with etidronate, fluoride, or calcitonin. A possible explanation for this greater increase in spine bone mineral density is that the women to whom we gave tibolone were older than those given estrogen. The skeletal response to agents that reduce bone resorption also depends on the degree of skeletal activation at the start of the treatment. A greater gain in bone mass

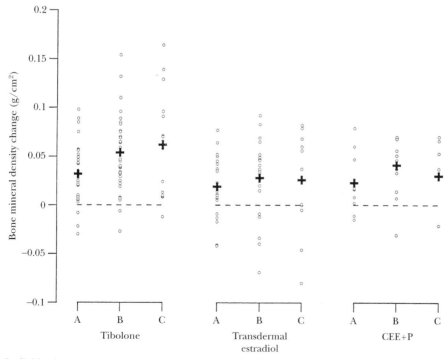

Figure 2 Individual net changes in spine bone mineral density (BMD) with tibolone, transdermal estradiol and conjugated equine estrogens with progestogen (CEE + P) over 1 year (A), 2 years (B) and 3 years (C) (reproduced from ref. 18, with permission)

would therefore be expected in women with a high turnover rate and a larger skeletal remodelling space, as is the case in older women who have more severe osteoporosis.

A randomized double-blind parallel group study showed that a lower dose of tibolone (1.25 mg) is effective in preventing bone loss in older women, i.e. more than 10 years after the menopause[24]. The effect of tibolone on bone mineral density is in fact dose dependent and 2.5 mg daily is more effective than 1.25 mg[25].

Increases in bone mineral density with tibolone should be clinically significant in reducing fracture rates since their magnitude is similar to that seen with other agents. However, there are as yet no studies that have specifically measured fracture reduction with tibolone.

Also, prevention of bone loss or a drug-induced increase in bone mineral density is not invariably associated with a proportionate decrease in risk of fracture. Our recent data have, however, shown that women on tibolone have better postural stability than women of corresponding age who are not on menopausal therapy[26]. This suggests that tibolone may provide additional benefit in terms of fracture prevention.

THE CARDIOVASCULAR SYSTEM AND TIBOLONE

The effect of tibolone on blood pressure

Our own clinical observation has shown no significant effect of tibolone on blood pressure in women even after years of treatment. The presence of hypertension is no contraindication to the administration of tibolone but clearly *any* woman with hypertension should receive effective hypotensive therapy.

The effect of tibolone on peripheral and cardiac flow

Tibolone causes a significant increase in forearm blood flow[27]. Hand flow is however unchanged. The fact that blood flow in the calf

also increases and the results of simultaneous measurement of flow by strain gauge plethysmography and water-filled venous occlusion plethysmography suggest that tibolone vasodilates skeletal muscle arterioles rather than those of forearm skin. The response to reactive hyperemia in the forearm showed a significant increase in both peak and overall forearm flow in women who had taken tibolone for only 8 weeks. This indicates a direct effect of tibolone on the vasculature since the vasodilatation associated with reactive hyperemia is a local response of the blood vessels unaffected by blood pressure. No change in the reactive hyperemic response is seen after estrogen treatment, either oral or transdermal, in menopausal women[28].

Stroke volume was overall unaffected by tibolone after 6–8 weeks of therapy in healthy subjects[27] but in women with diabetes mellitus who had received tibolone for 12 months there was an increase in stroke volume after 6 months[29], suggesting that in the long run tibolone may improve cardiac function. The fact that tibolone improved left ventricular relaxation in postmenopausal women with diabetes[29] could be of particular importance since impairment of left ventricular relaxation is thought to be the first sign of subclinical diabetic cardiomyopathy.

A recent study in a small number of post-menopausal women with coronary heart disease showed that tibolone might help to reduce ischemia and prolong the time to onset of angina[30].

The effect of tibolone on venous thromboembolism

There is no evidence of any increase in venous thromboembolism as occurs in women taking conjugated equine estrogens. Indeed the available information on the effects of the drug on parameters of blood fractions relevant to thromboembolism suggests the reverse – that the drug might even have a beneficial effect. Whilst short-term studies documented a decrease in fibrinogen and increases in anti-thrombin II, plasminogen and fibrinolytic activity[31], longer-term studies showed a significant reduction in plasminogen activator, plasminogen activator inhibitor-1 activity and fibrinogen with the standard (2.5 mg) and also with a lower (1.25 mg) dose of tibolone[32].

METABOLIC EFFECTS OF TIBOLONE

The effect of tibolone on serum lipid and lipoproteins

Several studies document that tibolone reduces serum triglycerides, high density lipoprotein (HDL) cholesterol and very low density lipoprotein (VLDL) cholesterol and also lipoprotein(a) (Lp(a)) and apoprotein A concentrations[33–37]. Reports of the effects of tibolone on low density lipoprotein (LDL) cholesterol and apoprotein B gave conflicting results – either no change[37] or a slight reduction in LDL[36] and also either an increase[37,38] or a decrease[36,39] in apoprotein B.

Since the specific protein component of Lp(a), apolipoprotein(a), is a mutant of plasminogen, it has been suggested that changes in Lp(a) induced by tibolone and other testosterone derivatives may be related to changes in plasminogen metabolism which might provide cardiovascular protection[40], although there are no corresponding clinical data

It must be emphasized that there are no controlled trials of the effects of lowering HDL on the incidence of coronary vascular disease in women. Hence the clinical significance of pharmacologically reduced circulating levels of HDL cholesterol and a possible association with increased risk of cardiovascular disease is unknown.

Longer-term studies are needed, at different dose levels, to establish the clinical relevance of lipid changes in relation to possible cardiovascular protection by different types of menopausal therapy. In the interim, the relationship between the observed lipid changes and possible long-term influences of tibolone and other drugs on the cardiovascular system, in terms of either beneficial or adverse clinical effects, must be speculative.

The effect of tibolone on carbohydrate metabolism

In intravenous glucose tolerance tests Cagnacci and associates[41] showed significant enhancement of insulin sensitivity after 3 months' tibolone treatment in healthy non-diabetic postmenopausal women.

We treated a group of postmenopausal women with type 2 diabetes with tibolone for 12 months and observed no change in fasting and postprandial blood glucose over the period of observation[42]. The most significant finding was however a reduction in fasting and postprandial serum insulin concentration, indicating an increase in insulin sensitivity, i.e. a decrease in insulin resistance (Figure 3). In theory, this reduced insulin concentration during tibolone treatment in postmenopausal women with non-insulin-dependent diabetes may have implications regarding possible alterations in cardiovascular risk in such women.

EFFECT OF TIBOLONE ON THE BREAST

By contrast with estrogens, tibolone does not stimulate the breast. Breast tenderness or swelling is virtually absent in women taking tibolone. Clinical reviews testify to the low incidence of breast symptoms with the drug,

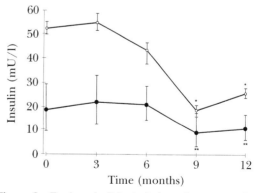

Figure 3 Fasting (solid circles) and postprandial (open circles) serum insulin concentrations (geometric means ± SE) during tibolone treatment in postmenopausal women with non-insulin-dependent diabetes mellitus (reproduced from ref. 42, with permission)

particularly in women who discontinued estrogen because of unacceptable breast swelling or tenderness.

Tissue studies have confirmed markedly reduced growth of breast cells, both human and animal, and even of neoplastic cell lines after tibolone[43,44]. Apoptosis is increased and in rats, growth of a dimethybenzanthracene-induced mammary carcinoma is inhibited[43]. There is also, as already mentioned, evidence of a tissue-specific effect of the drug in the breast, because of the inhibition by tibolone and its metabolites of estrone and estradiol formation[45].

Whilst inference from such studies to human neoplasia is tempting, there are, as yet, no studies of the potential influence of tibolone in women with breast cancer. Such studies are urgently needed. At present, whilst we may be using tibolone in selected cases referred for consideration of tibolone after treatment for breast carcinoma and where there are unacceptable hot flushes or other climacteric symptoms or severe osteoporosis, we urgently need data from comparative control studies of the effects of tibolone in such women.

VAGINAL BLEEDING IN WOMEN ON TIBOLONE

Despite the absence of endometrial stimulation by tibolone, vaginal bleeding has been reported in women taking the drug, albeit intermittently and only occasionally. The incidence of vaginal bleeding in our series is close on 12%[8]. Rymer and colleagues[46], however, reported a higher incidence, in the order of 20%. This occurred most frequently in younger women, i.e. those

who had only entered recently on the menopause and in whom consequently significant concentrations of endogenous estrogen were probably still present. The average age of women for whom we prescribed tibolone is higher than those seen by Rymer's group since we only gave tibolone to women after at least 1 years' amenorrhea and usually to those who had entered on the menopause some 5 or more years earlier.

In a recent double-blind study comparing bleeding and spotting in women on tibolone and on continuous combined estrogen/progestogen therapy, bleeding episodes on tibolone were one-third to one-half of those seen with a continuous combined preparation[47]. Also, while most of the bleeding episodes with tibolone occurred during the first 3 months of therapy it took up to 6 months for bleeding patterns to stabilize on the continuous combined regimen.

We investigated the cause of vaginal bleeding in some 500 postmenopausal women started on tibolone between 1987 and 1996[48] and who had taken tibolone for a mean duration of almost 3 years (range 2–75 months). Although a morphological change, such as a polyp or fibroid, was responsible for the bleeding in a significant proportion, there was no apparent intrauterine cause found to account for vaginal bleeding in over half the 47 women who bled in the course of tibolone treatment (Table 2). In the majority of those with no morphological cause for the bleeding, the endometrium was thin or atrophic. A thickened endometrium was however observed on ultrasound in a few cases but with no pathological features on subsequent

Table 2 Causes of vaginal bleeding in postmenopausal women on tibolone (reproduced from ref. 48, with permission)

	< 4 months of therapy*		> 12 months of therapy
	Previous E_2	No previous E_2	
Endometrial polyp	2	4	5
Fibroid	3	2	2
Endometrial carcinoma (*in situ*)	0	0	2
Benign endometrial hyperplasia	0	0	2
Thickened endometrium (no histological abnormality)	2	1	0
No apparent cause (inactive endometrium)	10	6	8

*E_2, estradiol

histological examination. Bleeding was never heavy and was not accompanied by severe pain. The duration of bleeding was rarely more than 2–3 days and generally was not repeated.

In younger women, intermittent ovarian activity with consequent estrogen secretion may be responsible for this bleeding. But at any age a switch from postmenopausal estrogen therapy to tibolone may result shortly thereafter in vaginal bleeding because of residual estrogen released from tissue depots.

A morphological abnormality may however be present even in women who have taken estrogens recently and experienced bleeding thereafter. Hence, bleeding after tibolone always requires investigation. It is not, however, necessary to discontinue the drug whilst investigation is in progress. The majority of our patients continued happily without incident on tibolone during and after the completion of investigation.

The incidence of carcinoma of the endometrium in women who bled on tibolone did not seem to be more than would be expected in postmenopausal women of that age. Even if carcinoma of the endometrium is found and hysterectomy then performed, tibolone may safely be continued.

SIDE-EFFECTS OF TIBOLONE THERAPY

The major side-effect of tibolone is weight gain and also a tendency to bloating and edema. However, this was reported in only 11% of women in our series[8].

Breast tenderness and/or breast enlargement was reported by 7.5%. But in a group of 70 women who had been switched to tibolone because of severe side-effects with estrogen, only one complained of breast tenderness, although 20% had experienced breast tenderness on estrogen.

Nausea was reported in 5% of our series. This occurred relatively soon after starting tibolone but tended to disappear within a few weeks. Our drop-out rate, overall, because of side-effects, was less than 3% in 301 women[8].

A small number of women reported a slight increase in facial hair growth after switching

from estrogen, which reflects the absence of estrogenic effects on facial hair.

WHY, WHEN AND FOR WHOM SHOULD TIBOLONE BE PRESCRIBED?

Tibolone is being increasingly used in the treatment of menopausal women, particularly in the older age groups.

It is not, however, suitable for younger women – not because it is harmful but because in the presence of significant amounts of circulating estrogens, as can occur in women shortly after the menopause and in the perimenopausal phase, the intake of tibolone, with its progestogenic potential, can result in irregular menstrual bleeding and hence the necessity to investigate. Ovarian activity can wax and wane in the perimenopause with corresponding variations in estrogen production, and significant amounts of circulating estrogens may be present for longer than is generally appreciated. It is therefore simpler not to give tibolone to women in the perimenopausal phase or within a few months of entering on the menopause, unless they no longer have a uterus. There are other preparations which can be given at that stage. In due course, when endogenous estrogen activity is thought to have ceased, the women can discontinue the exogenous estrogen. Ultrasound assessment of endometrial thickness should be made to confirm the absence of a thickened endometrium and circulating estrogen levels should be checked.

In our experience, the ideal candidate for the administration of tibolone is a women 2, 3 or more years postmenopause. If she has previously been treated with estrogens, these should have been discontinued for at least 6 months, unless the uterus is no longer *in situ*.

It should be emphasized that there is no age limit to the administration of tibolone. Unlike estrogens, where estrogen therapy in a woman of 70 or more can result in unacceptable breast stimulation or vaginal bleeding, tibolone is extremely useful for the older woman.

As far as osteoporosis is concerned, tibolone is particularly effective in the older woman with osteoporosis. Once an increase in bone mineral density has been effected, it seems that the dose required for maintenance of skeletal integrity is less. The dose for effective relief of hot flushes is 2.5 mg at night but for maintenance of skeletal integrity, half that dosage may be sufficient. At present, however, the only tablet marketed is the 2.5 mg. Women who bloat on that dosage or who require the drug for maintenance of skeletal integrity may in our experience achieve the desired effect by taking 2.5 mg on alternate nights.

References

1. Pasqualini JR, Gelly C, Nguyen B-L, Vella C. Importance of oestrogen sulfates in breast cancer. *J Steroid Biochem* 1989;34:155–63

2. Chetrite G, Kloosterboer HJ, Pasqualini JR. Effect of tibolone (Org OD14) and its metabolites on estrone sulphate activity in MCF-7 and T-47D mammary cancer cells. *Anticancer Res* 1997;17:135–40

3. Ederveen AGH, Kloosterboer HJ. Tibolone exerts an estrogenic effect on bone leading to prevention of bone loss and reduction in bone resorption in ovariectomised rats. *Osteoporosis Int* 1998;8(Suppl 3):95

4. Genazzani AR, Petraglia F, Facchinetti F, *et al.* Effects of OD14 on pituitary and peripheral β-endorpin in castrated rats and postmenopausal women. *Maturitas* 1987;S1:35–48

5. Kicovic PM, Cortes-Prieto J, Luisi M, *et al.* Placebo controlled cross-over study of the effects of Org OD 14 in menopausal women. *Reproduction* 1982; 6:81–91

6. Nevinny-Stickel J. Double-blind cross-over study with Org OD 14 and placebo in postmenopausal women. *Arch Gynecol* 1983;234:27–31

7. Benedek-Jaszmann LJ. Long-term placebo-controlled efficacy and safety study of Org OD 14 in climacteric women. *Maturitas* 1987;Suppl 1, 25–33

8. Ginsburg J, Prelevic G, Butler D, *et al.* Clinical experience with tibolone (LivialR) over eight years. *Maturitas* 1995;21:71–6

9. Crona N, Samsioe G, Lindberg UB, *et al.* A treatment of climacteric complaints with Org OD 14: a comparative study with estradiol valerate and placebo. *Maturitas* 1988;9:303–8

10. Nathorst-Boos J, Hammar M. Effects on sexual life – a comparison between tibolone and a continuous estradiol–norethisterone acetate regimen. *Maturitas* 1997;26:15–20

11. Rymer J, Chapman MG, Fogelman I, *et al.* A study of the effect of tibolone on the vagina in postmenopausal women. *Maturitas* 1994;18:127–33

12. Botsis D, Kassanos D, Kalogirou D, *et al.* Vaginal ultrasound of the endometrium in postmenopausal women with symptoms of urogenital atrophy on low-dose oestrogen or tibolone treatment: a comparison. *Maturitas* 1997;26:57–62

13. Netelenbos JC, Siregar-Emck MthW, Schot LPC, *et al.* Short-term effects of Org OD14 and 17 beta estradiol on bone and lipid metabolism in postmenopausal women. *Maturitas* 1991; 13:137–49

14. Schot LPC, Kloosterboer HJ, Deckers GHJ. Pharmacological profile of Org OD 14 in experimental animals. In Vermer H, van Duren D, eds. *Livial: The Current Status of Research and Therapy.* Carnforth: Parthenon Publishing, 1992:11–23

15. Lindsay R, McKay Hart D, Kraszewski A. Prospective double blind trial of synthetic steroid (Org OD 14) for preventing postmenopausal osteoporosis. *Br Med J* 1980;1:1207–9

16. Geusens P, Dequeker J, Gielen J, *et al.* Non-linear increase in vertebral density induced by a synthetic steroid (Org OD14) in women with established osteoporosis. *Maturitas* 1991;13: 155–62

17. Rymer J, Chapman MG, Fogelman I. Effects of tibolone on postmenopausal bone loss. *Osteoporosis Int* 1994;4:314–17

18. Prelevic GM, Bartram C, Wood J, *et al.* Comparative effects on bone mineral density of tibolone, transdermal oestrogen and oral oestrogen/progestogen therapy in postmenopausal women. *Gynecol Endocrinol* 1996;10:413–20

19. Lyritis GP, Karpathios S, Basdekis K, *et al.* Prevention of post-oophorectomy bone loss with tibolone. *Maturitas* 1995;22:247–53

20. Studd J, Arnala I, Zambhere P, *et al.* Tibolone increases bone mass in women with previous fractures in a placebo controlled bicentre study. *Osteoporosis Int* 1996; 6(Suppl 1):230

21. Pavlov PW, Ginsburg J, Kicovic P, *et al.* Double blind placebo-controlled study of the effects of tibolone on bone mineral density in postmenopausal osteoporotic women with and without

previous fractures. *Gynecol Endocrinol* 1999;in press

22. Compston JE, Yamaguchi K, Croucher PI, *et al.* The effects of GnRHa on iliac crest cancellous bone structure in women with endometriosis. *Bone* 1995;16:261–7

23. Lindsay PC, Shaw RW, Coelingh Bennink HJ, *et al.* The effect of add-back treatment with tibolone (Livial) on patients treated with the GnRHa triptorelin. *Fertil Steril* 1996;65:342–8

24. Bjarnason NH, Bjarnason K, Hassager C, *et al.* The response in spinal bone loss to tibolone treatment is related to bone turnover in elderly women. *Bone* 1997;20:151–5

25. Berning B, Kuijak CB, Kuiper JW, *et al.* Effects of two doses of tibolone on trabecular and cortical bone loss in early postmenopausal women: a two year randomized, placebo controlled study. *Bone* 1996;19:395–9

26. Brooke-Wavell K, Prelevic GM, Athersmith LE, *et al.* Tibolone use and physical activity associated with better postural stability in postmenopausal women. *26th European Symposium on Calcified Tissues*, 1999, Maastricht, the Netherlands

27. Hardiman P, Nihoyannopoulous P, Kicovic P, *et al.* Cardiovascular effects of Org OD 14 – a new steroidal therapy for climacteric symptoms. *Maturitas* 1991;13:235–42

28. Ginsburg J, Hardiman P. Cardiovascular effects of transdermal oestradiol in postmenopausal women. *Ann NY Acad Sci* 1990;592:424–5

29. Prelevic GM, Beljic T, Ginsburg J. The effect of tibolone on cardiac flow in postmenopausal women with non-insulin dependent diabetes mellitus. *Maturitas* 1997;27:85–90

30. Lloyd GWL, Patel NR, McGing EA, *et al.* Acute effects of hormone replacement with tibolone on myocardial ischaemia in women with angina. *IJCP* 1998;52:155–7

31. Cortes-Prieto J. Coagulation and fibrinolysis in post-menopausal women treated with Org OD14. *Maturitas* 1987;1:67–72

32. Bjarnason NH, Bjarnason K, Haarbo J, *et al.* Tibolone: influence on markers of cardiovascular disease. *J Clin Endocrinol Metab* 1997;82:1752–6

33. Kloosterboer HJ, Benedek-Jaszmann LJ, Kicovic PM. Long-term effects of Org OD 14 on lipid metabolism in postmenopausal women. *Maturitas* 1990;12:37–42

34. Crona N, Silfverstolpe G, Samsoie G. A double-blind cross over study on the effects of Org OD14 compared to estradiol valerate and placebo on lipid and carbohydrate metabolism in oophorectomized women. *Acta Endocrinol* 1983;102:451–5

35. Rymer J, Crook D, Sidhu M, *et al.* Effects of tibolone on serum concentrations of lipo-protein(a) in postmenopausal women. *Acta Endocrinol* 1993;128:259–62

36. Castelo-Branco C, Casals E, Figueras F, *et al.* A two year prospective and comparative study on the effects of tibolone on lipid pattern, behavior of apolipoproteins A1 and B. *Menopause* 1999;6:92–7

37. Farish E, Barnes JF, Fletcher CD, *et al.* Effects of tibolone on serum lipoproteins and apolipo-protein levels compared to a cyclical oestrogen/progestogen regimen. *Menopause* 1999;6:98–103

38. Haengi W, Lippuner K, Riesen W, *et al.* Long-term influence of different postmenopausal hormone replacement regimens on serum lipids and lipoprotein (a): a randomised study. *Br J Obstet Gynaecol* 1997;104:708–17

39. Millner MH, Sinnott MM, Cooke TM, *et al.* A two year study of lipid and lipoprotein changes in postmenopausal women with tibolone and estrogen–progestin. *Obstet Gynecol* 1996;87:593–9

40. Crook D, Cust MP, Gangar KF, *et al.* Comparison of transdermal and oral estrogen/progestin hormone replacement therapy: effects on serum lipids and lipoproteins. *Am J Obstet Gynecol* 1992;166:950–5

41. Cagnacci A, Mallus E, Tuveri F, *et al.* Effects of tibolone on glucose and lipid metabolism in postmenopausal women. *J Clin Endocrinol Metab* 1997;82:251–3

42. Prelevic GM, Beljic T, Balint-Peric LJ, *et al.* Metabolic effects of tibolone in postmenopausal women with non-insulin dependent diabetes mellitus. *Maturitas* 1998;28:271–6

43. Kloosterboer HJ, Schoonen WGEJ, Deckers GH, Klijn JGM. Effects of progestogens and Org OD14 in in vitro and in vivo tumour models. *J Steroid Biochem Molec Biol* 1994;49:311–18

44. Kandouz M, Lombet A, Perrot J-Y, *et al.* Proapoptotic effects of antiestrogens, progestins and androgens in breast cancer cells. *J Steroid Biochem Molec Biol* 1999;69:463–71

45. Chetrite GS, Kloosterboer HJ, Philippe J-C, Pasqualini JR. Effects of Org OD14 (Livial) and its metabolites on 17 β-hydroxysteroid dehydrogenase activity in hormone-dependent MCF-7 and T-47D breast cancer cells. *Anticancer Res* 1999;19:261–8

46. Rymer J, Fogelman I, Chapman MG. The incidence of vaginal bleeding with tibolone treatment. *Br J Obstet Gynaecol* 1994;101:53–6

47. Hammar M, Christau S, Nathorst-Boos J, *et al.* A double-blind, randomized trial comparing the effects of tibolone and continuous combined hormone replacement therapy in postmenopausal women with menopausal symptoms. *Br J Obstet Gynaecol* 1998;105:904–11

48. Ginsburg J, Prelevic GM. Cause of vaginal bleeding in postmenopausal women on tibolone. *Maturitas* 1996;24:107–10

8

Selective estrogen receptor modulators: a review for the clinician

N. Manassiev, F. Keating and M. Whitehead

INTRODUCTION

The menopause is recognized as a gender-specific risk factor affecting many aspects of women's health. The hormonal deficiency associated with ovarian failure has wide-ranging and unwelcome consequences and leads to diverse metabolic changes and symptomatology. Among the short-term effects are vasomotor instability and psychological symptoms; medium-term effects include urogenital atrophy. Long-term consequences are an increased risk of coronary artery disease, osteoporosis and possibly Alzheimer's disease. While the short- and medium-term effects of estrogen withdrawal can cause severe symptoms, the long-term consequences can be lethal. Traditionally, these consequences have been treated with hormone replacement therapy (HRT). It appears that HRT decreases the risk of coronary artery disease, prevents bone loss and possibly reduces the risk of Alzheimer's disease. Unfortunately, HRT has a number of side-effects, such as breast tenderness, bloatedness, headaches, muscle cramps and unscheduled vaginal bleeding, all of which lead to poor long-term compliance. There are data suggesting that HRT may increase the risk of venous thromboembolism and that long-term use of HRT may increase the risk of breast cancer slightly: current data suggest an approximate 2% increase in risk of incidence of breast cancer with each year of use of HRT.

A new class of drugs, selective estrogen receptor modulators (SERMs), is emerging which allows us to understand the mechanism of hormonal action better and which may open new indications for treatment. The term SERM has been suggested to define more precisely chemical compounds which can bind to and activate the estrogen receptor (ER), but which have effects on target tissues that are different from estradiol[1]. The fundamental concept behind SERMs is retention of the beneficial effects of HRT with avoidance of its drawbacks, especially with regard to endometrial stimulation, breast cancer and prothrombotic changes.

BACKGROUND

The search for an even safer alternative to HRT has led to the evaluation of several compounds, grouped together as 'antiestrogens'. Initially, these compounds were used for the treatment of hormonally responsive cancers, such as breast cancer. Therefore, they were termed 'antiestrogens'. However, after the realization that postmenopausal women with breast cancer treated with tamoxifen had lower cholesterol levels and increased spinal bone density compared with untreated controls, it became evident that the term 'antiestrogen' does not fully describe these compounds. It is now clear that 'antiestrogens' have a wide spectrum of activities, from being pure estrogen antagonists to mixed agonists/ antagonists.

The best known are the triphenylethylenes, such as clomiphene (Clomid®, Hoechst Marion Roussel, Denham, UK), tamoxifen (Nolvadex®, Zeneca, Wilmslow, UK), chlorotamoxifen (toremifene, Fareston®, Orion, Newbury, UK), 3-hydroxytamoxifen (droloxifene, Pfizer, Sandwich, UK), pyrrolidino-4-iodotamoxifen (idoxifene, SmithKline Beecham, Welwyn Garden City, UK) and miproxifene (TAT-59). The first two are in widespread clinical use, and recently toremifene (Fareston®) has been approved for the treatment of advanced breast cancer. Other agents with mixed agonist/antagonist properties include benzothiophenes, such as raloxifene (Evista®, Eli Lilly, Indianapolis, USA), and structurally distinct molecules such as ormeloxifene (centchroman) and levormeloxifene (Novo Nordisk, Glostrup, Denmark). ICI 182 780 (Zeneca, Wilmslow, UK) has been found to be a pure estrogen antagonist and is now under clinical investigation for the treatment of tamoxifen-resistant breast cancer. As

it is currently used, the SERM classification includes all compounds previously described excluding pure antiestrogens such as ICI 182 780. The structure of some SERMs is given in Figure 1.

MECHANISM OF ACTION OF ESTROGEN

To understand the mechanism of action of SERMs, a brief description of steroid hormone action and, in particular, estrogen action at cellular and molecular level is needed. The current understanding of the mode of action of steroid hormones is shown in Figure 2. Free unbound steroids are thought to diffuse passively to all cells, because there is no evidence as yet of an active transport mechanism. Steroids are preferentially retained in target cells as stable complexes with intracellular receptor proteins (e.g. estrogen receptor, ER), which are steroid- and tissue-specific. The receptor is thought to be a ligand-activated transcription factor, the steroid being the ligand. The receptor is also called a hormone-activated transcription factor. The

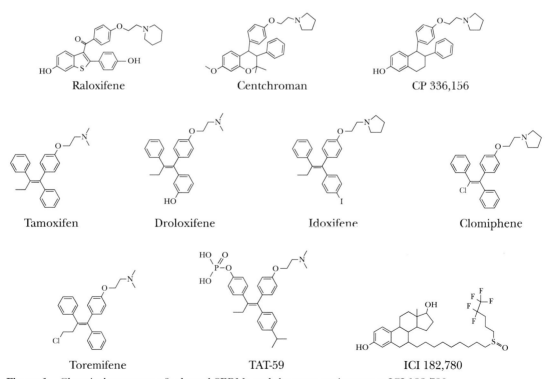

Figure 1 Chemical structure of selected SERMs and the pure antiestrogen ICI 182,780

terms are often used interchangeably. The ER has six structural domains of overlapping functions labelled A–F. Two important domains are the steroid-binding domain and the DNA-binding domain.

The receptor binds the hormone, i.e. estrogen, through its steroid-binding domain. The binding of the receptor by the steroid results in the activation of the receptor molecules, which, in turn, leads to conformational changes in the hormone–receptor complex, including its DNA-binding domain. This activation process allows the hormone–receptor complex to bind to specific sites in the DNA, termed nuclear acceptor sites. Once bound to the nuclear acceptor sites, the activated steroid–receptor complex acts as a transcription factor, which 'turns on' genes. Specific genes become acti-

vated by this process to produce nuclear RNA, and then messenger RNA (mRNA). This new mRNA codes for the production of new proteins in the ribosomes. The newly synthesized proteins change the metabolism of the target cell in a specific manner. The transfer of the steroid into the cell and nuclear binding of the steroid–receptor complex is rapid, occurring within minutes. Nuclear binding affects mRNA levels and synthesis within several hours, and finally changes in protein synthesis and turn-over occur within 12–24 h. The major physiological effects of steroids in cells are seen in 12–36 h[2,3].

Two estrogen receptors have been described so far: ER-α (classical ER) and ER-β (recently described). The classical ER has been cloned and sequenced from MSF-7 human breast

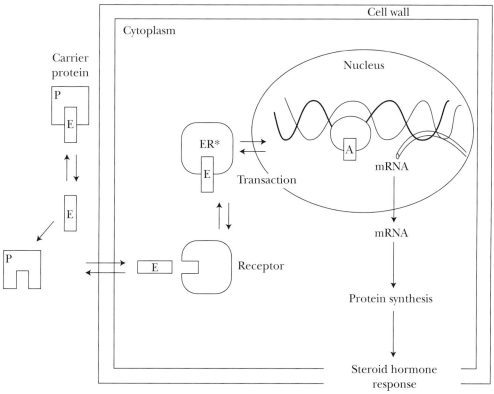

Figure 2 A schematic representation of the subcellular effects of estrogen (E) in estrogen target tissue. Estrogens dissociate from plasma proteins (P) and the complex becomes activated (ER*). Activated ER complex interacts with the nuclear acceptor site on the DNA. This results in the activation of DNA polymerase and RNA polymerase to initiate subsequent cell proliferation and protein synthesis, respectively. The receptor is then destroyed (processed), in which case a new cytoplasmic receptor is synthesized or recycled for subsequent ligand binding. Whether the binding of estrogen and the receptor occurs on the cytoplasm or the nucleus has been debated. It is currently thought that the interaction happens in the nucleus

cancer cells[4,5]. The ER-α consists of 595 amino acids with a molecular weight of 66 kDa. The ER-β was cloned in 1996 from rat prostate and ovary[6]. It consists of 485 amino acids and has a molecular weight of 54.2 kDa. ER-β is 95% homologous with ER-α in the DNA-binding domain and 55% in the hormone-binding domain. ER-α has a higher affinity for short-acting estrogens such as 17α-estradiol[7].

In some tissues, for example uterus, pituitary and epididymis, both types of receptor are present, but in others there is a predominance of one type of receptor. In the kidney, only ER-α is present, while the brain contains only ER-β. The ovary and the prostate seem to contain ER-α and -β in equal amounts. The physiological role of the different receptors is currently being studied. For example, ER-α knockout mice (mice which do not possess ER-α) develop to maturity, but are infertile and do not respond to estradiol[8].

SUGGESTED MECHANISM OF ACTION OF SERMS

During puberty and reproductive life, estrogen exerts its effects (via the mechanism just described) on all cells and tissues susceptible to its action. These include the reproductive system and breasts, the cardiovascular system (CVS), the central nervous system (CNS), the bone, and skin and connective tissues. After the menopause, the lack of estrogen leads to involutionary changes at some of these sites. When estrogen is given as HRT, it again starts to affect all these organs and systems indiscriminately. However, in postmenopausal women, not all its effects are desirable. This naturally leads to the concept of selective estrogen receptor modulating activation, where beneficial estrogen action on certain receptors is retained (CVS, the bone, CNS, skin and connective tissue, lower reproductive and urinary tracts), whilst leaving receptors in the breast and the upper reproductive tract (uterus) inactive.

It is possible that the estrogen agonist/antagonist properties of SERMs will find explanation, at least in part, in activation/deactivation of different classes of ERs.

Emerging evidence from several groups indicates the presence of multiple transcriptional pathways for ligand-bound estrogen receptor. The estrogen receptor contains multiple transcriptional activating functions (i.e. AF-1 and AF-2) that account for some of the tissue-selective effects of SERMs. At cellular and molecular level, agonist/antagonist activity may arise in one of several ways[9,10], which can be postulated thus:

(1) As competitive inhibitors which bind to the estrogen receptor but fail to activate it;

(2) By activating the estrogen receptor and binding to the nuclear acceptor site, but failing to initiate full gene transcription or expression;

(3) By binding to the ER but preventing its transport to the nucleus;

(4) By binding to the receptor and then destroying it;

(5) By binding to the cell DNA but without binding to the DNA-binding domain of the estrogen–receptor complex.

TAMOXIFEN

Background

Tamoxifen is a non-steroidal estrogen receptor agonist/antagonist which is widely used for palliative and adjuvant treatment of breast cancer. Tamoxifen was initially known as ICI 46 474 and was discovered in the late 1960s as part of the Fertility Control Programme at ICI Pharmaceuticals (now Zeneca)[11,12]. Although tamoxifen was developed as an antifertility agent[13] and was found to be an antiestrogen in the laboratory, like clomiphene it induced ovulation in subfertile women[14]. Preliminary clinical studies demonstrated efficacy of tamoxifen in the treatment of advanced breast cancer[15,16].

Effect of tamoxifen on breast cancer

From these early studies, it appears that tamoxifen has a high anti-tumor potency and a low incidence of side-effects. Its widespread long-term use as adjuvant therapy in breast cancer therapy and prevention of cancer in the contralateral breast with long-term treatment (2 or more years) has demonstrated a survival advantage in node-positive postmenopausal patients[17]. Its use soon became widespread as the antiestrogen drug of choice in the treatment of postmenopausal women with breast cancer. Several clinical trials showed the beneficial effects of tamoxifen in reducing tumor recurrence and in prolonging the disease-free interval and overall survival when administered after surgery for primary breast cancer. In postmenopausal women or those 50 years or older, the response rate is 30%, with a decrease in the risk of death of 20%. Tamoxifen is effective in advanced, metastatic breast cancer as well. It induces 10–50% regression of such cancers, depending on the receptor status[18]. Tamoxifen has also been shown to decrease the incidence of cancer in the contralateral breast significantly by 40–47%[19-21].

It is now being evaluated for the prevention of breast cancer in women with a strong family history of this disease[22], and interim results have already been published[23]. It appears that tamoxifen is an ineffective chemoprevention agent in this very high-risk group. However, when used as a prophylactic agent in healthy women with an average or moderately elevated risk for breast cancer, a different picture emerges. Tamoxifen (20 mg/day) or placebo was given to 13 388 women for 5 years in a double-blind, randomized clinical trial[24]. In this trial, tamoxifen led to a 49% reduction in the incidence of invasive breast cancer, and a 50% reduction in non-invasive breast cancer compared to placebo. Risk was also reduced in women with a history of lobular carcinoma *in situ* (56%) or atypical hyperplasia (86%). This decrease in risk was noted across a wide age group – 35–49 (44%), 50–59 (51%) and 60 years or older (55%). The reduction (69%) was in the incidence of estrogen receptor-positive cancers[24]. In a similar but smaller study, tamoxifen afforded protection to women taking HRT[25].

Effects of tamoxifen on menopausal symptoms

One of the commonest side-effects reported with the use of tamoxifen is the induction or worsening of vasomotor symptoms. Up to two-thirds of women treated with tamoxifen reported moderate to severe hot flushes[24,26].

Tamoxifen and bone

It was feared that the antiestrogenic effect of tamoxifen would lead to bone loss. However, these fears have not been realized in postmenopausal women because tamoxifen does not appear to have an antiestrogenic effect on bone. In a study involving iliac crest biopsy, it was shown that tamoxifen does not cause bone loss or defective bone formation[27]. The effect of tamoxifen on bone depends in part on the menopausal status. In postmenopausal women, 20–40 mg of tamoxifen administered daily leads to bone preservation or some increase in bone density of between 0.6 and 1.7% at 2 years[28,29]. In premenopausal women, it may lead to a slight bone loss[30]. The bone-preserving effects of long-term tamoxifen treatment (20 mg daily) are likely to be modest. At the end of one 5-year study, tamoxifen-treated patients had 2% more bone compared to the baseline level, while untreated patients had a 2.7% loss compared to baseline[31]. Another study found no increase in bone mineral density in postmenopausal women treated with 40 mg tamoxifen for 7 years, in comparison to the baseline[32].

The effects on fracture risks are controversial. One study reported that tamoxifen does not appear to offer protection against fracture[24], and may even increase the risk[33].

Tamoxifen and the endometrium

Endometrial polyps have been reported with tamoxifen use as both an incidental finding and as a pathological cause of uterine bleeding. The polyps tend to be multiple and larger than polyps in non-tamoxifen-exposed women. Several studies have reported on the increased incidence of endometrial polyps and carcinoma in postmenopausal women on tamoxifen therapy for breast cancer[34–36]. The relative risk for developing endometrial cancer amongst tamoxifen-treated women was between 1.1 (non-significant) and 6.5[37]. In spite of these disparate findings, most people would accept a link between tamoxifen and endometrial cancer as proven and advocate close surveillance for breast cancer patients treated with tamoxifen[38]. A recent large, prospective, randomized, controlled trial reported a relative risk of 2.53 for endometrial cancer in those taking tamoxifen compared to placebo[24].

Effects of tamoxifen on lipids

A number of studies investigating the effects of tamoxifen on serum lipids have been reported. It appears that tamoxifen leads to a decrease in total cholesterol, low density lipoprotein cholesterol (LDL-C) and lipoprotein(a), while high density lipoprotein cholesterol (HDL-C) and triglycerides remain unchanged. The fall was 10–12% in total cholesterol, 17–19% in the LDL-C and 37% in lipoprotein(a)[39–42]. Tamoxifen given for at least 5 years as adjuvant therapy for breast cancer has been reported to reduce the risk of myocardial infarction in postmenopausal women[43]. However, another study did not find such reduction[24].

Effects on venous thrombosis

It is traditionally taught that the use of tamoxifen is associated with an increase in venous thromboembolism. However, it is to be remembered that cancer *per se* increases the risk of venous thromboembolism[44]. The risk of venous thromboembolism in breast cancer victims varies from 0.1% in untreated early-stage disease to 17% in stage IV disease patients receiving chemotherapy[45]. There are conflicting reports on risk of venous thromboembolism with tamoxifen therapy, with some studies reporting an increase[46] and others[47] no change in incidence. The reported increase in the relative risk for pulmonary embolism was 3.01 and for deep vein thrombosis 1.6[24]. These

results are of similar magnitude to those reported for HRT. A number of studies have examined laboratory parameters of hemostasis and have consistently found a decrease in serum fibrinogen (14–18%), platelets (7–9%) and antithrombin III and little other significant changes in coagulation parameters[48–51].

Summary of the effects of tamoxifen

Tamoxifen has estrogenic effects on the uterus, antiestrogenic effects on the breast, neutral or weakly estrogenic effects on bone and weakly estrogenic effects on serum lipids. On coagulation and fibrinolysis it has a neutral or weakly estrogenic action and an antiestrogenic effect on vasomotor symptoms.

RALOXIFENE

Background

Raloxifene was originally called keoxifene, which was initially investigated as therapy for breast cancer. *In vitro* studies demonstrated the ability of raloxifene to prevent estrogen binding to ER and to exhibit antitumor activity which was carcinogen-induced in rodents[52], and to block estradiol-dependent proliferation of MCF-7 breast cancer cells[53]. However, it demonstrated a lack of antitumor effect in a small trial in postmenopausal women with breast cancer resistant to tamoxifen[54].

Animal studies

Through a number of animal studies, it became evident that raloxifene has a SERM profile distinct from that of tamoxifen. It is thought that the tissue selectivity of raloxifene may reside in its ability to occlude particular co-activator recruitment sites on the surface of the ER ligand-binding domain[54]. Raloxifene is also able to prevent transcriptionally competent AF-2 formation. It may be that, in some tissues, complete matching between the ER and the hormone is necessary for activation to occur, while in others partial matching may be sufficient[55]. There are data to show that the nitrogen in the raloxifene side-chain must specifically interact with aspartate 351 in the estrogen receptor to exert antiestrogenic activity[56]. This may explain the ability of raloxifene to 'switch on' some receptors but not others.

Raxolifene preserves bone tissue in ovariectomized rats. It preserves not only bone density but also the biomechanical properties of the bone (load to fracture in the vertebrae and shear to failure in the femoral neck)[57]. Interleukin-6 (IL-6) is a key cytokine involved in the bone loss associated with estrogen deficiency[58]. When IL-6 was used to stimulate the differentiation and resorptive activity of mammalian osteoclasts *in vitro*, raloxifene and estrogen had antiresorptive effects of similar potency and magnitude[59]. In the absence of IL-6, the antiresorptive activity of both raloxifene and estrogen was minimal with fully differentiated mammalian osteoclasts. In human studies, raloxifene and HRT behave similarly[60].

Raloxifene has been shown to lower serum cholesterol levels, and this effect was maintained for up to 1 year[61]. In ovariectomized, cholesterol-fed rabbits, raloxifene inhibits the process of atherogenesis by about one-third compared to the non-treated group, and is half as effective as estradiol[62]. The effect of raloxifene on the process of atherosclerosis is somewhat difficult to explain because there were no significant differences in the plasma lipid levels between the raloxifene-treated and sham-operated rabbits. The only difference between the placebo group and the raloxifene group was in the levels of LDL-C and triglycerides: both decreased in the raloxifene group. Raloxifene reduces the food consumption and produces weight loss in ovariectomized rats. It also decreases the total serum cholesterol and HDL cholesterol by 77%. Raloxifene had 77% of the potency of estrogen in this study[63]. These promising results on rats and rabbits were not, however, replicated in studies using the cynomolgus monkey model. When such monkeys were fed a moderately atherogenic diet and treated with placebo, two dosages of raloxifene or conjugated equine estrogens (Premarin, Wyeth-Ayerst, Philadelphia, USA), only those treated with estrogen showed a significant reduction in the coronary artery plaque size compared to placebo. Neither the lower nor the higher raloxifene dosage had any effect on the plaque size[64].

As a pharmacological antagonist of estrogen, raloxifene inhibits estrogen-induced stimulation of the rat uterus, which includes decreased uterine weight, myometrial thickness, epithelial cell height, endometrial stromal thickness and eosinophilic infiltration[65]. Raloxifene is a very potent antagonist of estrogen in the immature rat uterus assay (ED_{50} of approximately 0.4 mg/kg) and is unique among currently known SERMs in that it is able to block estrogen-induced uterine stimulation nearly completely because of its minimal intrinsic activity in the uterus[65,66]. Other compounds that antagonize estrogen in the uterus, such as tamoxifen, are more accurately described as partial estrogen agonists in this tissue, as they increase uterine weight and can only partially block estrogen's stimulatory effects[66]. Raloxifene also directly antagonizes the uterine stimulatory effects of tamoxifen in rats[67].

Human studies

Raloxifene is an antiresorptive drug. It, like estrogen, reduces bone remodelling in estrogen-deficient early postmenopausal women and induces a positive calcium balance shift. In one study, 60 mg/day of raloxifene was compared with sequential HRT consisting of 0.625 mg/day conjugated equine estrogen and 5 mg/day medroxyprogesterone acetate (Premique, Wyeth-Ayerst, Taplow, UK) from days 1 to 14. The study lasted 31 weeks and showed that raloxifene leads to improved intestinal calcium absorption, a fall in urinary calcium excretion and reduced bone resorption[60].

In another human experiment[68], 208 women were studied in four groups: raloxifene 200 or 600 mg/day or 0.625 mg/day conjugated equine estrogens or placebo were administered in a double-blind, randomized placebo-controlled trial (8 weeks). The study objective was to look for subtle morphological, endometrial changes. Endometrial biopsies were performed at the beginning and at the end of the study. At baseline, the estrogen effect was similar across the treatment groups. At the end, 77% of the estrogen-treated women had a moderate or marked estrogenic effect, whereas only 15% of the placebo group and none in the raloxifene-treated women showed this.

The results from a large clinical study[69] seem to be in agreement with data from lower mammals. This prospective, randomized study involved 601 postmenopausal women. The study subjects were assigned to 30, 60, or 150 mg of raloxifene or placebo daily for 24 months. At a 60 mg dose, raloxifene led to an increase of 2.4% of bone mineral density in the spine and the hip. The total cholesterol decreased by 6.4% and LDL-C by 10.1%. However, HDL-C also decreased by 3.7% and there was an elevation of 3.2% in triglycerides compared to baseline, which was not significant. The endometrial thickness was between 1.9 and 2.0 mm in both groups and did not change during the trial. Raloxifene was well tolerated and there was no significant difference in the total number of adverse events in both groups (breast pain or vaginal bleeding) or in the number of hot flushes.

There are two problems with this study. First is the high drop-out rate in both groups: about 25%. Second, the results of bone mineral density were reported as the difference between the study group and the placebo group. Statistically, this is absolutely correct but of clinical importance is the change with the active drug over time. The absolute gain of bone mineral density in the study group was relatively low

(1.6% in the lumbar spine and 1.2% in the femoral neck over 2 years).

Another controlled clinical trial specifically examined for the effect of raloxifene on markers of cardiovascular risk in postmenopausal women in comparison with placebo or continuous combined HRT (Prempro, Wyeth-Ayerst, Philadelphia, USA). The data revealed that raloxifene decreased LDL, lipoprotein(a) and fibrinogen, increased HDL-2, but not total HDL, and had no effect on triglycerides or plasminogen activator inhibitor-1[70] (see Tables 1 and 2). This confirms the results of an earlier study showing a 5–9% decrease in LDL and no endometrial stimulation[71].

Recently, the results of the largest study to date, the Multiple Outcomes of Raloxifene Evaluation (MORE) trial, were reported[72] (see Table 3). In this study, 60 mg/day or 120 mg/day raloxifene or placebo were given in double-blind randomized fashion to 7705 postmenopausal women with osteoporosis. All trial participants received calcium (500 mg/day) and vitamin D (400 IU/day) supplements. The mean age of the participants was 66.5 years and they were followed up for a median of 40 months between 1994 and 1998. The main outcome measures in this report were the number of new cases of breast cancer, the incidence of venous thromboembolism, the uterine effects and general adverse reactions (see Table 3).

Raloxifene reduced the risk of newly diagnosed invasive breast cancer by 76% during a median of 40 months of treating postmenopausal women for osteoporosis. This was

Table 1 Lipid/lipoprotein markers: median percentage change (baseline to end-point) during therapy with raloxifene, continuous combined HRT or placebo.

Lipoprotein	Placebo	Raloxifene 60 mg/day	HRT
LDL-cholesterol (mmol/l)	1 ± 3	−11 ± 2*	−13 ± 1*
Apolipoprotein B (mmol/l)	0 ± 2	−9 ± 2*	−4 ± 1
HDL-cholesterol (mmol/l)	1 ± 2	1 ± 2*	11 ± 2**
HDL$_2$-cholesterol (mmol/l)	0 ± 0	15 ± 6*	33 ± 4*
Apolipoprotein A$_1$ (mmol/l)	1 ± 2	2 ± 2**	12 ± 1*
Triglycerides (mmol/l)	0 ± 2	−4 ± 2**	20 ± 5*
Lipoprotein(a) (g/l)	3 ± 2	−4 ± 2*	−16 ± 3*

± values are medians ± standard errors of the medians. Changes refer to changes from baseline to end-point (i.e. the last completed visit). HRT, hormone replacement therapy with conjugated equine estrogen 0.625 mg/day and medroxyprogesterone acetate 2.5 mg/day. *$p < 0.05$ compared with placebo; **$p < 0.05$ compared with HRT. Adapted from reference 70 and reproduced with permission

Table 2 Coagulation markers: median percentage change (baseline to end-point) during therapy with raloxifene, continuous combined HRT or placebo

Coagulation factor	Placebo	Raloxifene 60 mg/day	HRT
Fibrinogen (g/l)	−2±1	−12±1*	−3±3
Plasminogen activator inhibitor-1 (U/ml)	−10±7	−2±3**	−29±3*
Prothrombin fragment 1 and 2 (nmol/l)	−3±4	2±2	16±7
Fibrinopeptide A (ng/ml)	13±8	9±3	16±7

±values are medians±standard errors of the medians. Changes refer to changes from baseline to end-point (i.e. the last completed visit). HRT, hormone replacement therapy with conjugated equine estrogen 0.625 mg/day and medroxyprogesterone acetate 2.5 mg/day. *$p < 0.05$ compared with placebo; **$p < 0.05$ compared with HRT. Adapted from reference 70 and reproduced with permission

Table 3 Summary of risks of breast cancer, endometrial cancer and thromboembolic disease in the Breast Cancer Prevention Trial and the MORE trial. Adapted from reference 72 and reproduced with permission

	Breast Cancer Prevention Trial	MORE Trial
Number randomized	13 175	7705
Daily treatment	tamoxifen 20 mg	raloxifene 60 mg or 120 mg
Median follow-up (months)	56.6	40.0

Breast cancer rates per 1000 woman-years and relative risk (RR) of cancer (95% CI)	invasive
	  placebo 6.8
	  tamoxifen 3.4
	  RR 0.51 (0.39–0.66)
	non-invasive
	  placebo 2.7
	  tamoxifen 1.4
	  RR 0.50 (0.33–0.77)
		all cases
		  placebo 4.3
		  raloxifene 1.5
		  RR 0.35 (0.21–0.58)
		invasive
		  placebo 3.6
		  raloxifene 0.9
		  RR 0.24 (0.13–0.44)

Number and RR (95% CI) of ER-positive breast cancer tumors	placebo 130 tamoxifen 41 RR 0.31 (0.22–0.45)	placebo 20 raloxifene 4 RR 0.10 (0.04–0.24)
Number and RR (95% CI) of endometrial cancers	placebo 15 tamoxifen 36 RR 2.53 (1.35–4.97)	placebo 4 raloxifene 6 RR 0.8 (0.2–2.7)

Number and RR (95% CI) of pulmonary embolisms and deep vein thromboses	pulmonary embolism
	  placebo 6
	  tamoxifen 18
	  RR 3.0 (1.2–9.3)
	deep vein thrombosis
	  placebo 22
	  tamoxifen 35
	  RR 1.60 (0.91–2.86)
		deep vein thrombosis and pulmonary embolism
		  placebo 8
		  raloxifene 49
		  RR 3.1 (1.5–6.2)

CI, confidence interval; RR, relative risk; ER, estrogen receptor

attributable to a 90% reduction in the risk of estrogen receptor-positive breast cancer. There was no apparent decrease in the risk of estrogen receptor-negative breast cancer. To prevent one case of breast cancer, 126 women will need to be treated for approximately 3.5 years. This supports the concept that raloxifene acts by interacting with estrogen receptors in the breast to inhibit estrogen-induced DNA transcription competitively[73]. Because breast cancers generally require several years to grow to a clinically or radiographically detectable size, the cancers that were diagnosed during the MORE trial were probably present when the study began. Therefore, the reduction in the risk of breast cancer within the first 40 months of treatment with raloxifene probably represents suppression or regression of subclinical cancer.

Table 4 Relative risk of new vertebral fracture: women with and without prevalent (baseline) fractures. Adapted from reference 72 and Evista® summary of product characteristics

	Placebo	Raloxifene 60 mg/day
No prevalent deformity present	n = 1454	n = 1388
Number with ≥ 1 new vertebral fracture (%)	39 (2.7)	18 (1.3)
Relative risk (95% CI) raloxifene vs. placebo		0.48 (0.28–0.84)
≥ 1 prevalent deformity present	n = 809	n = 832
Number with ≥ 1 new vertebral fracture (%)	132 (16.3)	84 (10.1%)
Relative risk (95% CI) raloxifene vs. placebo		0.62 (0.48–0.80)

CI, confidence interval

Bone data were not reported in detail. There was an unspecified decrease of the risk for vertebral fracture in the raloxifene group. Table 4 presents bone data taken from the raloxifene data sheet. Raloxifene did not increase or decrease the risk of endometrial cancer during the first 3 years of the MORE trial, but the total number of cases was small. The endometrial thickness was 5 mm in 4.1% more subjects in the raloxifene group than in the placebo group. Fluid in the endometrial cavity was seen in 2.7% more of the women taking raloxifene than placebo. However, there was no evidence of an increase in risk of endometrial hyperplasia among women who underwent endometrial biopsy. Therefore, routine monitoring of the endometrium with ultrasound or biopsy was not deemed necessary.

In the MORE trial, there was a 3.1-fold increase in the relative risk of venous thrombo-embolism in the group taking raloxifene. Translated into absolute risk, this means one case of venous thromboembolism occurred per 155 women treated with raloxifene for 3 years. In this study, significantly more women in the raloxifene-treated group (1.2%) reported new or worsening diabetes mellitus compared to the placebo-treated group (0.5%). Importantly, overall mortality rates did not differ between the placebo (1.0%) and raloxifene (0.8%) groups, and there were no differences in the causes of death.

Central nervous system effects

The effect of raloxifene on brain tissue has been the subject of laboratory studies[74]. The studies were set up to examine the impact of raloxifene on neurons derived from mammalian cerebral cortex, hippocampus and forebrain. Each of these brain regions is involved in memory function and is adversely affected in Alzheimer's disease. These studies used cultured neurons exposed to experimental substances in a serum-free medium and maintained in culture for 1–10 days. Results of these analyses indicated that raloxifene induced no significant effect on the outgrowth of cortical neurons across a wide range of concentrations. In contrast, studies involving 17β-estradiol and conjugated equine estrogens have shown that each induces significant neurotropic effects in cultured neurons. The impact of raloxifene in protecting against neurotoxic insult was complex. It protected against glutamate-induced toxicity, but not against hydrogen peroxide oxidative challenge. It appears to be exerting weaker estrogen-like properties on cultured brain cells, but, in certain instances (oxidative challenge), it can induce an effect opposite to that of an estrogen[74].

Adverse events

The adverse event profile of raloxifene has been extensively studied[75]. A large database, containing 2789 postmenopausal women who took part in randomized clinical trials, was analyzed. The comparison was between raloxifene 60 mg/day with placebo, HRT and unopposed estrogen (conjugated equine estrogens and 17β-estradiol). Overall discontinuation rates were not significantly different between treatment groups or placebo. Discontinuation rates due to adverse events were not significantly different between the treatment groups or placebo. The incidence of vaginal bleeding in women treated with raloxifene was low (less than 7%). This and the incidence of breast pain, abdominal pain, flatulence, vaginitis, leukorrhea, decreased libido or dyspareunia were not significantly different to that observed in placebo-treated women. An increased incidence of new hot flushes was observed among raloxifene-treated women in the placebo-controlled studies during the first 6 months of treatment, but after this there were no differences between the groups. The hot flushes in the raloxifene-treated women were mild to moderate and did not interfere with the sleeping pattern. The incidence of hot flushes was 7% and that of leg cramps was 4% more in the raloxifene-treated group compared to placebo; this difference was statistically significant.

Summary of the effects of raloxifene

Raloxifene has neutral or antiestrogenic effects on the uterus, and antiestrogenic effects on the breast. It has estrogenic effects on bone, serum lipids and coagulation/fibrinolysis. On vasomotor symptoms it has an antiestrogenic effect, while on brain (cell cultures) it has both weak estrogenic and antiestrogenic effects.

TOREMIFENE

Background

The research program which led to the development of toremifene was set up in Finland in 1978. In 1981, the triphenylethylene antiestrogen, toremifene, was first synthesized. It was found to bind to the estrogen receptor with an affinity of about 5% of that of tamoxifen[76].

Animal and human studies

Toremifene effectively reduces the growth of MCF-7 cells *in vitro* (breast cancer line cells) as well as dimethylbenzanthracene-induced rat mammary adenocarcinoma. *In vivo* studies on rat uterus have shown that toremifene is a weaker estrogen than tamoxifen and inhibits estrogen-induced uterine growth. Toremifene

appears to be well tolerated with a wide margin of safety in animal studies[77].

Toremifene was clinically tested in postmenopausal breast cancer patients in double-blind trials with tamoxifen, and the two drugs produced almost identical results. There were no significant differences in clinical response and side-effect profiles (hot flushes, nausea, vomiting and vaginal bleeding). The numbers of venous thromboembolism events and cardiac events were the same. There were more ocular abnormalities (cataracts) and more patients with elevated liver enzymes in the tamoxifen-treated group, but these differences were not statistically significant. There was one endometrial cancer and two ovarian cancers in the tamoxifen group and none in the toremifene group[77–79].

So far, there have been no reports of uterine cancer in patients treated with toremifene[80]. However, the similarities between tamoxifen and toremifene in chemical structure, clinical effectiveness and the side-effect profile mean that an association between toremifene and uterine cancer cannot be excluded.

In postmenopausal women, toremifene appears to be a bone-preserving agent at least as potent as tamoxifen[81]. Curiously, tamoxifen was better able to preserve bone in the femoral neck, whereas toremifene was more effective in the lumbar spine.

In a small study of 24 patients, toremifene was shown to decrease the serum total cholesterol and LDL levels with no change in HDL or triglycerides[82]. A larger and more detailed study of 49 patients confirmed these results and showed, in addition, a significant increase in HDL-C level with toremifene and a reduction of HDL-C with tamoxifen[83].

DROLOXIFENE

Background

The principle of an estrogen with high affinity for the ER has been exploited with the antiestrogens TAT-59 and 3-hydroxytamoxifen (droloxifene), which mimics the metabolites of tamoxifen. Droloxifene is derived from the tamoxifen metabolite 3,4 hydroxytamoxifen.

Animal and human studies

In preclinical testing, droloxifene has shown several potential advantages over tamoxifen. In particular, it has a 10–60-fold higher binding affinity to the estrogen receptor, a lower estrogenic to antiestrogenic ratio and faster absorption. It inhibits the growth of breast cancer cell lines and mammary tumors in rats. It is not carcinogenic in the rat liver[84].

One phase II trial reported a 44% response rate in postmenopausal women with metastatic, or inoperable, recurrent, or primary locoregional breast cancer treated with 100 mg droloxifene daily. The median response was 18 months[85]. There are currently phase II trials comparing droloxifene with tamoxifen. There are no human data on other metabolic aspects of droloxifene, but animal studies suggest that it prevents bone loss in rats.

IDOXIFENE

Background

Idoxifene (CB 7432) is a tamoxifen derivative originally discovered at the CRC Centre for Cancer Therapeutics, Institute of Cancer Research, UK. It was synthesized in an attempt to address some of the limitations of tamoxifen, namely:

(1) Only about a half of estrogen receptor-positive metastatic breast cancers exhibit regression with tamoxifen therapy;

(2) Acquired tamoxifen resistance eventually develops in previously responsive tumors;

(3) Tamoxifen also possesses estrogen agonist properties which are probably responsible for the increase in endometrial cancer seen following tamoxifen therapy.

Animal and human studies

It was found that idoxifene leads to significantly greater *in vitro* growth inhibition of MCF-7 cells compared to that observed for tamoxifen. Moreover, in *in vivo* studies using a nitrosomethylurea-induced rat mammary tumor, idoxifene caused regression of 92% of tumors, a number significantly greater than that suppressed by tamoxifen. Uterotropic studies, based upon measurement of uterine weight in immature rats and mice, showed that idoxifene also possessed a significantly weaker partial agonist activity compared to tamoxifen[86].

Idoxifene has been tested in ovariectomized rats, and the primary end-points were effects on bone loss, serum cholesterol, uterine wet weight and uterine histology. Idoxifene (0.5 mg/kg/day) completely prevented loss of lumbar and proximal tibial bone mineral density, whereas a significant loss occurred in the controls. It reduced total serum cholesterol levels. Myometrial and endometrial atrophy were observed in both the idoxifene and control groups[87].

One small clinical study, involving 20 subjects with metastatic breast cancer resistant to tamoxifen, has been reported. Idoxifene (in doses of 10–60 mg initially and subsequently 20 mg/day until disease progression) was well tolerated, with mild side-effects including tiredness, lethargy, weakness and nausea. No long-term side-effects were noted in the patients who continued to receive 20 mg/day for over a year. Of the 14 patients who remained on treatment, four showed stabilization and two achieved partial response.

The effect of idoxifene on the endometrium was assessed in a randomized control trial. The study involved 331 osteopenic postmenopausal women, who were treated with either placebo or idoxifene (2.5, 5 or 10 mg/day) for 12 weeks. Endometrial assessment was carried out by transvaginal ultrasound and endometrial biopsy at baseline and repeated at the end of treatment. Idoxifene use was associated with a dose-related increase in endometrial thickness, as measured by ultrasound. In 48 idoxifene patients (16% of total), the endometrial thickness was 5 mm or more over the study period. Of all women in the idoxifene arm, 19% developed intraluminal fluid. Of the women who underwent biopsy, 99% were reported to have either a benign or atrophic endometrium (85%) or insufficient tissue for diagnosis (14%). Proliferative features were reported in two cases (1%), both on 2.5 mg idoxifene, and atypical hyperplasia was noted in one patient on placebo[88]. Idoxifene has been studied for postmenopausal osteoporosis in phase III trials. The results did not match expectations and the trials were discontinued[89].

LEVORMELOXIFENE

Levormeloxifene (Novo Nordisk, Glostrup, Denmark) is the L-enantiomer of racemic centrochroman. Centrochroman has been used for about the past 20 years as a postcoital contraceptive, particularly in India, where it was originally developed. The L-enantiomer has a 7-fold higher binding affinity for ER as compared with the D-enantiomer and also has an approximately 7-fold higher uterotropic activity in sexually immature rats not treated with estrogen. When such rats were first treated with subcutaneous estrogen, levormeloxifene inhibited the maximal uterotropic activity of estrogen by only 40%. Thus, under these conditions, levormeloxifene is a partial agonist of ER in the rat uterus.

There are limited clinical data on levormeloxifene, none published in a peer-reviewed journal. It was until recently in phase III testing for prevention and treatment of osteoporosis. However, further development of levormeloxifene has been abandoned because of uterovaginal prolapse.

CONCLUSIONS

(1) The introduction of SERMs has helped with the understanding of the mode of action of estrogens and opens new opportunities for treatment of estrogen-dependent conditions. There is no doubt that development of new SERMs, which may be capable of precise targeting of specific estrogen receptors, will follow. This will result in the more effective treatment of gynecological conditions such as fibroids, endometriosis and estrogen-dependent cancer.

(2) As our knowledge about the basic mechanism of estrogen action improves, so too will our capabilities to modify such an action. This may lead to novel ways of tackling conditions such as osteoporosis and coronary artery disease in women.

(3) When developing, evaluating and using SERMs, it is to be remembered that they have the potential to affect any estrogen receptor-modulated function in either a positive or a negative way.

(4) For those with a 'Y' chromosome instead of two 'X' chromosomes, it is hoped that success with SERMs will lead to development of STERMs (selective testosterone receptor modulators) to tackle the more common causes of morbidity and mortality in men.

References

1. Sato M, Glasebrook AL, Bryant HU. Raloxifene: a selective estrogen receptor modulator. *J Bone Miner Metab* 1994;12(Suppl 2):519–20
2. Speroff L, Glass RH, Kase NG. Hormone biosynthesis, metabolism and mechanism of action. In Speroff L, Glass RH, Kase NG, eds. *Clinical Gynecological Endocrinology and Infertility.* Baltimore: Williams and Wilkins, 1978:19
3. Carr BR. The ovary. In Carr BR, Blackwell RE, eds. *Textbook of Reproductive Medicine.* Norwalk: Appleton & Lange, 1993:199–200
4. Green S, Walter P, Kumar V, *et al.* Human oestrogen receptor cDNA: sequence, expression and homology with v-erb. *Nature (London)* 1986; 320:134–9
5. Greene GL, Gilna P. Watefield M, *et al.* Sequence and expression of human estrogen receptor complementary DNA. *Science* 1986;231:1150–4
6. Kuiper GGJM, Enmark E, Pelto-Hulkko M, *et al.* Cloning of a novel estrogen receptor expressed in rat prostate and ovary. *Pros Natl Acad Sci* 1996; 93:5925–30

7. Kuiper GGJM, Carlsson B, Grandien K, *et al.* Comparision of the ligand binding specificity and transcript tissue distribution of estrogen receptor alpha and beta. *Endocrinology* 1997;138:863–70

8. Katzenellenbogen BS, Korach KS. Editorial: A new actor in the estrogen receptor drama – enter ER-beta. *Endocrinology* 1997;138:861–2

9. Macgregor JI, Jordan VC. Basic guide to the mechanisms of antiestrogen action. *Pharmacol Rev* 1998;50:152–95

10. Yang NN, Venugopalan M, Hardikar S, Glesebrook A. Identification of an oestrogen response element activated by metabolites of 17-beta estradiol and raloxifene. *Science* 1996;273:1222–5

11. Harper MJK, Walpole AL. Contrasting endocrine activities of CIS and transisomers in a series of substituted triphenylethylenes. *Nature (London)* 1966;212:87

12. Bedford GR, Richardson DN. Preparations and identification of *cis* and *trans* isomers of a substituted triarylethylene. *Nature (London)* 1966;212:133–4

13. Harper MJK, Walpole AL. A new derivative of triphenylethylene: effects of implantation and mode of action in rats. *J Reprod Fertil* 1967;13:101–19

14. Williamson JG, Ellis JP. The induction of ovulation by tamoxifen. *J Obstet Gynaecol Br Commonw* 1973;80:844–7

15. Cole MP, Jones CTA, Todd IDH. A new antioestrogenic agent in late breast cancer: an early clinical appraisal of ICI 46 474. *Br J Cancer* 1971;25:270–5

16. Ward HWC. Antioestrogen therapy for breast cancer: a trial of tamoxifen at two-dose levels. *Br Med J* 1973;1:13–14

17. Early Breast Cancer Trialists' Collaborative Group. Effect of adjuvant tamoxifen and cytotoxic therapy on mortality in early breast cancer. *N Engl J Med* 1988;319:1681–92

18. Early Breast Cancer Trialists' Collaborative Group. Systemic treatment of early breast cancer by hormonal, cytotoxic or immune therapy: 133 randomised trials involving 31 000 recurrences and 24 000 deaths among 75 000 women. *Lancet* 1992;339:1–15, 71–85

19. Fisher B, Redmond C. New perspective on cancer of the contra-lateral breast: a marker for assessing tamoxifen as a preventive agent. *J Natl Cancer Inst* 1991;82:1278–80

20. Rutqvist LE, Cedermark B, Glass V, *et al.* Contra-lateral primary breast tumours in breast cancer patients in a randomised trial of adjuvant tamoxifen therapy. *J Natl Cancer Inst* 1991;83:1299–306

21. Early Breast Cancer Trialists' Collaborative Group. Tamoxifen for early breast cancer: an overview of the randomised trials. *Lancet* 1998;351:1451–67

22. Powels TJ, Jones AL, Ashley SE. The Royal Marsden Hospital pilot chemoprevention trial. *Breast Cancer Res Treat* 1994;31:73–8

23. Powels TJ, Eeles R, Ashley S, *et al.* Interim analysis of the incidence of breast cancer in the Royal Marsden Hospital tamoxifen randomised chemoprevention trial. *Lancet* 1998;352:98–101

24. Fisher B, Constantino JP, Wickerham L, *et al.* Tamoxifen for the prevention of breast cancer: report of the National Surgical Adjuvant Breast and Bowel Project P-1 Study. *J Natl Cancer Inst* 1998;90:1371–88

25. Veronesi U, Malsonneuve P, Costa A, *et al.* Prevention of breast cancer with tamoxifen: preliminary findings from the Italian randomised trial among hysterectomised women. *Lancet* 1998;352:93–7

26. Love RR, Cameron L, Connell BL, Leventhal H. Symptoms associated with tamoxifen treatment in postmenopausal women. *Arch Intern Med* 1991;151:142–7

27. Wright CDP, Mansell RE, Gazet JS, Compston JE. Effect of long-term tamoxifen therapy on bone turnover in women with breast cancer. *Br Med J* 1993;306:429–30

28. Grey AB, Stapleton JP, Evans MC, *et al.* The effect of antioestrogen tamoxifen on bone mineral density in normal late postmenopausal women. *Am J Med* 1995;99:636–41

29. Love RR, Mazess RB, Barden HS, *et al.* Effects of tamoxifen on bone mineral density in postmenopausal women with breast cancer. *N Engl J Med* 1992;326:852–6

30. Powels TJ, Hickish T, Kanis JA, Tidy A, Ashby S. Effect of tamoxifen on bone mineral density measured by dual-energy X-ray absorptiometry in healthy premenopausal and postmenopausal women. *J Clin Oncol* 1996;14:78–84

31. Love RR, Barden HS, Mazess RB, Epstein S, Chappell RJ. Effects of tamoxifen on lumbar spine bone mineral density in postmenopausal women after 5 years. *Arch Intern Med* 1994;154:2585–8

32. Fornander T, Rutqvist LE, Sjoberg HE, *et al.* Long-term adjuvant tamoxifen in early breast cancer: effect on bone mineral density in postmenopausal women. *J Clin Oncol* 1990;8:1019–24

33. Andersen HT, Kristensen B, Ejiertsen B, Andersen KW, Lauritsen JB. Fractures in postmenopausal breast cancer patients treated with adjuvant tamoxifen. *Breast* 1995;4:245–6

34. Fornander T, Rutqvist LE, Cedermark B, *et al.* Adjuvant tamoxifen therapy in early breast cancer: occurrence of new primary cancers. *Lancet* 1980;1:117–20

35. Rudqvist LE, Sedemark B, Glass V, *et al.* The Stockholm trial of adjuvant tamoxifen in early

breast cancer. *Breast Cancer Res Treat* 1987;10: 255–66

36. Rutqvist LE, Johansson H, Signomllao T, *et al.* Adjuvant tamoxifen therapy for early stage breast cancer and second primary malignancies. *J Natl Cancer Inst* 1995;87:645–51

37. Anderson M, Storm HH, Mouridsen HT. Carcinogenic effect of adjuvant tamoxifen treatment and radiotherapy for early breast cancer. *Acta Oncol* 1992;31:259–63

38. Neve P, Vergote I. Should tamoxifen users be screened for endometrial lesions? *Lancet* 1998; 351:155–6

39. Morales M, Santana N, Soria A, *et al.* Effects of tamoxifen on serum lipids and apolipoprotein levels in postmenopausal women with breast cancer. *Breast Cancer Res Treat* 1996;40:265–70

40. Grey AB, Stapleton JP, Evans MC, Reid IR. The effect of the antioestrogen tamoxifen on cardiovascular risk factors in normal postmenopausal women. *J Clin Endocrinol Metab* 1995;80:3191–5

41. Love PR, Wiebe DA, Feyzi JM, Newcomb PA, Chapell PJ. Effects of tamoxifen on cardiovascular risk factors in postmenopausal women after 5 years of treatment. *J Natl Cancer Inst* 1994;86: 534–9

42. Dewar JA, Horobin JM, Preece PE, *et al.* Long-term effect of tamoxifen on blood lipid values in breast cancer. *Br Med J* 1992;305:225–6

43. McDonald CC, Steward HJ. Fatal myocardial infarction in the Scottish adjuvant tamoxifen trial. *Br Med J* 1991;303:435–7

44. Rickles FR, Levine M, Edwards RL. Haemostatic alterations in cancer patients. *Cancer Metastases Rev* 1992;11:237–48

45. Goodnought LT, Saito H, Manni A. Increased incidence of thromboembolism in stage IV breast cancer patients treated with 5 drugs chemotherapy regimen – a study of 159 patients. *Cancer* 1984;54:1264–8

46. Saphner T, Dormay DC, Gray R. Venous and arterial thrombosis in patients who receive adjuvant therapy for breast cancer. *J Clin Oncol* 1991;9:286–94

47. Rutqvist LE, Mattson A. Cardiac and thromboembolic morbidity among postmenopausal women with early stage breast cancer in a randomised trial of tamoxifen. The Stockholm Breast Cancer Study Group. *J Natl Cancer Inst* 1993;85:1398–406

48. Grey AB, Stapleton JP, Evans MC, Reid IR. The effect of the antioestrogen tamoxifen on cardiovascular risk factors in normal postmenopausal women. *J Clin Endocrinol Metab* 1995;80:3191–5

49. Chang J, Powels TJ, Ashley SE, *et al.* The effects of tamoxifen and hormone replacement therapy on serum cholesterol, bone density and coagulation factors in healthy postmenopausal women participating in a randomised, controlled

tamoxifen prevention study. *Ann Oncol* 1996;7: 671–5

50. Mannucei PM, Bettega D, Chantaranykul, *et al.* Effects of tamoxifen on measurement of haemostasis in healthy women. *Arch Intern Med* 1996; 156:1806–10

51. Love RR, Surawicz TS, Williams EC. Antithrombin III level, fibrinogen level and platelet count changes with adjuvant tamoxifen therapy. *Arch Intern Med* 1992;152:317–20

52. Clements JA, Bennett DR, Black LJ, Jones CD. Effects of a new antioestrogen, keoxifene (LY1567758) on carcinogen-induced mammary tumours and on LH and prolactin levels. *Life Sci* 1983;32:2869–75

53. Wakeling AE, Valcaccia B, Newboult E, Green LR. Non-steroidal antioestrogens: receptor binding and biological response in rat uterus, rat mammary carcinoma and human breast cancer cells. *J Steroid Biol Chem* 1984;20:111–20

54. Buzdar AU, Marcus C, Holmes F, Hug V, Hortobagyi G. Phase II evaluation of LY156758 in metastatic breast cancer. *Oncology* 1988;45: 344–5

55. Brzozowski AM, Pike ACW, Dauter Z, *et al.* Molecular basis of agonism and antagonism in the oestrogen receptor. *Nature (London)* 1997; 389:753–8

56. Levenson AS, Jordan VC. The key to the antiestrogenic mechanism of raloxifene is aminoacid 351 (aspartate) in the estrogen receptor. *Cancer Res* 1998;58:1872–5

57. Sato M, Rippy MK, Bryant HU. Raloxifene, tamoxifen, nafoxidine or estrogen effects on reproductive and non-reproductive tissues in ovariectomized rats. *FASEB J* 1996;10:1

58. Jilka RL, Hangoc G, Girasole G, *et al.* Increased osteoclast development after estrogen loss: medication by interleucin-B. *Science* 1992;257:88–91

59. Sato M, Bryant HU, Helterbrand J, *et al.* Advantages of raloxifene over alendronate or estrogen on nonreproductive and reproductive tissues in the long-term dosing of ovariectomized rats. *J Pharmacol Exp Ther* 1996;279:298–305

60. Heany RP, Draper MW. Raloxifene and estrogen: comparative bone remodelling kinetics. *J Clin Endocrinol Metab* 1997;82:3425–9

61. Bryant HU, Turner CH, Frolik CA, *et al.* Long-term effect of raloxifene (LYI 39478 HCl) on bone, cholesterol and uterus in ovariectomised rats. *Bone* 1995;16(Suppl):116 S

62. Bjarnason NH, Haarbo J, Byrjalsen I, Kaufman RF, Christiansen C. Raloxifene inhibits aortic accumulation of cholesterol in ovariectomised cholesterol-fed rabbits. *Circulation* 1997;96:1964–9

63. Kaufman RF, Bensch WR, Roudebush RE, *et al.* Hypocholesterolemic activity of raloxifene (LY 139481): pharmacological characterization

as a selective estrogen receptor modulator. *J Pharmacol Exp Ther* 1997;280:146–53

64. Clarkson TB, Anthony MS, Jerome CP. Lack of effect of raloxifene on coronary artery atherosclerosis of postmenopausal monkeys. *J Clin Endocrinol Metab* 1998;83:721–6

65. Black LJ, Sato M, Rowley ER, *et al.* Raloxifene (LY 139481 HCl) prevents bone loss and reduces serum cholesterol without causing uterine hypertrophy in ovariectomised rats. *J Clin Invest* 1994;93:63–9

66. Bryant HU, Wilson PK, Adrian MD, *et al.* Selective estrogen receptor modulators: pharmacological profile in the rat utcrus. *J Soc Gynecol Invest* 1996; 3:152A

67. Fuchs-Young R, Magee DE, Adrian MD, *et al.* Raloxifene, a selective estrogen receptor modulator, inhibits the uterotrophic effect of tamoxifene over 21-day course. *J Soc Gynecol Invest* 1996;3:153A

68. Moss SM, Huster WJ, Neild JA, *et al.* Effects of raloxifene hydrochloride on the endometrium of postmenopausal women. *Am J Obstet Gynecol* 1997;117:1458–64

69. Delmas PD, Bjarnason NH, Mitlak BH, *et al.* Effects of raloxifene on bone mineral density, serum cholesterol concentration, and uterine endometrium in postmenopausal women. *N Engl J Med* 1997;337:1641–7

70. Walsh BW, Kuller LH, Wild RA, *et al.* Effect of raloxifene on serum lipids and coagulation factors in healthy postmenopausal women. *J Am Med Assoc* 1998;279:1445–51

71. Draper MW, Flowers DE, Huster WJ, *et al.* A controlled trial of raloxifene (LY 139481) HCl: impact on bone turnover and serum lipid profile in healthy postmenopausal women. *J Bone Miner Res* 1996;11:835–42

72. Cummings SR, Eckert S, Krueger KA, *et al.* The effect of raloxifene on risk of breast cancer in postmenopausal women. Results from the MORE randomized trial. *J Am Med Assoc* 1999; 281:2189–97

73. Grese TA, Sluca JP, Bryant HU, *et al.* Molecular determinant of tissue selectivity in estrogen receptor modulators. *Proc Natl Acad Sci USA* 1997; 94:14105–10

74. Brinton RD, Zhang S, Chen S, Oji G. Effect of raloxifene on neuronal outgrowth and protection against neurotoxic insult: comparative analysis with oestrogenic steroids. *Fertil Steril* 1998;69:582

75. Davies GC, Huster WJ, Lu Y, *et al.* Adverse events reported by postmenopausal women in controlled trials with raloxifene. *Obstet Gynecol* 1999; 93:558–65

76. Kangas L. Introduction to toremifene. *Breast Cancer Res Treat* 1990;16(Suppl):53–7

77. Kangas L. Review of pharmacological properties of toremifene. *J Steroid Biochem* 1990;36:191–5

78. Stenbygaard LE, Herrstead J, Thomsen JF, *et al.* Toremifene and tamoxifen in advanced breast cancer – a double blind cross-over trial. *Breast Cancer Res Treat* 1993;25:57–63

79. Pyrhonen S, Valavaara R, Modig H, *et al.* Comparison of toremifene and tamoxifen in postmenopausal patients with advanced breast cancer: a randomised double-blind 'nordic' phase III study. *Br J Cancer* 1997;76:270–7

80. Hayes DF, Van Zyl JA, Hacking A, *et al.* Randomized comparison of tamoxifen and two separate doses of toremifene in postmenopausal patients with metastatic breast cancer. *J Clin Oncol* 1995; 13:2556–66

81. Maenpaa J, Ala-Fossi SL. Toremifene in postmenopausal breast cancer – efficacy, safety and cost. *Drugs Aging* 1997;11:261–70

82. Gylling H, Pyrhonen S, Mamtyla E, *et al.* Tamoxifen and toremifene lower serum cholesterol by inhibition of delta 8 – cholesterol conversion to lanosterol in women with breast cancer. *J Clin Oncol* 1995;13:2900–5

83. Saourto T, Blomqvist C, Ehnholm C, *et al.* Antiatherogenic effects of adjuvant anti-estrogens. A randomized trial comparing the effects of tamoxifen and toremifene on plasma lipid levels in postmenopausal women with node positive breast cancer. *J Clin Oncol* 1996;14: 429–33

84. Hosmann M, Ratel B, Loser R. Preclinical data for droloxifene. *Cancer Lett* 1994;84:101–16

85. Rauschining W, Pritchard KI. Droloxifene, a new antioestrogen: its role in metastatic breast cancer. *Breast Cancer Res Treat* 1994;31:83–94

86. Kelland LR, Jarman M. Idoxifene. *Drugs Future* 1995;20:666–9

87. Nuttall ME, Bradbeer JN, Stroup GB, *et al.* Idoxifene: a novel selective estrogen receptor modulator prevents bone loss and lowers cholesterol levels in ovariectomized rats and decreases uterine weight in intact rats. *Endocrinology* 1998;139:5524–34

88. Fleischer AC, Wheeler JE, Yeh IT, Kravitz B, Jensen C, MacDonald B. Sonographic assessment of the endometrium in osteopenic postmenopausal women treated with idosifene. *J Ultrasound Med* 1999;18:503–12

89. Smith Kline Beecham. Data on file

9

The molecular biology of the action of SERMs

M. L. Brandi

BACKGROUND

Estrogen is involved in a number of physiological processes in the body, with highly tissue-selective responses. After cessation of menses (menopause), average circulating estrogen levels eventually fall to less than 10% of premenopausal levels. This state of estrogen deficiency contributes to the acceleration of several age-related health problems in women, including cardiovascular disease, osteoporosis and, possibly, dementia[1-3]. With an increasing fraction of a woman's life occurring after the menopause, these disorders have collectively become urgent medical, economic and social concerns[4]. Despite a large and growing body of information on the use of long-term hormone replacement therapy (HRT) to prevent or treat some of the disorders associated with menopause, HRT for disease prevention remains an area of significant therapeutic controversy[5]. In part, this controversy reflects a lack of clear answers to fundamental questions such as when to initiate HRT and how long to continue it to best balance the benefits and risk of treatment. The reproductive tissue-related adverse effects associated with estrogen replacement therapy and the increased risk (either real or perceived) of various tumors (particularly of the breast or uterus) markedly reduce compliance with this therapy. Women with a uterus who choose to take HRT must necessarily be prescribed progestin therapy concomitantly with estrogens in order to avoid the endometrial hyperplasia resulting from sustained, unopposed estrogen therapy. Progestins may cause breast pain or tenderness,

fluid retention, mood fluctuations and resumption of menses (when used cyclically) or temporary spotting (when used continuously). Understandably, some physicians are reluctant to continue to prescribe HRT for disease prevention due to these side-effects and a low rate of long-term compliance.

Given these limitations of HRT for disease prevention, optimal disease prevention therapy for postmenopausal women might be better realized by estrogen-like compounds which can mimic the actions of estrogen on the skeleton, the cardiovascular system (including serum lipids) and the central nervous system, while at the same time minimizing, or perhaps eradicating, estrogenic effects on reproductive tissues. Such compounds would seemingly be ideally suited to the long-term health maintenance of women in their non-reproductive years. Therefore, the ideal agent should have a high therapeutic index or safety margin, because it would likely be used for an extended length of time in a prophylactic manner. There is currently great interest in identifying compounds that possess this 'ideal' estrogen profile and several agents have been considered in female reproductive tissue cell lines. Such a profile is tantamount to a selective reversal of estrogen deficiency in certain desired tissues, while at the same time bypassing or failing to act in tissues in which estrogen produces adverse effects. Such a selective estrogen profile might be achieved by one of two means. The first possibility would involve exploitation of a preferential tissue distribution (i.e. in the bone and/or cardio-vascular system, but not in reproductive tissue), resulting in an improved therapeutic index. Because estrogen effects, both beneficial and adverse, are mediated in multiple tissues, the feasibility of achieving desirable estrogen selectivity based on tissue distribution is considered low. The second possible approach to achieving estrogen selectivity involves developing compounds that activate estrogen receptors only in desired tissues, while remaining inactive or acting as an antagonist in reproductive tissues. The success of this general approach depends on the existence and differential distribution of receptor subtypes throughout the body.

THE SERM CONCEPT

Recently, the search for a safer, more acceptable form of HRT has led to the evaluation of several classes of organic compounds grouped together as 'antiestrogens'. The term 'antiestrogen' reflected the first uses of these drugs as treatments for hormonally responsive breast cancer. Antiestrogens compete with estradiol for binding to the estrogen receptor but can be either steroidal or non-steroidal in structure. The term 'antiestrogen' covers a wide range of compounds which demonstrate a spectrum of estrogen receptor activity, ranging from that of 'pure' estrogen antagonists to mixed estrogen agonist/antagonists. The evaluation of antiestrogens as potential HRT substitutes followed from observations that tamoxifen-treated, postmenopausal breast cancer patients had lower serum cholesterol and preservation of bone mass during treatment as compared with untreated control patients[6,7]. Thus, tamoxifen appeared to act as an estrogen agonist in bone and liver but as an estrogen antagonist in the breast.

Today, a number of synthetic compounds generally display a mixed estrogen agonist/antagonist profile. The best known are the triphenylethylenes, examples of which include clomiphene, tamoxifen and tamoxifen derivatives (3-hydroxytamoxifen (droloxifene), chlorotamoxifen (toremifene), 4-iodo-pyrrolidinotamoxifen (idoxifene) and TAT-59).

Other compounds with mixed agonist/antagonist properties include benzothiophenes such as raloxifene (formerly keoxifene), currently being evaluated for the prevention and treatment of osteoporosis[8], benzopyrans[9], tetrahydronaphthylenes such as CP 336,156, and structurally distinct molecules such as ormeloxifene (centchroman)[10]. Of interest, a recent report suggests that one of the plant-derived estrogenic substances, the phyto-estrogen coumesterol, can be modified to act as an estrogen agonist/antagonist[11]. Pure antiestrogens include the 7α-alkyated steroids, e.g. ICI 164,384 and 182,780[12,13]. ICI 182,780 has shown early promise in the treatment of tamoxifen-refractory advanced breast cancer[13].

The term 'selective estrogen receptor modulator' (SERM) has been suggested to more precisely characterize those compounds that can bind to and activate the estrogen receptor but which have tissue-specific effects distinct from estradiol[14]. A selective estrogen receptor modulator is defined as a compound that produces estrogen agonism in one or more desired target tissues such as bone, liver, etc., together with estrogen antagonism and/or minimal agonism (i.e. clinically insignificant) in reproductive tissues such as the breast or uterus.

Based on its pattern of tissue specificity, raloxifene was deemed representative of a second-generation SERM, the first-generation represented by tamoxifen and its derivatives, which demonstrate estrogen-agonist properties in the endometrium[14]. It is fair to say that tamoxifen must now be viewed as a successful example of a first-generation selective estrogen receptor modulator for treatment of all stages of breast cancer. Raloxifene, by contrast, has been developed for a much broader application as a prevention maintenance therapy for postmenopausal women[15]. Although raloxifene will be used by millions of women as a preventive for osteoporosis, its antiestrogenic effects in the breast and the uterus are predicted to prevent breast and endometrial cancers[16,17]. Clearly, it is the targeted antiestrogenic action of raloxifene that will generate the most interest.

MOLECULAR BIOLOGY OF ACTION OF SERMS

SERMs represent a structurally diverse group of compounds which interact with the estrogen receptor (ER) but which elicit agonist or antagonist activity, depending on the organ system and physiological context (e.g. dose delivered, target tissue, hormonal milieu). Evaluation of the actions of these compounds has led researchers to a fuller understanding not only of estrogens but also of steroid signalling in general. Based on their evolving clinical profiles, SERMs have the potential to address long-term health maintenance needs of women in their non-reproductive years, while overcoming some of the limitations associated with currently available HRT. However, the mechanism by which antiestrogens interact with estrogen receptors but display a gene activation profile differing from the prototypic estrogen, estradiol, is not fully understood. While the estrogen antagonist properties of antiestrogens were originally ascribed to simple competition for estrogen receptor binding, it is now believed that estrogen antagonism is an active process, derived from estrogen receptor- and, perhaps, non-estrogen receptor-mediated events[18,19]. Importantly, the relationship between the agonist and antagonist properties of antiestrogens appears to depend on the cellular context in which the observation is made, giving rise to an apparent tissue-specific pattern of action unique to each compound.

The estrogen receptor is a ligand-activated transcription factor with six structural domains of overlapping function (labelled A–F). The two transcription activation functions (AF-1 and AF-2) are located in domains A/B and E, respectively[20,21]. Binding of ligand to the latent estrogen receptor induces conformational changes which favor dissociation of heat shock proteins, followed by estrogen receptor dimerization and, later, binding of cell-specific adapter proteins to the active, dimerized complex[18]. It is believed that the strength of the ligand–estrogen receptor-induced activating function is modulated by these cell-specific adapter proteins and, perhaps, by other signalling pathway transcription factors, e.g. AP-1[22].

The role of the promoter element, AP-1, a binding site for proteins from the Jun/Fos family, was recently defined[22]. In the presence of an estrogen response element, tamoxifen acts as an estrogen antagonist. In contrast, when the estrogen response element is replaced by an AP-1 site, tamoxifen is converted to an estrogen agonist in cell lines of diverse tissue origin, excluding breast cells. This mechanism involves direct interaction of estrogen receptor with AP-1 proteins and utilizes the AP-1 DNA response element. In some cell lines, activation from these sites does not require the DNA-binding domain of estrogen receptor (ER).

A new dimension to interaction of ER with AP-1 proteins was unveiled with the discovery of ERβ[23]. The interaction of AP-1 with ERα, as described above, was diametrically opposite to its interaction with ERβ: while estradiol stimulated activity from an ERα complexed with AP-1, estradiol diminished the transcriptional activity of AP-1 associated with ERβ[24]. Importantly, raloxifene was a partial agonist on an AP-1 coupled ERα, yet a complete agonist on an AP-1 coupled ERβ. Together, these findings indicate that the cellular response to SERMs is determined by the expression of estrogen receptor subtypes, by a repertory of accessory DNA-bound proteins (such as AP-1) and by co-activators and corepressors, all interacting in a promoter-specific manner. The relative contribution of each of these components to the cellular response to SERM administration *in vivo* remains to be determined.

By examining the susceptibility of the estrogen receptor–antiestrogen complexes to protease degradation, structural (conformational) distinctions between the complexes were deduced which could account for the observed divergent genomic actions[25]. Indeed, antiestrogens could form distinct estrogen receptor–ligand complexes representing different points along a continuum of potential estrogen receptor activation (i.e. intrinsic estrogenicity). Consistent with this model, tamoxifen binding to the estrogen receptor distinctly affects the two transcription activation functions of the estrogen receptor compared with estradiol, such that AF-2 (the hormone-dependent transcription activation function) is usually enhanced by estradiol binding, while it may be suppressed by tamoxifen in a dose- and cell-specific manner[20,21]. Therefore, the estrogen agonist/antagonist profile of tamoxifen in a given tissue results from the relative strength of AF-2 inhibition versus constitutive (hormone-independent) AF-1 activation, both of which may be modulated by cell-specific adapter proteins and transcription factors[26]. The conformation of the estrogen receptor–ligand complex could impose structural specificity on these putative protein–protein and protein–DNA interactions[25].

Another cellular mechanism likely to play a role in cell- and promoter-specific actions of antiestrogens has been elucidated through the ability of estrogen and antiestrogens to initiate transcription of the *TGF-β3* gene in an *in vitro* system[27]. Raloxifene and some estradiol metabolites, but not estradiol itself, interacted with estrogen receptor and activated the *TGF-β3* gene, even when the estrogen receptor region containing the DNA-binding domain (domain C) was muted. These findings suggested the presence of a novel pathway for estrogen receptor-mediated gene activation not requiring direct estrogen receptor–DNA contact. Indeed, a region of the *TGF-β3* gene promoter, distinct from the canonical estrogen response element (ERE) and which recognized the raloxifene-bound estrogen receptor, was identified and termed the raloxifene response element (RRE)[27]. Further evidence of novel, non-ERE promoter sequences able to mediate antiestrogen genomic actions has been reported for the human retinoic acid receptor-α1 gene[28].

The resolution of the crystal structure of the ligand-binding domain of the estrogen receptor, bound to either estradiol or raloxifene, provided the molecular basis for interaction of ligand-bound estrogen receptor with selective coregulators[29]. While the ligand-binding pocket of estrogen receptor absolutely requires that its ligand possesses an aromatic ring, the relatively large size of this pocket can accommodate a variety of hydrophobic side-groups. When bound by estradiol, discrete helices within the ligand-binding domain are packed in a manner that directs the charged activation function domain of estrogen receptor away from the body of the protein, allowing it to interact with coactivators. In contrast, the hydrophobic side-chain of raloxifene prevents this alignment of the activation domain, hindering its correct alignment with other regions within the ligand-binding domain of estrogen receptor, thereby impeding interaction with particular coactivators. These data are important because they support the notion that individual ligands for estrogen receptor do not all exhibit the same effects. The alkylaminoethoxy side-chain is the essential structural feature of the non-steroidal antiestrogens[30]. The distance between the nitrogen and the oxygen must be optimal[31], the conformations available to the side-chain must not be restricted[32], and the basicity of the nitrogen must be correct[33]. Removal of the side-chain results in loss of all activity or exclusive estrogenic properties[34]. The side-chain was originally predicted[35,36] to bind to an 'antiestrogenic region' in the ligand-binding domain of the estrogen receptor. Simply stated, the antiestrogen was perceived to act like a stick to prevent the jaws of the estrogen receptor from closing around the ligand. An estrogenic complex would only be created by protein enveloping the ligand. Resolution of the crystal structure of the estrogen receptor also showed that the alkylaminoethoxy side-chain of raloxifene binds to Asp351. Therefore, this is the key to the antiestrogenic properties of raloxifene. This single critical interaction forces all the other changes to occur. On the basis of this knowledge, it is now possible to confirm the biological relevance of the crystal structure by tying together the cancer research literature. Indeed, an estrogen receptor signal transduction pathway can be naturally converted from inhibitory to stimulatory and establishes that a mutant receptor can confer drug resistance to tamoxifen. Clearly, it will be important to examine crystal structures of several different antiestrogens complexed with the estrogen receptors to build a picture of conformational possibilities and to compare the shapes with efficacy.

CONCLUSIONS

The ultimate genetic response to estrogens and antiestrogens is a result of a tripartite interaction between the ligand, receptor and effector system. Diversity in the response is provided by the existence of gene- and/or cell-specific effectors (e.g. co-activators, transcription factors, chromatin remodelling proteins), receptors (e.g. ERα, ERβ), additional hormone response elements (e.g. estrogen response element, raloxifene response element) and, of course, unique ligands, including endogenous steroid hormones and their metabolites. As the complexity of the steroid/antisteroid signalling pathway is further unravelled, we will likely witness a wide array of therapies based on selective modulation of steroid receptor activity. Our expanding body of knowledge of the molecular details of estrogenic regulation provides the potential for design or development of other compounds that might possess similar regulatory profiles to raloxifene, but which have a higher affinity for estrogen receptor or increased bioavailability. An example is LY353381 HCl, a new member of the benzothiophene family, with potency advantages over raloxifene in a prevention model of osteoporosis in ovariectomized rats[37]. The third generation of SERMs is behind the door.

References

1. Colditz GA, Willett WC, Stampfer MJ, *et al.* Menopause and the risk of heart disease in women. *N Engl J Med* 1987;316:1105–10
2. Kiel DP, Felson DT, Anderson JJ, *et al.* Hip fracture and the use of estrogen in post menopausal women: the Framingham Study. *N Engl J Med* 1987;317:1169–74
3. Paganini-Hill A, Henderson VW. Estrogen deficiency and risk of Alzheimer's disease in women. *Am J Epidemiol* 1994;140:256–61
4. US Congress, Office of Technology Assessment. *Effectiveness and Cost of Osteoporosis Screening and Hormone Replacement Therapy.* Washington: US Government Printing Office, 1995
5. Lindsay R, Bush TL, Grady D, *et al.* Therapeutic controversy: estrogen replacement in the menopause. *J Clin Endocrinol Metab* 1996;81:3829–38
6. Love RR, Mazess RB, Barden HS, *et al.* Effects of tamoxifen on bone mineral density in postmenopausal women with breast cancer. *N Engl J Med* 1992;326:852–6
7. Love RR, Newcomb PA, Wiebe DA, *et al.* Effects of tamoxifen therapy on lipid and lipoprotein levels in postmenopausal patients with node-negative breast cancer. *J Natl Cancer Inst* 1990;82:1327–32
8. Draper MW, Flowers DE, Huster WJ, *et al.* A controlled trial of raloxifene (LY 139481 HCl): impact on bone turnover and serum lipid profile in healthy postmenopausal women. *J Bone Miner Res* 1996;11:835–42
9. Grese TA, Sluka JP, Bryant HU, *et al.* Benzopyran selective estrogen receptor modulators (SERMs): pharmacological effects and structural correlation with raloxifene. *Bioorg Med Chem Lett* 1996;6:903–8
10. Kamboj VP, Ray S, Dhawan BN. Centchroman. *Drugs Today* 1992;28:227–32
11. Grese TA, Cole HW, Magee DE, *et al.* Conversion of the phytoestrogen coumestrol into a selective estrogen receptor modulator (SERM) by attachment of an amine-containing sidechain. *Bioorg Med Chem Lett* 1996;6:2683–6
12. Wakeling AE, Dukes M, Bowler J. A potent specific pure antiestrogen with clinical potential. *Cancer Res* 1991;51:3867–73
13. Howell A, DeFriend DJ, Robertson JF, *et al.* Pharmacokinetics, pharmacological and antitumor effects of the specific antiestrogen ICI 182780 in women with advanced breast cancer. *Br J Cancer* 1996;74:300–8
14. Sato M, Glasebrook AL, Bryant HU. Raloxifene: a selective estrogen receptor modulator. *J Bone Miner Metab* 1994;12:S9-20
15. Jordan VC, MacGregor JI, Tonetti DA. Tamoxifen: from breast cancer therapy to the design of a post menopausal prevention maintenance therapy. *Osteoporos Int* 1997;7:S52–7
16. Jordan VC, Phelps E, Lindgren JU. Effects of anti-estrogen on bone in castrated and intact female rats. *Breast Cancer Res Treat* 1987;10:31–5

17. Lerner LJ, Jordan VC. Development of anti-estrogen and their use in breast cancer: Eighth Cain Memorial Award Lecture. *Cancer Res* 1990; 50:4177–89

18. Katzenellenbogen BS, Montano MM, LeGoff P, *et al*. Antiestrogens: mechanisms and actions in target cells. *J Steroid Biochem Mol Biol* 1995;53:387–93

19. Colletta AA, Benson JR, Baum M. Alternative mechanisms of action of anti-oestrogens. *Breast Cancer Res Treat* 1994;31:5–9

20. Berry M, Metzger D, Chambron P. Role of the two activating domains of the oestrogen receptor in the cell-type and promoter-context dependent agonistic activity of the anti-oestrogen 4-hydroxytamoxifen. *EMBO J* 1990;9:2811–18

21. Danielian PS, White R, Lees JA, *et al*. Identification of a conserved region required for hormone dependent transcriptional activation by steroid hormone receptors. *EMBO J* 1992;11: 1025–33

22. Webb P, Lopez GN, Uht RM, *et al*. Tamoxifen activation of the estrogen receptor/AP-1 pathway: potential origin for the cell-specific estrogen like effects of antiestrogens. *Mol Endocrinol* 1995; 9:443–56

23. Kuiper GGJM, Enmark E, Pelto-Huikko M, *et al*. Cloning a novel estrogen receptor expressed in rat prostate and ovary. *Proc Natl Acad Sci USA* 1996;93:5925–30

24. Paech K, Webb P, Kuiper GGJM, *et al*. Differential ligand activation of estrogen receptors ERα and ERβ at AP-1 site. *Science* 1997;277:1508–10

25. McDonnell DP, Clemm DL, Hermann T, *et al*. Analysis of estrogen receptor function *in vitro* reveals three distinct classes of antiestrogens. *Mol Endocrinol* 1995;9:659–69

26. Katzenellenbogen JA, O'Malley BW, Katzenellenbogen BS. Tripartite steroid receptor pharmacology: interaction with multiple effector sites as a basis for the cell- and promoter-specific action of these hormones. *Mol Endocrinol* 1996;10:119–31

27. Yang NN, Venugopalan M, Hardikar, *et al*. Identification of an estrogen response element activated by metabolites of 17beta-estradiol and raloxifene. *Science* 1996;273:1222–5

28. Elgort MG, Zou A, Marschke KB, *et al*. Estrogen and estrogen receptor antagonists stimulate transcription from the human retinoic acid receptor-alpha1 promoter via a novel sequence. *Mol Endocrinol* 1996;10:477–87

29. Brzozowski AM, Pike ACW, Dauter Z, *et al*. Molecular basis of agonism and antagonism in the oestrogen receptor. *Nature (London)* 1997;389:753–8

30. Jordan VC. Biochemical pharmacology of anti-estrogen action. *Pharmacol Rev* 1984;36:245–76

31. Lednicer D, Lyster SC, Duncan GW. Mammalian antifertility agents. IV. Basic 3,4-dihydro-naphthalenes and 1,2,3,4-tetrahydro I naphthols. *J Med Chem* 1967;10:78–84

32. Clark ER, Jordan VC. Oestrogenic, anti-oestrogenic and fertility effects of some triphenylethenes and triphenylethylenes related to athamoxytriphenol (MER25). *Br J Pharmacol* 1976;57:487–93

33. Robertson DW, Katzenellenbogen JA, Hayes, *et al*. Antiestrogen basicity–activity relationship: a comparison of estrogen receptor binding and antiuterotrophic potencies of several analogues of (Z)-1,2 diphenyl-1(4(-(dimethylamino) ethoxy)phenyl)-1 butene (tamoxifen, Nolvadex) having altered basicity. *J Med Chem* 1982;25: 167–71

34. Jordan VC, Gosden B. Importance of the aminoethoxy side chain for the estrogenic and anti-estrogenic actions of tamoxifen and trioxifene in the immature rat uterus. *Mol Cell Endocrinol* 1982; 27:291–306

35. Lieberman ME, Gorski J, Jordan VC. An estrogen receptor model to describe the regulator of prolactin synthesis by antiestrogens *in vitro*. *J Biol Chem* 1983;258:4741–5

36. Tate AC, Greene GL, DeSombre ER, *et al*. Differences between estrogen and antiestrogen–estrogen receptor complexes from human breast tumors identified with an antibody raised against the estrogen receptor. *Cancer Res* 1984;44: 1012–18

37. Sato M, Zeng GQ, Rowley E, *et al*. LY353381 HCl: an improved benzothiophene analog with bone efficacy complementary to parathyroid hormone-(1-34). *Endocrinology* 1998;139:4642–51

10

When hormone replacement therapy is not possible

M. Neves-e-Castro

INTRODUCTION

Hormone replacement therapy (HRT) has been one of the more convincing approaches to add quality and years to the life of postmenopausal women. The concept of HRT is open to discussion[1].

After the onset of menopause many women complain of disturbing symptoms that may adversely affect their quality of life. Vasomotor symptoms (hot flushes), irritability, depressive mood, insomnia, sexual dysfunction, bone and joint pains, weight gain, etc., are among those that more often cause discomfort and determine that a woman seeks medical support.

Alternatively, it is well established that after the menopause there is a clear increase in the risk for cardiovascular diseases and osteoporosis.

Both the often incapacitating symptoms and the risk for diseases later in life are accepted to be mainly due to the pronounced fall in circulating estrogens that is a characteristic of the primary ovarian failure, a landmark of the physiological menopause, in middle-aged women. Treatment with estrogens is effective in the relief of most symptoms and in the favorable modification of the above-mentioned risk factors.

Hormones have long been considered by many women either as wonder drugs or as very dangerous medications that may be related to cancer, hirsutism, weight gain, etc. Conversely, there are a few absolute and relative medical contraindications that may prevent the use of HRT by some women. However, in the majority of cases, HRT may be not possible because it is not wanted by the women, who are negatively affected by the 'bad news' that is often inaccurately transmitted by the media. Unfortunately, in many cases, 'bad news is good news' and that is what sells best.

The symptomatology of menopausal women is not universal. In a number of studies, among several ethnic and cultural groups in the world, it was found that there are 'important differences in women's experiences of symptoms and their responses to them, reflecting cultural influences on explanatory models of menopause, lifeways, and in turn, biology' . . . 'Their lifeways, including exercise and nutritional intake, affect symptom experiences and symptom distress'[2]. Filipino American midlife women consider the perimenopausal transition in a positive light, as part of normal life that does not warrent concern[3].

The 1998 North American Menopause Society Survey concluded that the majority of women viewed the menopause and midlife as the beginning of many positive changes in their lives and health[4]. Thus, some women may not feel the need for HRT, whereas others may not want to take it.

In a recent study involving 3000 women > 50 years old, 1350 were not on HRT. Of those, 82% were menopausal out of which only 21% had been treated with HRT in the past. The reasons for not taking HRT included the following: 49% no longer had menopausal symptoms, 45% did not want to take HRT, 33% were not offered it by their doctors, 28% were afraid to use it[5].

Therefore, HRT is sometimes not possible, either because women do not feel the need, or because they are afraid. Often this is due to lack of information for which health providers are responsible.

OBJECTIVES

Assuming that, no matter why, HRT is either not possible or not wanted, which are the goals of the attending physician and what can be offered to a menopausal woman who seeks support?

Basically, with or without HRT, there are always three fundamental objectives:

(1) Relief of symptoms,

(2) Maintenance and improvement of health,

(3) Prevention (primary or secondary) of diseases.

The assessment of health is far more difficult than the diagnosis of disease. However, the World Health Organization (WHO) has given a definition of health that can be very useful as a guide line: 'Health is a condition of physical, mental and social well-being and not only the absence of disease'.

Thus, the attending physician must adopt a holistic vision of the middle-age woman who comes to him for support. He must be concerned and involved in all the aspects that define health. If he is a gynecologist he should be aware of the etymology of this word, of Greek origin (*gyneka* – woman/*logos* = science). Gynecology in its broader dimension means the science or the knowledge of women, and not only the treatment of the diseases of the reproductive tract. Perhaps one should invent another designation (hybrid from Latin and Greek) like *feminology* or *holistic feminology* to better define the role of a modern gynecologist. As a matter of fact, if he is only a good specialist, with an average knowledge of internal medicine and little time or talent to establish a good

empathic relationship with a human being, he is certainly not a good gynecologist.

Middle-aged women do not routinely visit a cardiologist or a rheumatologist, but they go regularly to their gynecologists for a routine pelvic examination, a Papanicolaou smear, mammography, etc.

It is the responsibility of the modern gynecologist to take advantage of this opportunity to perform the necessary screenings to identify risks (cardiovascular, osteoporosis, cancer, etc.) and to attempt to modify them to the extent of his capacities and possibilities.

THE WOMAN

She may be defined as:

(1) A menopausal woman – if one considers that the shut down of ovarian function and the consequent hypoestrogenism is the key problem; or as

(2) A middle-aged woman – in whom natural aging is already playing a role, both from a biological and a psychological perspective.

In both cases she may suffer from a lack of estrogens and from aging. Biological age and chronological age run in parallel. She may complain of somatic and of psychic symptoms. For practical purposes one must accept that there is a biological syndrome and a psychological syndrome that affect these women. The purpose of the anti-aging interventions is to dissociate the biological age from the chronological age[6] and thus to compress morbidity as late as possible in the life time[7]. Adding life to the years and years to life is the target to hit. That is to say longer life but with greater quality.

The biological syndrome

Estrogens have profound effects in almost every organ and tissue of the body. Be it through genomic (α and β receptors) or non-genomic mechanisms the fact is that estrogen deprivation may cause dysfunctions and that treatment with estrogens may have corrective effects.

With aging and lack of estrogens the development of insulin resistance, increase in blood pressure, changes in lipid metabolism, a decrease in immune function, and increase in stored fat are almost universal phenomena.

These are the major factors for the high cardiovascular morbidity from which women were protected until the onset of menopause.

Insulin resistance (with hyperinsulinemia) seems to be one of the major factors of aging. It has profound impact on other hormonal systems, in particular eicosanoids, considered to be the molecular foundation of aging[6]. Insulin causes the production of more 'bad' (vasoconstrictor) than 'good' (vasodilator) eicosanoids. Insulin also increases the fat stores in the body.

Besides hyperinsulinemia there is also an excess in free radicals and cortisol, both with dangerous effects in the aging process. According to Sears[6], excessive insulin, excess in glucose, excess in free radicals and excess in cortisol, cause increased caloric consumption, increased DNA turnover, increased formation of advanced glycosylated end products (AGEs), neural death in some areas of the brain and an imbalance in eicosanoid synthesis, considered to be the molecular nature of chronic diseases.

From the above it can already be inferred that nutrition, exercise and life-style are closely related to these problems, as will be discussed later.

The lack of estrogens, lower amounts of vitamin D, lack of exercise and poor calcium intake are some of the factors that contribute to osteopenia and osteoporosis. Therefore, osteoclasts become more active (due to increased parathyroid hormone secretion resulting from a lesser negative feedback of calcium) and osteoblasts are not stimulated by the low levels of estrogens and androgens.

These woman seek help mostly because of the following:

(1) Weight gain,

(2) Different body fat distribution,

(3) Increased appetite,

(4) Asthenia, tiredness,

(5) Pain in the bones and joints,

(6) Precordial pressure,

(7) Hypertension,

(8) Dyspareunia (dry vagina),

(9) Stress incontinence,

(10) Breast tenderness (in early menopause).

The following are markers of good health[6,8,9]:

(1) Fasting insulin levels less than 10 μU/ml,

(2) Fasting glucose/insulin ratio (mg/dl : μU/ml) greater than 4.5,

(3) Glycosylated hemoglobin less than 5%,

(4) Fasting triglycerides less than 140 mg/dl,

(5) Low total cholesterol (less than 200 mg/dl),

(6) Low-density lipoprotein less than 130 mg/dl and high density lipoprotein greater than 50 mg/dl,

(7) Triglycerides/HDL ratio less than 2,

(8) Total cholesterol/HDL less than 4.5,

(9) BMI (body mass index) 20–25 kg/m^2,

(10) Body fat less than 22%,

(11) Blood pressure: diastolic less than 90 mmHg and systolic less than 140 mmHg,

(12) Bone mineral density: T above –1.0 SD.

The psychic and neurovegetative syndromes

Vasomotor symptoms (hot flushes),
Insomnia,
Irritability,
Depressive mood,
Frigidity,
Headaches and migraine,
Poor memory.

These symptoms are not necessarily estrogen related, other than the hot flushes. However, since the brain is a target for estrogens that act via several neurotransmitters, it is likely that its lower levels after the menopause may have an impact on mood, sleep and memory.

Since in industrialized countries the menopause has for many women (and men, too) a negative connotation, being considered the beginning of the end, the lack of femininity, etc., it is conceivable that menopausal women consider themselves very insecure (feelings of jealousy, need of reaffirmation, etc.). The unhappiness they may feel needs compensatory gratification (food, sweets, etc.). The 'empty nest' syndrome does not help them to reformulate their lifestyles; they do not feel any interest in life, they became inactive and do not want to exercise, and they may often feel miserable.

Estrogens also act on the arterial wall and stimulate the synthesis of nitric oxide (NO) by the endothelium. NO is a potent vasodilator. The lack of nitric oxide may cause vasospasm and cause headaches and migraine.

STRATEGIES

It is obvious that despite the fact that HRT is very important to help in the maintenance of health, the prevention of diseases and the relief of symptoms, there are many other possibilities, other than the use of hormones, to help those women who cannot or do not want to take HRT.

It is beyond the scope of this chapter to go through all the steps that are applicable to all women who are in this phase of their lives. Instead, reference will be made to a number of interventions that are usually omitted despite their proven efficacy as anti-aging, anti-cardiovascular disease, anti-osteoporosis and even anti-cancer. The following topics deserve far greater attention than they have had so far. As a matter of fact it is easier and less time consuming to prescribe pills than to persuade a woman to change her lifestyle, nutrition, etc.

Time to listen

The most important single measure is to have time to listen and to talk. Many of the problems faced by these women can be solved or greatly alleviated if the attending physician believes that he is capable of understanding and supporting and giving, sometimes for the first time, the information those women are lacking. If a woman is properly informed about the physiology of this change in her life, and that most other women do have similar complains, then the mystery starts fading and doors can be opened to establish a positive dialog. Sometimes if one explains to them the meaning of some clinical trials they may understand what is a benefit–risk analysis, or a relative risk, and eventually change their minds. But, assuming that HRT is out of question what should be the next step?

Physical activity

It is well established that well-planned physical exercise has very positive effects on mood and on the sense of well being (due to the release of beta-endorphins by the brain). It helps to develop motivation. It contributes to weight loss, to muscle strength, to a better cardiovascular function, and it helps the bone and joint function. It also decreases stress.

Women who took part in moderate exercise, as little as once a week, were 24% less likely to die prematurely than women who did not exercise. Women who took part in vigorous exercise (jogging, swimming, etc) more than four times a week had 43% lower risk of premature death[10].

Anti-stress

The attending physician, with time (!) is often in a better position than a psychotherapist to give the support and advice that may help to decrease psychological stress and distress. Explaining how the central and autonomic nervous systems and the adrenal glands may cause vasospasm (headaches, migraine, hypertension), increase cortisol secretion (with all the metabolic consequences) and make one feel unhappy, is one of the first steps to help that woman look into herself, in the mirror, to start equating her problems and maybe solving some of them. Stress is a major risk for coronary heart disease. If needed, the attending physician should not refrain from complementing his mild psychotherapy with mild tranquillizers or antidepressants. It is expected that he knows how to manipulate these psychopharmacological medicines and that he is also capable of identifying mental disorders that should be treated by another specialist.

Vasomotor symptoms

Sometimes these are intense and require treatment. Antidopaminergics (veralipride) and α2 blockers (clonidine) have been used with some success. However, even when HRT is not possible, an injection of 150 mg medroxyprogesterone acetate is more effective. The side-effect to be considered is on mood.

Insomnia

There is no problem in prescribing mild sedatives and hypnogens.

Headaches and migraine

If acetylsalicylic acid is well tolerated, for short periods, it is acceptable since it also has anti-aggregating effects, preventing atheromatous plaque formation. Otherwise, other mild analgesics are to be recommended. Ergot derivatives should be used with caution. A balanced diet may help. Smoking should be proscribed, since it causes vasoconstriction.

Dyspareunia and frigidity

Only later in the menopause is the vaginal epithelium atrophic enough to cause dyspareunia. In the majority of cases, in the early menopause, dyspareunia is psychogenic and due to perineal muscle spasm. The same with frigidity and anorgasmia, which are seldom hormone-related. Lubricant jellies are effective. Even when HRT is not possible there is no reason to avoid estrogen vaginal suppositories or creams. When possible it is advisable to have a joint conversation with the partner to demystify the problem and to propose some techniques that may be less traumatic and more gratifying.

Nutrition and weight control

There is a significant association between younger age at menopause and higher risk of coronary heart disease among women who experienced natural menopause and never used hormone therapy[11]. Therefore, particular attention must be paid to this group of women, particularly if they are obese. Obesity is a significant independent predictor of cardiovascular disease[12].

Aerobic exercise plays an important role in preventing obesity in most persons. Genetic factors do not predispose to obesity as has sometimes been accepted. In a study conducted in 970 healthy female twins (mean age 55.5 years) it was concluded that physical activity is the strongest independent predictor of total body fat and central abdominal fat, far greater than other environmental factors[13].

Higher levels of physical activity lessen total body and abdominal fat, prevent insulin resistance, hypertension and cardiovascular diseases. This can be achieved with 2 hours of sport or 15 km of walking per week. Weight-bearing sport of any intensity was related to lower fat deposits and greater muscle strength. Therefore, physical activity seems to be, according to this study, the strongest determinant of body fat, more than diet. It should be, together with physical activity, another leg of the tripod that supports good health and longevity. (The third leg, pharmacological intervention, will be discussed later.)

This does not mean, of course, that the food intake is not extremely important both quantitatively and qualitatively.

One should never talk about a diet. The woman has already followed many of them and is frustrated by not achieving what she expected.

What is important is to explain how the body functions. How much protein, fat and carbohydrate are needed for that particular person, with that type of energy consumption. It is mandatory to take measures to determine the body mass index, the percentage of body fat and to set the objectives.

One must take the time to explain the nutritional value of food and its content of substances that are health protective. This may be reinforced by the information of the high or low prevalence of several diseases in different areas of the world as a function of their nutrition.

Many women ignore that excessive weight and a high consumption of animal fat raises the risk for breast cancer more than does HRT. A high consumption of vegetables, fruit and fiber is linked with a lesser prevalence of cardiovascular events, cancer of the colon and breast.

It can be stated that modern nutritional advice is very effective for the prevention of cancer and cardiovascular diseases. It is this type of information that motivates a woman to change her dietary habits. The objective is not to start on a diet but to change and incorporate the change. This is fundamental for behavior support.

Antioxidants

It was previously mentioned that a typical marker of aging is an increase in oxygen free radicals that damage cells. Antioxidants prevent free radicals from damaging the cells. Aging appears to be due, in good part, to the oxidants produced by mitochondria as by-products of normal metabolism. Vitamins C, E and betacarotene are good antioxidants which are contained in certain foods (fruit, vegetables). Olive oil is a powerful antioxidant, too. Oxygen free radicals oxidize low density lipoprotein cholesterol particles, which are atherogenic. Antioxidants may prevent heart disease, and also cancer[14].

Tomatoes are rich in antioxidants (lycopene and carotenoids) and do protect from coronary heart disease and cancer[15].

In a recent study involving 2400 Greek women it was shown that the incidence of breast cancer dropped with a higher intake of olive oil, certain vegetables and fruits[16].

Similar conclusions were reported in other studies[17,18].

Frequent nut consumption is associated with a reduced risk of both fatal coronary heart disease and non-fatal myocardial infarction (relative risk 0.65, 95% confidence interval 0.47–0.89, p for trend = 0.0009). Adjustment for intakes of dietary fats, fiber, vegetables and fruit did not alter these results derived from the Nurses' Health Study[19].

Phytoestrogens

Red clover and soy are particularly rich in phytoestrogens[20]. Green split peas, chick peas and broad beans are also rich in some isoflavones (genistein, daidzein, biochamin, formononetin) that have special estrogenic effects. Perhaps this is why traditional legume based diets used by Asiatic populations are associated with reduced heart disease and also breast cancer.

Some commercial preparations containing these isoflavones are available and have been tested in clinical trials[21,22]. Isoflavones are also strong antioxidants.

Dietary fiber

Wolk and colleagues[23] examined the association between long-term intake of total dietary fibre and the risk of coronary heart disease in women aged 37–64 years, followed for 10 years, without evidence of heart disease, hypercholesterolemia or diabetes at base line. The age-adjusted relative risk (RR) for major coronary heart disease was 0.53 for highest quintile of total dietary fibre intake (median, 22.9 g/ day) compared with women in the lowest quintile (median, 11.5 g/day). After controlling for age, cardiovascular risk factors and multivitamin supplement use, the RR was 0.77. Only cereal fiber was strongly associated with a reduced risk of coronary heart disease. These fiber-rich diets may also increase insulin sensitivity (reduce insulin resistance) and lower triglyceride levels. The recommended daily intake of fiber is 20–35 g. Rich in fiber are: wholegrain bread, oatmeal, brown rice, apple (with skin), avocado, oranges, prunes, raspberries, kidney beans, etc.

Vitamins (C, A and β-carotene)

Vegetables and fruit are very good vitamin sources, namely, broccoli, Brussels sprouts, chicory, tomatoes, carrots, kiwi fruit, citrus fruits, raspberries and strawberries, water-melons and many others.

The natural micronutrients contained in food seem to be more protective than in their pure form. Deficiency of vitamins B12, folic acid, B6, niacin, C, or E, or iron, or zinc appears to mimic radiation in damaging DNA by causing single and double strand breaks, oxidative lesions, or both.

Micronutrient deficiency may explain, in good part, why the quarter of the North American population that eats the fewest fruits and vegetables (five portions a day is advised) has approximately double the cancer rate for most types of cancer when compared to the quarter with the highest intake[24].

Whole foods and fibers

Even if one takes tablets, daily, with vitamins and minerals, a balanced diet with whole foods must be a centerpiece. An orange or a glass of milk supply much more than vitamin C or protein.

Dietary fibers are important for digestion. Soluble fiber (in most fruits, certain beans and grains, some vegetables) may help prevent heart diseases and diabetes. Insoluble fibers, found in most vegetables, some fruits and breakfast cereals, can prevent constipation and colon cancer.

A diet high in fruits and vegetables reduces the risk of cancer, heart diseases and stroke.

High intake of whole-grain products is linked to reduced mortality among older women by 15% compared to non-users[25].

Fish

The more fish one eats the less coronary artery disease one has. Salmon, tuna fish and sardines are particularly rich in omega 3 polyunsaturated fatty acids. Eating these fish can reduce triglycerides and cholesterol because of their content of omega 3 fatty acids. The American Heart Association recommends eating fish two or three times a week.

It is of interest to note that a reduction in total or saturated fat intake, or cholesterol intake, is significantly associated with a reduction in area of breast density on mammography.

A dense breast tissue is a risk for breast cancer, i.e. because it may disguise occult minor atypical lesions[26].

MORE SPECIFIC INTERVENTIONS

Again the targets for primary and secondary prevention will be the cardiovascular system and the bones. Cancer is not the women's big killer. They live and suffer with their heart, and it is ultimately the heart that will kill most of them!

(1) What to do to prevent coronary heart disease?

(2) What to do to decrease insulin resistance?

(3) What to do in cases of resistant obesity?

(4) What to do to prevent osteoporosis?

Coronary heart disease

Reducing cholesterol and blood pressure, as well as stopping smoking, are effective strategies to prevent cardiovascular disease. There are many convincing coronary primary prevention trials, all showing that either with diet or with lipid-lowering agents (cholestyramine, gemfibrozil, nicotinic acid, simvastatin, pravastatin, pravachol) there was a decrease in mortality due to coronary heart disease. Unfortunately, these trials were conducted only in men. It is hoped that the same conclusions may apply to women; this seems to be the case at least with the statins[27,28].

There are some new preventive strategies that include the liberal use of antioxidants, the use of angiotensin-converting enzyme inhibitors and homocystein lowering[29].

Cholesterol lowering by pharmacological means prevents atherosclerotic plaque progression and it has been shown to reduce both fatal and non-fatal coronary events in patients with or without coronary heart disease. Simvastatin for secondary prevention and lovastatin for primary prevention have a very favorable cost-effect profile[30].

Vitamin E seems to be a good choice in doses of 200 mg/day although the final proof in terms of death reduction is not yet known since the ongoing trials have not yet been reported[31].

Vitamin E, besides being a powerful antioxidant (inhibiting the oxidation of low-density lipoprotein cholesterol), also has a biological anti-inflammatory effect that contributes to the prevention of fatty plaque formation on the arterial walls. Recent studies suggest that plaque formation is an inflammatory process.

Of greater interest seem to be the angiotensin-converting enzyme inhibitors that are anti-proliferative, improve endothelial function, may act as antioxidants, decrease platelet aggregation and enhance fibrinolysis.

Homocysteine, an amino acid, can experimentally induce vascular damage. It was demonstrated that there is a non-linear relation between homocysteine concentration and cardiovascular risk[32].

Low circulating concentrations of folic acid and vitamins B6 and B12 increase the risk of cardiovascular disease and cause a rise in homocysteinemia. Administration of folic acid and those vitamins rapidly decreases the levels of homocysteine. Clinical trials are underway to determine if these strategies are cardioprotective. It has been suggested that even people with normal levels of homocysteine might benefit from its reduction. Elderly patients taking vitamin B6 supplements of 100–200 mg/day showed a 73% reduction in the risk of angina and myocardial infarction with an average increase in lifespan of 8 years[33]. In the Nurses' Health Study it was found that the intake of folate and vitamin B6 above the current recommended dietary allowance may be important in the primary prevention of coronary heart disease among women[34].

The understanding of coronary artery disease risk and atherogenesis has changed very much in recent years. It is the unstable soft plaque, that cannot been seen in angiography, that is prone to rupture and result in infarction. There are also important changes in vascular reactivity that result from diet. Most infarctions occur in patients who have normal total cholesterol levels. At risk patients can be identified using the ratios of total cholesterol to high density lipoprotein, and triglycerides to high density lipoprotein. Primary prevention trials demonstrate that coronary artery disease risk can be lowered dramatically with diet and drug therapy[35].

Insulin resistance

A fasting glucose/insulin (G : I) ratio (md/dL : μU/ml) less than 4.5 is the single best screening measure for detecting insulin resistance[36].

Strong physical activity and a properly balanced diet are the best initial approaches. The so called insulin sensitizers can be used, with caution, as if these women had type 2 diabetes. For this purpose, biguanides (like metformin) have been widely used. A new class of compounds, the glitazones[37], was recently introduced in the market; but they may have some liver toxicity.

Obesity

In most cases, obesity is psychogenic in its origin. If general measures[38] (physical exercise, balanced nutrition) do not work it is essential to refer the woman to a behavioral psychotherapist. Two new compounds have been introduced in the market. Orlistat[39] decreases the intestinal absorption of dietary fat. Sibutramine[40] inhibits the reuptake of both serotonin and norepinephrine; it reduces food intake and increases thermogenesis, thus contributing to weight loss.

Obesity, per se, is a cause of insulin resistance which, in turn, can also cause obesity. In such cases, when hyperinsulinemia is present, these cases should be managed as in insulin resistance.

Osteopenia and osteoporosis

In a recent study[41] it was concluded that subclinical vitamin D deficiency may contribute to increased fractures. Low levels of vitamin D are associated with high levels of parathyroid hormone, may cause a parathyroid hormone-mediated bone loss. Vitamin D and calcium therapy reduce parathyroid hormone and decrease bone resorption, with a consequent decrease in fractures. It is estimated that 800 IU of vitamin D and 1 g elemental calcium per day are needed to reduce fractures. This is a recommendation for the primary prevention of bone loss.

Fatty fish is a good source of vitamin D. Too much protein in the diet can result in increased loss of calcium in the urine; the same is true of too much sodium, caffeine and alcohol. Smoking increases the risk for osteoporosis.

If one has to complement these measures with drugs, specific estrogen receptor modulators like raloxifene cannot be considered as being hormones and may safely be used. Besides increasing bone mineral density and preventing osteoporosis, they also have a positive effect in lipid metabolism, they do not stimulate the endometrium and may even protect against breast cancer[42,43]. Bisphosphonates[44] have a very positive effect on the bone and are used with success for the treatment of osteoporosis.

Breast cancer

Other important information from the Nurses' Health Study suggests that folates, which are involved in DNA synthesis, may reduce breast cancer risk, particularly among women with greater alcohol consumption (at least 15 g/day of alcohol)[45]. (The relative risk of breast cancer for current users of folate supplements versus never users was RR 0.74; 95% CI, 0.59–0.93). It is also known that alcohol increases breast cancer risk.

This study did not show any association between total folate intake and breast cancer risk among women who consumed less than 15 g/day of alcohol. Thus, a decrease in alcohol, and also in animal fat consumption, seems a wise measure to decrease the risk of breast cancer, even more so if one also eats more fruits and vegetables containing isoflavones.

CONCLUDING REMARKS AND PRACTICAL GUIDELINES

There seems to be little doubt that Hippocrates was right when he said 2500 years ago 'Let food be your Medicine, and let Medicine be your food'. Barry Sears[7] has made a monumental contribution to the science of nutrition with a very comprehensive and highly scientific logical approach to anti-aging. Public Health authorities are concerned with the little attention that is paid to the urgent need to change alimentary habits and lifestyles, as a cheap and very effective strategy to prevent many diseases. Health-care providers are also not motivated to implement and reinforce such life-saving strategies.

There is nowadays an abuse of drug consumption. Most people do not know, or do not believe, that many a time proper nutrition, good physical exercise and changes in lifestyle can achieve more, in terms of disease prevention and health maintenance, than some tablets taken by mouth.

When HRT is not possible, what can be done for menopausal women? It is unquestionable that estrogens can be of great help during the early and late postmenopausal phases of a woman's life. Nevertheless one can often achieve as much with non-hormonal medication or even without drugs. It may take longer but, in the long run, it pays.

The following suggestions and recommendations should be made to *all* middle-aged women whether or not they are on HRT.

(1) Start a Mediterranean diet[46] or a 'zone' diet[6], eating:

    (a) More whole breads and cereals,

    (b) More root vegetables, green vegetables and legumes (beans, peas, carrots, broccoli, tomatoes, etc.),

    (c) More fish (salmon, tuna, etc.),

    (d) More fresh fruit (apples, citrus etc.),

    (e) Replace beef with poultry,

    (f) No butter,

    (g) Plenty of olive oil,

    (h) Some red wine,

    (i) Plenty of black or green tea,

    (j) Nuts;

(2) Start a program of physical fitness, and exercise as much as possible;

(3) Keep mentally active;

(4) Reformulate the life-style;

(5) Take the following nutrients (essential)

    (a) Vitamin A 4.000 IU/day,

    (b) Vitamin B6 5–10 mg/day,

    (c) Vitamin C 500–1000 mg/day,

    (d) Vitamin D 400–800 IU/day,

    (e) Vitamin E 200–400 IU/day,

    (f) Folic acid 0.5–1.0 mg/day,

    (g) Calcium 500–1000 mg/day,

    (h) Magnesium 250–400 mg/day,

    (i) β-carotene 5000 IU/day;

(6) For the prevention of atherosclerosis (advisable)

    (a) Lovastatin or simvastatin (for primary and secondary prevention, respectively),

    (b) Aspirin (50–100 mg/day),

    (c) Angiotension-converting enzyme inhibitors.

References

1. Speroff L. It's time to stop using the word 'replacement'. *Maturitas* 1999;in press
2. Woods NF. Symptoms among midlife women: cultural lenses, research, and health care. Editorial. *Menopause* 1999;6:90–1
3. Berg DA, Taylor DL. Symptom experience of Filipino American midlife women. *Menopause* 1999;6:105–14
4. Utian WH, Boggs PP. The North American Menopause Society 1998 Menopause Survey. Part I: Postmenopausal women's perception about menopause and midlife. *Menopause* 1999; 6:122–8
5. Rabin DS, Cipparrone N, Linn ES, *et al.* Why menopausal women do not want to take hormone replacement therapy. *Menopause* 1999; 6:61–7
6. Sears, B. *The Anti-aging Zone.* New York, NY: Harper Collins Publisher Inc., 1999
7. Speroff L. Women's health care in the 21st century. *Maturitas* 1999;in press
8. Notelovitz M, Tonnessen D. *The Essential Heart Book for Women.* New York: St. Martin's Griffin, 1997.
9. Byyny RL, Speroff L. *A Clinical Guide for the Care of Older Women.* Baltimore: Williams and Wilkins, 1990
10. Kushi LH, Fee RM, Fulson AR, *et al.* Physical activity and mortality in postmenopausal women. *J Am Med Assoc* 1997;227:1287–92
11. Hu FB, Grodstein F, Hennekens CH, *et al.* Age at natural menopause and risk of cardiovascular disease. *Arch Intern Med* 1999;159:1061–6
12. Tamaka K, Nakamishi T. Obesity as a risk factor for various diseases: necessity for lifestyle changes for healthy aging. *Appl Human Sci* 1996;15:139–48
13. Samaras K, Kelly PJ, Chiano MN, *et al.* Genetic and environmental influences on total-body and central abdominal fat: the effect of physical activity in female twins. *Ann Intern Med* 1999; 13:873–82
14. Stampfer MJ, Hennekens CH, Manson JE, *et al.* Vitamin E consumption and the risk of coronary disease in women. *N Engl J Med* 1993; 328:1444–9
15. Giovannuci E. Tomatoes, tomato-based products, lycopene and cancer: review of the epidemiological literature. *J Natl Cancer Inst* 1999;91: 317–31
16. Trichopoulou A, Katsouyanni K, Stuver S, *et al.* Consumption of olive oil and specific food groups in relation to cancer in Greece. *J Natl Cancer Inst* 1995;87:110–16
17. Block G, Patterson B, Subar A. Fruit, vegetables and cancer prevention: a review of epidemiological evidence. *Nutr Cancer* 1992;18:1–29
18. Tavani A, La Vechia C. Fruit and vegetable consumption and cancer risk in a Mediterranean

population. *Am J Clin Nutr* 1995;61(Suppl) 1374S–7S

19. Hu FB, Stampfer MJ, Manson JE, *et al.* Frequent nut consumption and risk of coronary heart disease in women: prospective cohort study. *Br Med J* 1998;317:1341–5

20. Reinil K, Block G. Phytoestrogen content of food – a compendium of literature values. *Nutr Cancer* 1996;26:123–48

21. Nachtigall L, Fenichel R, Lagregal L, *et al.* The effects of isoflavone derived from red clover on vasomotor symptoms, endometrial thickness and reproductive hormone concentrations in menopausal women. Poster 2–59, The 81st Hormonal Meeting of the Endocrine Society, USA, 1999

22. Washbuen S, Burke GL, Morgan T, *et al.* Effect of soy protein supplement on serum lipoproteins, blood pressure, and menopausal symptoms in perimenopausal women. *Menopause* 1999;6:7–13

23. Wolk A, Manson JE, Stampfer MS, *et al.* Long-term intake of dietary fiber and decreased risk of coronary heart disease among women. *J Am Med Assoc* 1999;281:1998–2004

24. Ames BN. Micronutrients prevent cancer and delay aging. *Toxicol Lett* 1998;102–3:5–18

25. Jacobs DR Jr, Meyer KA, Kushi LH, *et al.* Is whole grain intake associated with reduced total and cause-specific death rates in older women? The Iowa Women's Health Study. *Am J Public Health* 1999;89:322–9

26. Knight JA, Martin LJ, Greenberg CV, *et al.* Macronutrient intake and change in mammography density at menopause: results from a randomised trial. *Cancer Epidemial Biomarkers Prev* 1999;8:123–8

27. Williamson DR, Pharand C. Statins in the prevention of coronary heart disease. *Pharmacotherapy* 1998;18:242–54

28. Downs JR, Clerfield M, Weis S, *et al.* Primary prevention of acute coronary events with lovastatin in men and women with average cholesterol levels. *J Am Med Assoc* 1998;279:1615–22

29. Lonn EM, Yusuf S. Emerging approaches in preventing cardiovascular disease. *Br Med J* 1999;318:1337–41

30. Hay JN, Yu WM, Ashraf T. Pharmacoeconomics of lipid-lowering agents for primary and secondary prevention of coronary artery disease. *Pharmacoeconomics* 1999;15:47–74

31. Devaraj S, Jialal I. Alpha-tochophero 2 decreases interleukin 1 beta release from activated human monocytes by inhibition of 5-lipoxygenase. *Arterioscler Thromb Vasc Biol* (United States) 1999; 19:1125–33

32. Boushey CJ, Beresford SAA, Omenn GS, *et al.* A quantitative assessment of plasma homocysteine as a risk factor for vascular disease. Probable benefits of increasing folic acid intakes. *J Am Med Assoc* 1995;274:1049–57.

33. Ellis JM, Mckully KS. Prevention of myocardial infarction by vitamin B6. *Res Comm Mol Pathol Pharmacol* 1995;89:208–20

34. Rimm EB, Willett WC, Hu FB, *et al.* Folate and vitamin B6 from diet and supplements in relation to risk of coronary heart diseases among women. *J Am Med Assoc* 1998;279:359–64

35. Castelli WP. The new pathophysiology of coronary artery disease. *Am J Cardiol* 1998;82: 60T–65T

36. Legro RS, Finegood D, Dunaif A. A fasting glucose to insulin ratio is a useful measure of insulin sensitivity in women with polycystic ovary syndrome. *J Clin Endocrinol Metab* 1998;83:2694–8

37. Nolan JJ, Ludvik B, Beerdsen P, *et al.* Improvement in glucose tolerance and insulin resistance in obese subjects treated with troglitazone. *N Engl J Med* 1994;331:1188–93

38. Anderson DA, Wadden TA. Treating the obese patient. Suggestions for primary care practice. *Arch Fam Med* 1999;8:156–67

39. Sjöström L, Rissanen A, Andersen T, *et al.* Controlled trial of Orlistat for weight loss and prevention of weight regain in obese patients. *Lancet* 1998;352:167–72

40. Bray GA, Blackburn GL, Fergunson JM *et al.* Sibutramine produces dose-related weight loss. *Obesity Res* 1999;7:189–98

41. LeBoff MS, Kohlmeier L, Hurwitz S, *et al.* Occult vitamin D deficiency in postmenopausal US women with acute hip fracture. *J Am Med Assoc* 1999;281:1505–11

42. Delmas P, Bjarnason NH, Mitlak BH, *et al.* Effects of raloxifene on bone mineral density, serum cholesterol concentrations, and uterine endometrium in postmenopausal women. *N Engl J Med* 1997;337:1641–7

43. Walsh BW, Kuller LH, Wild RA, *et al.* Effects of raloxifene on serum lipids and coagulation in healthy post-menopausal women. *J Am Med Assoc* 1998;279:1445–50

44. Ensrud K, Black DM, Palermo L, *et al.* Treatment with alendronate prevents fractures in women at highest risk: results from the Fracture Intervention Trial. *Arch Intern Med* 1997;157:2617–24

45. Zhang S, Hunter DJ, Hankinson SE, *et al.* A prospective study of folate intake and the risk of breast cancer. *J Am Med Assoc* 1999;281:1632–7

46. Greenwood S. The Mediterranean diet: acceptable and effective for Americans? *Menopause Management* (NAMS) 1999;8:16–19

Suggested reading

Notelovitz M, Tonnessen D. *Menopause and Midlife Health.* New York: St. Martin's Press, 1993

Neves-e-Castro M, Birkhäuser M, Clarkson TB, Collins P, eds. *Menopause and the Heart.* Carnforth, UK: Parthenon Publishing, 1999

Web sites

Mayo Clinic – http:// *www.mayo.health.org/* (women's health and diets)

Tufts University – http:// *www.navigator.tufts.edu/* (excellent for nutrition)

11

Hormone replacement therapy and the brain

D. Robertson, T. van Amelsvoort and D. Murphy

INTRODUCTION

By the year 2010, the proportion of people aged over 65 years will have increased by 30%, and an increasing number of people will experience age-related cognitive decline and late-onset neuropsychiatric disorders, such as Alzheimer's disease, stroke, late-onset forms of anxiety and affective disorders, and psychotic disorders. Significant gender differences in the prevalence, symptomatology and prognosis of these age-related brain disorders implicate sex steroids/sex chromosomes in their pathophysiology. Moreover, a large body of literature documents the effects of gonadal hormones, particularly estrogen, on brain structure, function and metabolism. An understanding of the effects of estrogens is therefore important. This chapter reviews:

(1) The effects of estrogen and the X chromosome on normal brain development and aging;

(2) How estrogens modulate brain structure and function;

(3) The actions of estrogen replacement therapy on mood (including depressive disorder) and cognition in postmenopausal women;

(4) The role of estrogen replacement therapy in neurological disorders, including Alzheimer's disease, stroke and schizophrenia.

NORMAL BRAIN DEVELOPMENT AND AGING

Sexual dimorphism in brain aging

Aging of the normal brain is accompanied by changes in brain structure, function and metabolism. Moreover, there are significant gender differences in brain aging. For example, a precipitous increase in ventricular volume begins in the fifth decade in men[1] and in the sixth decade in women, suggesting that brain atrophy begins earlier in men than in women. However, once started, the velocity of the atrophy process increases with age more rapidly in women[2]. Murphy and co-workers[3] reported that age-related loss of brain tissue was significantly greater in males than females in whole brain, frontal and temporal lobes, whereas the loss was greater in females than males in the hippocampus and parietal lobes. Further investigation using positron emission tomography (PET) and 18F-2-fluoro-2-deoxy-D-glucose (FDG) reported significant sex differences in age-related effects on glucose metabolism in the temporal and parietal lobes, Broca's area, thalamus and hippocampus[3]. For example, males had no age-related decline in hippocampal metabolism, whereas women did. Furthermore, age-related decline in brain metabolism was greater on the left than the right hemisphere in males, but in females it was generally symmetrical. These gender differences in brain aging implicate sex chromosomes and sex steroids in healthy brain aging. In addition, because they occur in brain regions associated with cognitive function and neuropsychiatric disease (see below), they may underlie gender differences in the prevalence and symptomatology of neuropsychiatric disorders, such as autism, dyslexia, schizophrenia and Alzheimer's disease.

Effects of estrogens on human brain development

Turner's syndrome provides a biological model by which to investigate the effects of the X chromosome and sex steroids on the brain. Most women with Turner's syndrome have the 'pure' karyotype (45,X), whilst others are mosaic (45,X/46,XX or 45,X/47,XXX). In both pure and mosaic Turner's syndrome there is no ovarian estrogen production because of a failure of ovarian development. Neuropsychological studies have shown a typical pattern of deficit in people with Turner's syndrome which includes better verbal than visuospatial skills and abnormalities of social interaction[4]. Also, a quantitative magnetic resonance imaging (MRI) study of women with pure and mosaic Turner's syndrome reported significant bilateral decreases in the volume of hippocampus, parieto-occipital brain matter and lenticular and thalamic nuclei compared to controls (46,XX)[5]. However, in mosaics the volumes of cerebral hemisphere, caudate nucleus and lenticular and thalamic nuclei showed 'X-chromosome dosage effects', suggesting that these structures depend upon the X chromosome to develop normally. Whilst hippocampal volume was decreased in all Turner's syndrome subjects, it did not show such 'X-chromosome dosage effects', suggesting that hippocampal development depends to a greater degree on sex steroids. Resting brain glucose metabolism has also been compared in Turner's syndrome females and controls, using FDG-PET. Clark and colleagues[6] reported decreased metabolism in occipital and parietal cortices, and recently Murphy and colleagues[7] reported that Turner's syndrome was associated with relative bilateral hypometabolism in association neo-cortices and insulae. In women with Turner's syndrome there were also significant differences in cortical functional relationships originating bilaterally in the occipital cortices, and within the right hemisphere. There were 'X-chromosome dosage' effects in language ability and left middle temporal lobe metabolism, and in neuropsychological test scores and asymmetry of parietal metabolism, indicating that the X chromosome is involved in the function of the left and right association neocortices, and that brain metabolic abnormalities in Turner's syndrome are associated with cognitive deficits.

Thus, sex steroids and the X chromosome have differential effects on brain structure and function in humans. In addition to explaining some of the neuropsychological and social deficits seen in Turner's syndrome, such studies demonstrate that sex steroids affect brain regions involved in age-related cognitive decline and neuropsychiatric disorders (e.g. the hippocampus).

Effects of estrogens on dendrites

Estrogens increase synaptic and dendritic spine density in the hippocampus – a brain region which is crucial to memory function and which is severely affected in Alzheimer's disease. For example, in rats following bilateral oophorectomy there is a significant decrease in dendritic spine density in CA1 pyramidal cells. However, this is prevented by administration of estrogens, and synaptic spine density is significantly related to circulating estradiol levels[8]. Until recently it was unclear how these estrogen-induced dendritic changes affected neuronal function. However, it has now been demonstrated that estrogen induces an increase in NMDA receptors in rat hippocampal neurons in the same region where an increase in dendritic spines is found. This is of importance because the NMDA receptor is a membrane protein that detects incoming signals from the excitatory neurotransmitter glutamate. Thus, the 'new' estrogen-induced spines are now thought to be related to NMDA-type synapses[9,10].

Effects of estrogen on neurotransmitter systems

The cholinergic system

Cholinergic receptor and enzyme systems are influenced directly and indirectly by estrogens. The basal forebrain nuclei (which are a major source of cholinergic innervation to the brain and are implicated in the pathology of Alzheimer's disease[11]) contain receptors for sex steroids, and in ovariectomized rats muscarinic cholinergic receptors are up-regulated by 48–72 hours of estradiol priming[12]. Furthermore, activities of choline acetyltranferase (CAT) and acetylcholinesterase (AChE), which respectively synthesize and degrade acetylcholine, are responsive to the levels of circulating estrogen hormones. In ovariectomized rats, estrogen increases the activity of CAT by inducing *de novo* enzyme synthesis in the basal forebrain, with subsequent axonal transport to the CA1 region of the hippocampus and the frontal cortex[13,14].

The noradrenergic system

Alpha-[15] and beta-adrenergic[16] receptors are up-regulated by estradiol in ovariectomized female rats. However, beta-adrenergic receptors are eventually down-regulated due to a hormone-dependent increase in noradrenergic activity. The effects of estrogen on reuptake at receptor sites may be influenced by post-treatment with progesterone – when administered alone, estrogen inhibits synaptic reuptake of noradrenaline in rats[17], but when estrogen is followed by progesterone the uptake of noradrenaline is increased[15].

The effect of estrogens on the synthesis and breakdown of noradrenaline is disputed. For example, estrogens have been reported to inhibit the enzyme tyrosine hydroxylase (which is responsible for a step in dopamine, adrenaline and noradrenaline synthesis) activity in the hypothalamus and striatum[18]. However, others reported that estrogens increase tyrosine hydoxylase activity[19], facilitate noradrenaline release[20], and decrease monoamine oxidase (a catabolic enzyme) activity in rats[13] and postmenopausal women[21]. Thus, there is general support for the suggestion that estrogens can enhance adrenergic activity. This is of relevance because there is a link between the adrenergic system and human cognition[22]. For example, inhibition of human noradrenergic neuron firing and noradrenaline turnover is associated with reduced mental performance[23] and learning[24]. Therefore, it is possible that estrogens may improve human memory ability via the noradrenergic system as well as the cholinergic system.

The dopaminergic system

Both human and animal research indicate that estrogens modulate some aspects of dopaminergic function. Estradiol inhibits dopamine release from the median eminence[25] and induces an increase in the release and turnover of striatal dopamine[15,26]. Reuptake of dopamine is increased in rat preoptic–septal tissue but is decreased in hypothalamus[16]. In female rat striatum, ovariectomy and chronic 17β-estradiol administration decrease dopamine D1 and D2 receptor concentrations[27], and in humans estrogens reduce the symptoms of L-dopa-induced tardive dyskinesia[28]. However, the mechanism by which estrogens affect the dopaminergic receptor is unknown and it is controversial if estrogens enhance or suppress the dopamine system in the corpus striatum (decreased dopaminergic neurotransmission in these deeply buried gray matter nuclei is responsible for Parkinson's disease and the parkinsonian effects of many antipsychotic drugs). In the rat, relatively high doses of estrogen can induce dopamine receptor hypersensitivity and increase D2 receptor binding[29]. However, lower estrogen doses and a shorter lagtime between steroid treatment and killing/ testing of the animal can lead to dopamine receptor hyposensitivity, indicating that this dopamine receptor hypersensitivity may be due to a rebound effect[30].

The serotonergic system

Estrogens have both rapid and long-term effects on serotonergic receptors due to non-competitive stereospecific interaction; serotonin receptors are up-regulated by estradiol in ovariectomized female rats[31], but long-term *in vivo* estrogen treatment does not alter serotonin receptor density more than a 1–2 hour treatment[32]. However, the long-term effects of estrogens on the serotonergic system in humans are unknown; in particular no data are available concerning the effects on the serotonin type 2A receptors which are implicated in human neuropsychiatric disorder.

The effects of estrogen on neurotransmitters are important because neurotransmitter systems are implicated in the pathology of neuropsychiatric disorders. For example, a deficit in cholinergic function is well described in Alzheimer's disease, decreased serotonergic activity is implicated in depression, and increased dopaminergic activity is a feature of schizophrenia. Therefore, in postmenopausal women low circulating estrogen levels may predispose to late-onset schizophrenia because of effects on the dopaminergic system, and to Alzheimer's disease because of effects on the cholinergic system. The estrogen-induced enhancement of the cholinergic system may be of particular relevance in Alzheimer's disease because some of the cognitive impairments in Alzheimer's disease are probably secondary to significant cholinergic deficits[33].

Neuroprotective actions of estrogen

In addition to direct effects on neurons, estrogens also act with neurotrophins (such as nerve growth factor) to stimulate nerve cell growth indirectly. Receptors for estrogen and neurotrophins are located on the same neurons in rodent basal forebrain, hippocampus and cerebral cortex, and this co-localization may be important for the survival of neurons[34]. Estrogen also has a neuroprotective action[35] against several toxins that boost production of free radicals, including glutamate (which is toxic in high concentrations), and recently it has been shown that estrogen can reduce the neuronal generation of β-amyloid[36]. Estrogen may also act as an antioxidant[37] and recent findings suggest that the neuroprotective antioxidant activity of estrogens is dependent on the presence of the hydroxyl group in the C3 position on the A ring of the steroid molecule[37]. Furthermore, Green and colleagues[38] reported that the estrogen molecule also needs a phenolic ring A and at least three rings of the steroid nucleus for its neuroprotective actions.

Other indirect beneficial effects of estrogens on the brain include prevention of glucocorticoid-induced hippocampal neuronal damage[39,40] enhancement of cerebral blood flow[41] and an interaction with apolipoprotein E (see below)[42,43].

ESTROGEN REPLACEMENT THERAPY: EFFECTS ON COGNITION

Whilst there are no significant sex differences in overall cognitive performance (as measured by full-scale IQ), sex differences in cognition can be found at a more fine-grained level. For example, on average males perform better than females in tests of visuospatial function, but females perform better in verbal tests[44]. These differences suggest that sex-determining factors, including sex hormones, modulate specific aspects of cognition. Moreover, women with congenital adrenal hyperplasia (21-hydroxylase deficiency), who are exposed to high levels of adrenal androgens during prenatal life, have superior spatial abilities[45], poor verbal abilities[46], and an increased frequency of specific cognitive deficits, such as dyscalculia[47]. This suggests that androgens can reverse the characteristic pattern of sex differences in cognition. In contrast, males with idiopathic hypogonadotrophic hypogonadism have significantly impaired spatial ability[48]. Women with Turner's syndrome, who do not produce endogenous estrogens, have decreased verbal memory, implicating estrogens in cognition. Moreover, in normal women cognitive abilities vary with phase of menstrual cycle, with improved fine motor and articulatory skills but decreased spatial ability[49] and improved memory performance[50,51] during the high estrogen and low progesterone phase of the cycle.

In humans, most[52–55], but not all[56,57], of the early studies on the cognitive effects of estrogen replacement therapy on cognition in postmenopausal women supported a positive effect on verbal performance and memory. More recently, Sherwin[58,59] assessed women before, and 3 months after, total abdominal hysterectomy and bilateral salpingo-oophorectomy; both estrogens and progestogens helped women to maintain the ability to recall newly learned verbal material, whilst this decreased in a control group who received placebo. Moreover, verbal recall deteriorated during a 1-month placebo-only wash-out period prior to the start of the cross-over phase of the study. Other prospective studies of women who have had total abdominal hysterectomy and bilateral salpingo-oophorectomy also support a positive effect of estrogens on verbal memory[51,60,61]. Barret-Connor and Silverstein[62] reported that women who had used hormone replacement therapy for more than 20 years had better verbal fluency than those who had not. Carlson and Sherwin, found improved forward and backward digit span in estrogen users compared to age-matched non-users (but see ref. 63).

A novel experimental design was recently employed to assess the effects of estrogens on cognitive function[64]. A gonadotropin releasing hormone agonist (GnRHa) was given to a group of premenopausal women with uterine myomas in doses high enough to suppress ovarian estrogen production. The women underwent a deterioration in verbal memory after 12 weeks of GnRHa compared with a pretreatment baseline. Women treated with 'add-back' estrogen (estrogen in combination with the GnRHa) regained their preGnRHa treatment scores, whereas those treated with 'add-back' placebo did not, suggesting that estrogens have postive effects on verbal memory, and that deterioration in performance due to estrogen deficiency may be reversible with the addition of exogenous estrogens.

Thus, the weight of evidence suggests that estrogens have beneficial effects on verbal memory, and possibly some other aspects of verbal functioning. Also, it has been reported

that estrogen affects visual memory[65], and the new learning of visual material[50,60].

ESTROGEN REPLACEMENT THERAPY: EFFECTS ON MOOD

Depressive disorders are characterized by decreased activity in the noradrenergic and serotonergic neurotransmitter systems. Moreover, these systems are down-regulated by the menopause and up-regulated by exogenous estrogens, suggesting that estrogens may have an antidepressant effect[66]. However, contrary to received wisdom, and in conflict with this hypothesis, most epidemiological studies fail to find excess depressive disorder in postmenopausal compared to premenopausal women (e.g. ref. 67). In addition, it is important to appreciate that low mood and depressive disorder are not the same entity at different degrees of severity and that estrogens may have differential effects on low mood and on depressive disorder.

Low mood

Estrogen replacement is associated with positive effects on mood and well-being in healthy postmenopausal women. For example, a 2-year treatment with estrogen or estrogen and testosterone improved mood in oophorectomized women compared to controls[58], and when estrogen, testosterone, combined estrogen and testosterone, or placebo were administered to premenopausal women who underwent bilateral salpingo-oophorectomy, there was an increase in depression scores in women who took placebo[68]. Moreover, depression scores increased during a placebo wash-out period prior to a cross-over phase of the study and were related to falling levels of steroid hormones. In addition, Ditkoff and colleagues[63] reported improved mood in postmenopausal women taking conjugated equine estrogens compared to placebo. These studies suggest the doses of estrogen found in hormone replacement therapy are capable of improving mood in healthy postmenopausal women.

Recently, Klaiber and colleagues[69] related mood changes to serum estradiol levels during estrogen treatment, and found these to be related to duration of menopause prior to receiving hormone replacement therapy, with longer duration of untreated menopause leading to less beneficial effect. Platelet monoamine oxidase levels (a marker of adrenergic and serotonergic function) were negatively correlated with serum estradiol levels, supporting the notion that changes in serotonin and noradrenaline metabolism are the mechanism by which estrogens affect mood.

In contrast to estrogens, progestins increase monoamine oxidase levels and thereby lead to lower brain serotonin concentration. Thus, progestins are generally thought to decrease some of estrogen's positive effects on mood[70–73] and have been associated with frank dysphoria. In addition, women with longer pretreatment duration of menopause may experience significantly more dysphoria when taking both progestins and estrogens than those with short pretreatment duration of menopause[73].

Depressive disorder

In support of studies that find positive effects on mood in women without depressive disorder, Schneider and co-workers[74] reported that women who were only 'mildly' depressed improved when treated with conjugated equine estrogen. Remarkably, those who were 'clinically' depressed became worse, suggesting that estrogens may have different effects in low mood and depressive disorder. Other work also suggests that estrogen is an ineffective treatment for depressive disorder in postmenopausal women[75–79]. On the other hand, transdermal estrogen may be an effective treatment in women with postnatal depression[80], and when large doses of estrogen were administered to postmenopausal women with refractory depression, 90% improved after 3 months of treatment[81], suggesting a possible role for estrogens in refractory depression.

ESTROGEN REPLACEMENT THERAPY AND NEUROPSYCHIATRIC DISORDER

Alzheimer's disease

The prevalence of Alzheimer's disease increases dramatically with age, from less than 1% at age 65 years to about 15% of people in their 80s[82]. Alzheimer's disease is accompanied by progressive cognitive impairment, and this has an enormous impact on the quality of life of patients and their caregivers. Risk factors for Alzheimer's disease include a positive family history, presence of Down's syndrome, head injury, female sex, hypothyroidism, depression[83] and the possession of the apolipoprotein E epsilon 4 allele[84]. In contrast, education, smoking and non-steroidal anti-inflammatory agents may be protective factors[85]. At a cellular level, the disease is characterized by neuronal loss, accumulation of intracellular neurofibrillary tangles, and extracellular senile plaques in the hippocampus and association neocortex[86]. Much progress has been made in understanding the etiology and pathology of Alzheimer's disease (including the identification of susceptibility genes[87]. Nevertheless, no major success has been gained so far with respect to its treatment. The search for pharmacological treatments of Alzheimer's disease has mainly focused on the major deficits in the cholinergic system, including selective loss of basal forebrain cholinergic neurons, a decreased activity of the synthetic enzyme ChAT, and a decreased activity of the catabolic enzyme AChE. Trials with precursors of acetylcholine and cholinesterase inhibitors have demonstrated only limited cognitive improvement, and many have significant unwanted side-effects.

Estrogens have significant effects on the brain systems that are pathophysiologically implicated in Alzheimer's disease, and may offer new therapeutic potential. *In vivo* studies using single photon emission tomography demonstrated that people with Alzheimer's disease have a significant reduction in cholinergic receptor density in both the temporal and parietal lobes and a significant decrease in brain cholinergic terminals compared to controls.

However, long-term use of hormone replacement therapy in healthy, post-menopausal women protects against age-related loss of cholinergic terminals and cholinergic responsivity (for a review of acetylcholine and Alzheimer's disease, see ref. 33). Thus, one mechanism by which hormone replacement therapy could reduce the risk and delay the onset of Alzheimer's disease in postmenopausal women may be by preservation of cholinergic neuronal density. An alternative mechanism may be by up-regulation of the serotonergic system. Serotonergic dysfunction has been reported in Alzheimer's disease in post-mortem and SPECT studies and serotonin affects memory and learning (possibly by modulating cholinergic neuronal activity). Furthermore, long-term use of hormone replacement therapy has been shown to enhance serotonergic function in postmenopausal women, and this may interact with the effects of estrogen on the cholinergic system to improve cognitive function and decrease the risk of Alzheimer's disease.

Epidemiological studies have reported that the prevalence of Alzheimer's disease is significantly decreased in females on hormone replacement therapy, and that those women with Alzheimer's disease who were taking it had a significantly milder disease than those who were not[88]. A recent longitudinal study reported that prolonged use of hormone replacement therapy decreases the risk, and delays the onset, of Alzheimer's disease; moreover, use of estrogen for longer than 1 year reduced the risk of developing Alzheimer's disease by 5% annually[89]. For example, one clinical trial reported that three of seven women with Alzheimer's disease improved on measures of attention, orientation, mood and social interaction after 6 weeks of low-dose estradiol treatment, but suffered loss of improvement after estradiol was discontinued[90]. In another study, women with Alzheimer's disease who were using estrogen had significantly better scores on the Alzheimer's Disease Assessment Scale (ADAS-Cog, a standard instrument used in AD clinical trials) than women with Alzheimer's disease who did not take estrogens[91].

The results of the studies described above are promising and point to the need for further prospective studies of hormone replacement therapy in postmenopausal women with and without Alzheimer's disease. Results of early clinical trials of hormone replacement therapy in people with Alzheimer's disease are also promising but require replication. Thus, whilst experience from prospective clinical trials is still limited, epidemiological, neuropsychological and biological studies support the hypothesis that estrogens have a role in the genesis and treatment of Alzheimer's disease. The effect on the central nervous system of the new selective estrogen receptor modulators (SERMS), which have fewer side-effects on breast and endometrium, is not yet known.

Stroke

Whilst the incidence of stroke has remained essentially unchanged in recent years, the ratio of non-fatal to fatal stroke has been increasing, and this effect is more marked in women than in men[92]. The incidence of first stroke in women aged from 45 to 65 years is 1–2 per thousand per annum, and fatal stroke remains the third most common cause of death in postmenopausal women[93]. Estrogens are known to protect against coronary artery disease[94], relax arterial smooth muscle, increase high-density lipoprotein (HDL) cholesterol levels[95], improve cardiac output and reduce platelet aggregation[96]. On the other hand, estrogens increase thrombogenicity[97] and progestins significantly attenuate estrogen-induced effects on HDL cholesterol levels, arterial dilatation and blood flow. Therefore, hormone replacement therapy could plausibly either increase or decrease the risk of suffering from ischemic or hemorrhagic stroke.

A substantial body of observational data on the use of hormone replacement therapy and risk of stroke now exists[98–111]. However, interpretation of available data is complicated by differences in study design, particularly the inclusion of different hormone replacement therapy types, failure to differentiate between ischemic and hemorrhagic stroke, and status of replacement therapy use ('current use' versus 'ever use'). Early studies of the current use of estrogens present a confused picture, with relative risk for stroke reported as decreased[99] and slightly increased[101]. Similarly, Falkeborn and colleagues[111] reported significantly decreased risk of stroke in users of combined hormone replacement therapy, and Grodstein reported increased risk in current users of estrogen compared to never users. Recent studies have failed to demonstrate a relationship between replacement therapy use and non-fatal stroke[112] and ischemic stroke.

Overall, these data suggest that the current or past use of estrogen replacement therapy, alone or with progestins, has little or no effect on the risk of ischemic or hemorrhagic stroke. Despite this disappointing conclusion, Dubal and colleagues[113] have recently reported that physiological doses of estrogen protect against artificially induced ischemic brain lesions in rat cerebral cortex. If a similar protective effect exists in humans, estrogens may yet have a role in decreasing post-stroke mortality and morbidity, but this remains to be established.

Schizophrenia

Gender differences in the premorbid functioning, age of onset, symptomatology and outcome of schizophrenia suggest a possible role for estrogens. Women are more likely to have a family history of schizophrenia, atypical or affective features and to show a seasonal pattern of hospital admission. Moreover, age at onset is gender dependent: men show a distribution about a single peak in their early 20s, women have a later age of onset and a second peak in

incidence between the ages of 45 and 55 years. Because of their putative antidopaminergic/antipsychotic action, estrogens may be responsible for the delay in the onset of the first peak, and the second peak may be due to the decline in estrogen levels at menopause. An antipsychotic action of estrogens is supported by clinical studies which report that women have increased admission rates for psychosis around the menses[114], and that psychotic symptomatology varies with the phase of menstrual cycle[115]. Also, women with schizophrenia may have reduced estradiol levels compared to controls[116]. However, when women with schizophrenia were given adjunctive treatment with exogenous estrogen there was a slight increase in speed of recovery, but no improvement overall compared to antipsychotic medication alone[117]. Despite the lack of clear evidence for the efficacy of estrogen as an antipsychotic, it remains plausible that estrogen replacement therapy might protect against late-onset schizophrenia in postmenopausal women by inhibiting the development of predisposing age-related changes in brain structure and neurochemistry.

CONCLUSION

Estrogens interact with neuronal networks at many different levels and affect brain development and aging. This multiplicity of action implicates estrogens in the etiology, and possibly treatment, of age- and sex-related neuropsychiatric disorder. In particular, estrogens offer exciting new possiblities for the treatment of Alzheimer's disease.

References

1. Kaye JA, DeCarli CD, Luxenberg JS, Rapoport SI. The significance of age-related enlargement of the cerebral ventricles in healthy men and women measured by quantitative computed X-ray tomography. *J Am Geriatr Soc* 1992;40: 225–31

2. Takeda S, Matsuzawa T. Age-related brain atrophy: a study with computed tomography. *J Gerentol* 1985;40:159–63

3. Murphy DGM, DeCarli C, McIntosh A, *et al.* Sex differences in human brain morphometry and metabolism: an *in vivo* quantitative magnetic

resonance imaging and positron emission tomography study on the effect of aging. *Arch Gen Psychiatry* 1996;53:585–94

4. Murphy DGM, Allen G, Haxby JV, *et al*. The effects of sex steroids, and the X chromosome, on female brain function: a study of the neuropsychology of adult Turner syndrome. *Neuropsychologia* 1994;32:1309–23

5. Murphy DGM, DeCarli C, Daly E, *et al*. X-chromosome effects on female brains: a magnetic resonance imaging study of Turner's syndrome. *Lancet* 1993;342:1197–200

6. Clark C, Klonoff H, Hayden M. Regional cerebral glucose metabolism in Turner syndrome. *Can J Neurol Sci* 1990;17:140–4

7. Murphy DGM, Mentis MJ, Pietsini P, *et al*. A PET study of Turner's syndrome: effects of sex steroids and the X chromosome on the brain. *Biol Psychiatry* 1997;41:285–98

8. Gould E, Woolley CS, Frankfurt M, McEwen BS. Gonadal steroids regulate dendritic spine density in hippocampal pyramidal cells in adulthood. *J Neurosci* 1990;10:1286–91

9. Gazzaley AH, Weiland NG, McEwen BS, Morrison JH. Differential regulations of NMDAR1 mRNA and protein by estradiol in the rat hippocampus. *J Neurosci* 1996;16:6830–8

10. Woolley CS, Weiland NG, McEwen BS, Schwartzkroin PA. Estradiol increases the sensitivity of hippocampal CA1 pyramidal cells to NMDA receptor-mediated synaptic input: correlation with dendritic spine density. *J Neurosci* 1997;17:1848–59

11. Coyle JT, Price DL, DeLong MR. Alzheimer's disease: a disorder of cortical cholinergic innervation. *Science* 1983;219:1184–90

12. Rainbow TC, DeGroff V, Luine VN, McEwen GS. Estradiol 17beta increases the number of muscarinic receptors in hypothalamic nuclei. *Brain Res* 1980;198:239–43

13. Luine VN, McEwen BS. Effects of oestradiol on turnover of type A monoamine oxidase in brain. *J Neurochem* 1977;28:1221–7

14. Luine V. Estradiol increases choline acetyltransferase activity in specific basal forebrain nuclei and projection areas of female rats. *Exp Neurol* 1985;89:484–90

15. McEwen BS. Gonadal steroids: humoral modulators of nerve-cell function. *Psychoneuroendocrinology* 1980;16:151–64

16. Vacas MI, Cardinelli. Effect of estradiol on alpha and beta-adrenoceptor density in medial basal hypothalamus, cerebral cortex and pineal gland of ovariectomized rats. *Neurosci Lett* 1980;17:73–7

17. Janowsky DS, Davis JM. Progesterone–estrogen effects on uptake and release of norepinephrine by synaptosomes. *Life Sci* 1970;9:525–31

18. Hersey RM, Llojd T, MacLusky NJ, Weisz J. The catecholestrogen, 2-hydroxyestradiol-17 alpha, is formed from estradiol-17 alpha by hypothalamic tissue *in vitro* and inhibits tyrosine hydroxylase. *Endocrinology* 1982;111:1734–6

19. Beattie CW, Rodgers CH, Soyka LF. Influence of ovariectomy and ovarian steroids on hypothalamic tyrosine hydroxylase activity in the rat. *Endocrinology* 1972;91:276–86

20. Paul SM, Axelrod J, Saavedra JM, Skolnick P. Estrogen-induced efflux of endogenous catecholamines from the hypothalamus *in vitro*. *Brain Res* 1979;178:499–505

21. Klaiber EL, Kobayashi Y, Broverman DM, Hall F. Plasma monoamine oxidase activity in regularly menstruating women and in amenorrhoeic women receiving cyclic treatment with estrogens and progestin. *J Clin Endocrinol Metab* 1971;33:630–8

22. Walsh B, Schiff I. Vasomotor flushes. *Ann NY Acad Sci* 1990;592:34–356

23. Kugler J, Seus R, Krauskopf R, Brecht HM, Raschig A. Differences in psychic performance with guanfacine and clonidine in normotensive subjects. *Br J Clin Pharmacol* 1980;10:1S–80S

24. Frith CD, Dowdy J, Ferrier IN, Crowe TJ. Selective impairment of paired associate learning after administration of a centrally-acting adrenergic agonist (clonidine). *Psychopharmacology* 1985;87:490–3

25. Cramer OM, Parker CRJ, Porter JC. *Endocrinology* 1979;104:419–21

26. DiPaolo T, Rouillard C, Bedard P. 17beta-estradiol at physiological dose acutely increases dopamine turnover in rat brain. *Eur J Pharmacol* 1985;117:197–203

27. Tonnaer JADM, Leinders T, Van Delft AML. Ovariectomy and subchronic oestradiol – 17beta administration decrease dopamine D1 and D2 receptors in rat striatum. *Psychoneuroendocrinology* 1989;14:469–76

28. Villneuve A, Czaejust T, Cote M. Estrogens in tardive dyskinesia in male psychiatric patients. *Neuropsychobiology* 1980;6:145–51

29. Gordon JH, Perry KO. Pre- and postsynaptic neurochemical alterations following estrogen induced dopamine hypersensitivity. *Brain Res Bull* 1983;10:425–8

30. Gordon JH. Modulation of apomorphine induced stereotypy by estrogen: time course and dose response. *Brain Res Bull* 1980;5:679–82

31. Biegon A, McEwen BS. Modulation by estradiol of serotonin receptors in brain. *J Neurosci* 1982;2:199–205

32. Biegon A, Resches A, Snyder L, McEwen BS. Serotonergic and noradrenergic receptors in the rat brain: modulation by chronic exposure to ovarian hormones. *Life Sci* 1983;32:2015–21

33. Muire JL. Acetylcholine, aging, and Alzheimer's disease. *Pharmacol Biochem Behav* 1997;56:687–96

34. Toran-Allerand CD. The estrogen/neurotrophin connection during neural development: is co-localization of estrogen receptor with the neurotrophins and their receptors biologically relevant? *Dev Neurosci* 1996;18:36

35. Simpkins JW, Singh M, Bishop J. The potential role for estrogen replacement therapy in the treatment of the cognitive decline and neurodegeneration associated with Alzheimer's disease. *Neurobiol Aging* 1994;15(Suppl 2): S195–7

36. Xu H, Guoras GK, Greenfield JP, *et al.* Oestrogen reduces neuronal generation of Alzheimer β amyloid peptides. *Nature Med* 1998;4:447–51

37. Behl C, Skutella T, Lezoualc'h F, *et al.* Neuroprotection against oxidative stress by estrogens: structure–activity relationship. *Mol Pharmacol* 1997;51:535–41

38. Green PS, Gordon K, Simpkins JW. Phenolic ring requirement for the neuroprotective effects of steroids. *J Steroid Biochem Mol Biol* 1997;63:229–35

39. Mizoguchi K, Tatshuhide T, De-Hua C, Tabira T. Stress induces neuronal death in the hippocampus of castrated rats. *Neurosci Lett* 1992;138: 157–60

40. Sapolsky RM, Plotsky PM. Hypercortisolism and its possible neural bases. *Biol Psychiatry* 1990;27: 937–52

41. Ohkura T, Isse K, Akazawa K, *et al.* Evaluation of estrogen treatment in female patients with dementia of the Alzheimer type. *Endocr J* 1994: 41:361–71

42. Honjo H, Tanaka K, Kashiwagi T, *et al.* Senile dementia Alzheimer's type and estrogen. *Hormone Metab Res* 1995;27:204–7

43. Stone D, Rozovsky I, Morgan T, Anderson C, Finch C. Increased synaptic sprouting in response to estrogen via an apolipoprotein E-dependent mechanism – implications for Alzheimer's disease. *J Neurosci* 1998;18:3180–5

44. Jarvik LF. Human intelligence: sex differences. *Acta Genet Med Gemellol (Rome)* 1975;24:189–211

45. Perlman S. Cognitive abilities of children with hormone abnormalities: screening by psychoeducational tests. *J Learn Disabil* 1973;6:24–34

46. Resnick S, Berenbaum S, Gottesman R, Bouchard T. Early hormonal influences on cognitive functioning in congenital adrenal hyperplasia. *Dev Psychol* 1986;22:191–8

47. Nass R, Baker S. Androgen effects on cognition: congenital adrenal hyperplasia. *Psychoneuroendocrinology* 1991;16:189–201

48. Hier DB, Crowley WF. Spatial ability in androgen-deficient men. *N Engl J Med* 1982;306: 1202–5

49. Hampson E. Estrogen-related cognitive abilities across the menstrual cycle. *Brain Cogn* 1990; 14:26–43

50. Phillips S, Sherwin BB. Effects of estrogen on memory function in surgically menopausal women. *Psychoneuroendocrinology* 1992;17: 485–95

51. Phillips SM, Sherwin BB. Variations in memory function and sex steroid hormones across the menstrual cycle. *Psychoneuroendocrinology* 1992; 17:497–506

52. Caldwell BM, Watson RI. An evaluation of psychologic effects of sex hormone administration in aged women. Results of therapy after six months. *J Gerontol* 1952;7:228–44

53. Campbell S, Whitehead M. Oestrogen therapy and the menopausal syndrome. *Clin Obstet Gynaecol* 1977;4:31–47

54. Hackman BW, Galbraith D. Six month study of oestrogen therapy with piperazine oestrone sulphate and its effects on memory. *Curr Med Res Opin* 1977;4:21–7

55. Feydor-Freybergh P. The influence of oestrogen on wellbeing and mental performance in climacteric and postmenopausal women. *Acta Obstet Gynecol Scand* 1977;64:5–69

56. Rauramo L, Lagerspetz K, Engblom P, Punnonen R. The effect of castration and peroral estrogen therapy on some psychological functions. *Front Horm Res* 1975;3:94–104

57. Vanhulle R, Demol R. A double blind study into the influence of estriol on a number of psychological tests in post-menopausal women. In van Keep PA, Greenblatt RB, Albeaux-Fernet M, eds. *Consensus on Menopausal Research*. London: MTP Press, 1976:94–9

58. Sherwin BB. Estrogen and/or androgen replacement therapy and cognitive functioning in surgically menopausal women. *Psychoneuroendocrinology* 1988;13:345–57

59. Sherwin BB. Affective changes with estrogen and androgen replacement therapy in surgically menopausal women. *J Affect Disord* 1988;14: 177–87

60. Sherwin BB, Phillips S. Estrogen and cognitive functioning in surgically menopausal women. *Ann NY Acad Sci* 1990;592:474–5

61. Kampen D, Sherwin BB. Estrogen use and verbal memory in healthy postmenopausal women. *Obstet Gynecol* 1994;83:979–83

62. Barrett-Connor E, Silverstein D. Estrogen replacement therapy and cognitive function in older women. *JAMA* 1993;269:2637–41

63. Ditkoff EC, Crary WG, Cristo M, Lobo RA. Estrogen improves psychological function in asymptomatic postmenopausal women. *Obstet Gynecol* 1991;78:991–5

64. Sherwin BB, Tulandi T. 'Add-back' estrogen reverses cognitive deficits induced by a

gonadotropin releasing-hormone agonist in women with leiomyomata uteri. *J Clin Endocrinol Metab* 1996;81:2545–9

65. Resnick SM, Metter EJ, Zondermann AB. Estrogen replacement therapy and longitudinal decline in visual memory: a possible protective effect? *Neurology* 1997;49:1491–7

66. Halbreich U. Role of estrogen in postmenopausal depression. *Neurology* 1997;48(Suppl 7): S16–S20

67. Kessler RC, McGonagle KA, Swartz M, Blazer DG, Nelson CB. Sex and depression in the National Comorbidity Survey. I: Lifetime prevalence, chronicity and recurrence. *J Affect Disord* 1993;29:85–96

68. Sherwin BB, Gelfand MM. Sex steroids and the effect of the surgical menopause: a double blind cross over study. *Psychoneuroendocrinology* 1985;10:325–35

69. Klaiber E, Broverman D, Vogel W, Peterson LG, Snyder M. Relationships of serum oestradiol levels, menopausal duration and mood during hormonal replacement therapy. *Psychoneuroendocrinology* 1997;22: 549–58

70. Dennerstein L. Depression in the menopause. *Obstet Gynecol Clin North Am* 1987;4:33–48

71. Dennerstein L, Burrows GD, Hyman G, Sharope K. Hormone therapy and affect. *Maturitas* 1979; 1:247–54

72. Holst J, Backstrom T, Hammerbach S, Von Schoultz B. Progestogen addiction during oestrogen replacement therapy – effects on vasomotor symptoms and mood. *Maturitas* 1989;11:13–19

73. Magos AL, Brewster E, Singh R, O'Dowd R, Bruncart M, Studd JWW. The effects of norethisterone in postmenopausal women on oestrogen replacement therapy: a model for the premenstrual syndrome. *Br J Obstet Gynaecol* 1986;93:1290–6

74. Schneider MA, Brotherton PL, Hailes J. The effect of exogenous oestrogens on depression in menopausal women. *M J Aust* 1977;2: 162–70

75. Oppenheim G. Estrogen in the treatment of depression: neuropharmacological mechanisms. *Arch Gen Psychiatr* 1986;43:569–73

76. Schapira B, Oppenheim G, Zohar J, *et al.* Lack of efficacy of oestrogen supplementation to imipramine in resistant female depressives. *Biol Psychiatr* 1985;20:576–9

77. Coope J. Is oestrogen therapy effective in the treatment of menopausal depression? *J R Coll Gen Pract* 1981;31:134–40

78. Coope J, Thomsom J, Poller L. Effects of 'natural estrogen' replacement therapy on menopausal symptoms and blood clotting. *Br Med J* 1975;4:139–43

79. Prange AJ. Estrogen may well affect response to antidepressant. *JAMA* 1972;219:143–4

80. Gregoire AJP, Kumar R, Everitt B, Henderson AF, Studd JWW. Transdermal oestrogen for treatment of severe postnatal depression. *Lancet* 1996;347:930–3

81. Klaiber EL, Broverman DM, Vogel W, Kobayashi Y. Estrogen therapy for severe persistent depression in women. *Arch Gen Psychiatr* 1979;36:742–4

82. Skoog I, Nilsson L, Palmertz B, *et al.* A population based study of senile dementia in 85 year olds. *N Engl J Med* 1993;328:153–8

83. van Duijn CM, Hofman A. Risk factors for Alzheimer's disease: the EURODEM collaborative re-analysis of case–control studies. *Neuroepidemiology* 1992;11(Suppl 1):106–13

84. Corder EH, Saunders AM, Strittmatter WJ, *et al.* Gene dose of apolipoprotein E type 4 allele and risk of Alzheimer's disease in late onset families. *Science* 1993;261:921–3

85. Burns A, Murphy D. Protection against Alzheimer's disease? *Lancet* 1996;348:420–1

86. Cummings JL, Vinters HV, Cole GM, Khachaturian ZS. Alzheimer's disease: etiologies, pathophysiology, cognitive reserve and treatment opportunities. *Neurology* 1998;51 (Suppl 1):S2–S17

87. Lendon CL, Ashall F, Goate AM. Exploring the etiology of Alzheimer disease using molecular genetics. *JAMA* 1997;277:825–36

88. Henderson V, Paganini-Hill A, Emanuel C, Dunn M, Buckwalter J. Estrogen replacement therapy in older women. *Arch Neurol* 1994;51: 896–900

89. Tang M, Jacobs D, Stern Y, *et al.* Effects of oestrogen during menopause on risk and age at onset of Alzheimer's disease. *Lancet* 1996;348:429–32

90. Fillit H, Weinreb H, Cholst I, *et al.* Observations in a preliminary open trial of estradiol therapy for senile dementia-Alzheimer's type. *Psychoneuroendocrinology* 1986;11:337–45

91. Doraiswamy PM, Krishen A, Martin WL, *et al.* Gender, concurrent oestrogen use and cognition in Alzheimer's disease. *Int J Geriatr Psychopharmacol* 1997;40:34–7

92. Falkeborne M, Persson I, Terent A, Bergstrom R, Lithell H, Naessen T. Long term trends in incidence of and mortality from acute myocardial infarction and stroke in women: analyses of total first events and of deaths in the Uppsala Health Care Region, Sweden. *Epidemiology* 1996;7:67–74

93. Lindstrøm E, Boysen G, Nyboe J, Appleyard M. Stroke incidence in Copenhagen, 1976–1988. *Stroke* 1992;23:28–32

94. Grodstein F, Stampfer MJ. The epidemiology of coronary heart disease and oestrogen

replacement in postmenopausal women. *Prog Cardiovasc Dis* 1995;38:199–210

95. Postmenopausal Estrogen/Progestin Interventions Trial Writing Group. Effects of estrogen or estrogen/progestin regimens on heart disease risk factors in postmenopausal women. *J Am Med Assoc* 1995;273:199–208

96. Speroff L. The effect of oestrogen–progestogen postmenopausal hormone replacement therapy on the cardiovascular system. *Eur J Menopause* 1996;3:151–63

97. Salomaa V, Rasi V, Pekkanen J, *et al.* Association of hormone replacement therapy with hemostatic and other cardiovascular risk factors: the FINRISK hemostasis study. *Arterioscler Thromb Vasc Biol* 1995;15:1549–55

98. Pfeffer RI. Estrogen use, hypertension and stroke in postmenopausal women. *J Chron Dis* 1978;31:389–98

99. Pettinin DB, Wingerd J, Pellegrin F, Ramcharan S, Risk of vascular disease in women: smoking, oral contraceptives, noncontraceptive estrogens and other factors. *J Am Med Assoc* 1979; 242:1150–4

100. Hammond CB, Jelovsek FR, Lee KL, Creasman WT, Parker RT. Effects of long-term estrogen replacement therapy: metabolic effects. *Am J Obstet Gynecol* 1979;133:525–36

101. Rosenberg SH, Fausone V, Clark R. The role of estrogens as a risk factor for stroke in postmenopausal women. *West J Med* 1980;133:292–6

102. Wilson PWF, Garrison RJ, Castelli WP. Postmenopausal estrogen use, cigarette smoking and cardiovascular morbidity in women over 50: the Framingham Study. *N Engl J Med* 1958; 313:1038–43

103. Busch TL, Barrett-Connor E, Cowan LD, *et al.* Cardiovascular mortality and noncontraceptive use of estrogen in women: results from the Lipid Research Clinics Program Follow-up Study. *Circulation* 1987;75:1102–9

104. Boysen G, Nyboe J, Appleyard M, *et al.* Stroke incidence and risk factors for stroke in Copenhagen, Denmark. *Stroke* 1988;19:1345–53

105. Paganini-Hill A, Ross RK, Henderson BE. Postmenopausal oestrogen treatment and stroke: a prospective study. *Br Med J* 1988;297:519–22

106. Thompson SG, Meade TW, Greenberg G. The use of hormonal replacement therapy and the risk of stroke and myocardial infarction in women. *J Epidemiol Commun Health* 1989;43:173–8

107. Hunt K, Vessey M, McPherson K. Mortality in a cohort of long-term users of hormone replacement therapy: an updated analysis. *Br J Obstet Gynaecol* 1990;97:1080–6

108. Stampfer MJ, Colditz GA, Willett WC, *et al.* Postmenopausal estrogen therapy and cardiovascular disease: ten-year follow-up from the Nurses Study. *N Engl J Med* 1991;325:756–62

109. Finucane FF, Madans JG, Busch TL, Wolf PH, Kleinman JC. Decreased risk of stroke among postmenopausal hormone users: results from a national cohort. *Arch Intern Med* 1993;153:73–9

110. Falkeborne M, Persson I, Terent A, Adami HO, Lithell H, Bergstrom R. Hormone replacement therapy and the risk of stroke: follow-up of a population-based cohort in Sweden. *Arch Intern Med* 1992;153:1201–9

111. Longstreth WT, Nelson LM, Koepsell TD, van Belle G. Subarachnoid hemorrhage and hormonal factors in women: a population-based case control study. *Ann Intern Med* 1994;121:168–73

112. Pedersen AT, Lidegaard Ø, Kreiner S, Ottesen B. Hormone replacement therapy and risk of non-fatal stroke. *Lancet* 1997;350:1277–83

113. Dubal DB, Kashon ML, Pettigrew C, *et al.* Estradiol protects against ischaemic injury. *J Cerebral Blood Flow Metab* 1998;18:1253–8

114. Hallonquist J, Seeman MV, Lang M, Rector NA. Variation in the symptom severity over the menstrual cycle of schizophrenics. *Biol Psychiatr* 1993;33:207–9

115. Harris AH. Menstrually related symptom changes in women with schizophrenia. *Schizophrenia Res* 1997;27:93–9

116. Reicher-Rossler A, Hafner H, Stumbaum M, Maurer K, Schmidt R. Can oestradiol modulate schizophrenic symptomatology? *Schizophrenia Bull* 1994;20:203–14

117. Kulkarni J, Castella A, Smith D, *et al.* A clinical trial of the effects of estrogen in acutely psychotic women. *Schizophr Res* 1996;20:247

12

Sex steroid hormones and central nervous system: neuroendocrine effects of Δ5 androgens in postmenopausal women

M. Stomati, F. Bernardi, P. Monteleone, A. D. Genazzani, G. D'Ambrogio, M. Luisi and A. R. Genazzani

INTRODUCTION

Brain development and functions are modulated by several endogenous and exogenous stimuli. Among endogenous factors, sex steroid hormones have a relevant role in modulating the brain's activities. In fact, the action of sex hormones is not limited to the regulation of endocrine functions and mating behavior; the identification of estrogen, progestin and androgen receptors in numerous regions of the central nervous system (CNS) is the confirmation that sex steroids are involved in modulating several functions. The mechanism of action of sex steroid hormones in the brain is similar to that observed in the peripheral target organs, with genomic and non-genomic effects[1-3]. Through classical genomic mechanisms, steroids induce slow, long-term actions on neurons by activating specific intracellular receptors that modulate gene transcription and protein synthesis. Thus, gonadal steroids modulate the synthesis, release and metabolism of many neuropeptides and neuroactive transmitters and the expression of their receptors (Figure 1)[1-4]. On the other hand, steroid hormones exert very

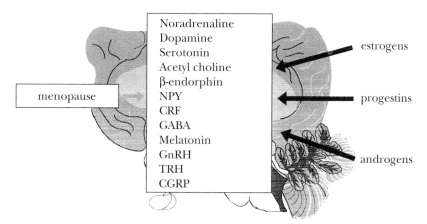

Figure 1 Gonadal steroids modulate the synthesis, release and metabolism of neuroactive transmitters; NPY, neuropeptide Y; CRF, corticotropin releasing factor; GABA, gamma-aminobutyric acid; GnRH, gonadotropin releasing hormone; TRH, thyrotropin releasing hormone; CGRP, calcitonin gene-related peptide

rapid effects that cannot be attributed to genomic mechanisms. In fact, through specific non-genomic mechanisms estrogens, androgens and progestogens modulate electrical excitability, synaptic functioning and morphological features[5–8]. The interplay of genomic and non-genomic mechanisms allows for a wide range of sex steroid actions in the regulation of cerebral functions.

Classical knowledge and recent developmental data regarding the effects of sex steroid hormones on the brain have been acquired by *in vitro* and *in vivo* studies. Only a few clinical trials are available regarding the effects of exogenous sex steroids on the CNS in humans. In postmenopause, neuroactive transmitters undergo important modifications as a consequence of the failure of gonadal hormone production, bringing on specific symptoms due to CNS function rearrangement. Hot flushes, sweat, obesity and hypertension that occur during menopause transition are consequences of the neuroendocrine changes in the hypothalamus. Mood changes, anxiety, depression, insomnia, headaches/migraine and alterations of cognitive functions are related to postmenopausal alterations of the limbic system.

Therefore estrogen, progestin and androgen administration in postmenopausal women represents a valid tool to clarify the role of sex steroid hormones in the modulation of the neuroendocrine system and CNS function.

ESTROGENS, PROGESTINS AND THE BRAIN

The increased use of sex steroid hormone therapies has led to studies on the biochemical and metabolic properties of different estroprogestin molecules available in hormonal therapies. In particular, the attention has been focused on the interactions between estrogens and progestins in the neuroendocrine control of brain functions and its clinical implications. In fact, each molecule is able to bind to different receptors and exert specific effects. Moreover, the different kinds of molecules may either interfere with other steroid hormones or other receptors, or be metabolized inside or outside the brain into other neuroactive steroids, thus exerting multiple effects in each target tissue.

Sex steroid hormones modulate the noradrenergic, dopaminergic and serotoninergic systems of the hypothalamus, as well as of the superior areas of the brain, controlling movement and behavior in both animals and humans. Animal studies showed an increase in norepinephrine and dopamine turnover rate induced by estrogens during proestrous[3,9]. On the other hand, in castrated female rats an impairment of catecholaminergic neurons has been demonstrated, with an increase in noradrenaline release and a decrease in dopamine release[3,9]. Estrogen administration decreases noradrenaline hypothalamic release, while increasing dopaminergic neuronal activity and the dopamine release in medio-basal hypothalamus[9]. Regarding the modulation of the different subtypes of adrenergic receptors, *in vitro* studies suggest that estrogens upregulate α1-adrenergic and down-regulate β-adrenergic receptors' activity[9]. Studies in ovariectomized female rats have demonstrated that estrogen effects on the noradrenergic neurons in the pineal gland are suppressed when progesterone is associated[3]. In an animal model, estradiol and progesterone enhance noradrenaline release, leading to an increase in the excitability of ventromedial hypothalamic neurons and in lordosis behavior[9]. Regarding the serotoninergic system, several findings have indicated a sex-related difference in the central serotoninergic system: female rats have elevated synthesis, turnover rate and concentration of serotonin in the hypothalamus, cortex, hippocampus, forebrain and raphe compared to male rats[10]. Brain serotonin concentration and activity are modified during the estrous cycle[11]. Estrogen positively affects the serotoninergic system in ovariectomized rats[12]. Estrogens can also modify the concentration and the availability of serotonin, by increasing the rate of degradation of monoamine oxidase, the enzyme that catabolizes serotonin[13]. Experimental data have demonstrated that estrogen displaces tryptophan from its binding sites to plasma albumin; in this manner tryptophan is more available in the brain to be metabolized into serotonin[14].

At the hypothalamic level, the principal target of sex steroid hormones for the modulation of reproductive function is the group of neurons producing a pulsatile release of the gonadotropin releasing hormone (GnRH), localized into the mediobasal hypothalamus and the arcuate nucleus. The GnRH release depends upon the complex and co-ordinated interrelationships among these peptides, gonadal steroids and other neurotransmitter systems, such as the dopaminergic, opiatergic and noradrenergic systems[12]. The interplay of these control mechanisms is governed by feedback of peripheral signals, and signals from the higher brain centers could also modify the GnRH secretion. Experimental studies on female rats show a significant increase in hypothalamic concentration of GnRH after surgical ovariectomy when compared to control fertile rats[15,16]. Estradiol benzoate treatment induces a significant reduction in GnRH concentration to values similar to the ones found in fertile rats. Moreover, the treatment of ovariectomized female rats with estradiol benzoate in association with different types of progestins (progesterone, norethisterone enanthte, desogestrel, medroxyprogesterone acetate (MAP)) induced different results with respect to estradiol alone[15,16]. However, the final effects of the steroid hormones on the GnRH synthesis and release may occur directly on the gonadotropic neurons but also indirectly, mediated by other neuroendocrine systems and neuroactive transmitters.

At the pituitary level, the amount of luteinizing hormone (LH) was significantly higher in ovariectomized than in control fertile rats. The administration of estradiol benzoate alone in ovariectomized rats induces a significant increase in LH. The chronic treatment of ovariectomized rats with progesterone or norethisterone enanthate alone significantly reduced LH concentration. Desogestrel and medroxyprogesterone acetate administration did not induce significant changes. All progestins, given in association with estradiol benzoate in ovariectomized rats, blocked the increase in LH induced by estradiol benzoate alone[15,17]. Surgical ovariectomy induced a significant increase in plasma LH levels in fertile female rats, while estradiol benzoate administration reduced circulating LH to values similar to the fertile control group. Progesterone and different progestins were inactive in counteracting the effects of estradiol benzoate on plasma LH levels[15–18]. Desogestrel and medroxyprogesterone acetate did not influence the inhibitory effects of estradiol benzoate at the hypothalamic level, but all gestagens were able to modulate the estrogen effects on pituitary cells.

Among the neuropeptides regulated by gonadal steroids our attention is focused on endogenous opioids[19]. Experimental evidence shows that β-endorphin reduces circulating LH levels by inhibiting LH releasing hormone secretion and decreases sexual activity[20]. The injection of β-endorphin is able to decrease circulating LH levels by inhibiting the release of GnRH. Chronic treatment with progesterone or different progestins (medroxyprogesterone acetate, norethisterone enanthate, desogestrel), with or without estradiol benzoate administration, induces different effects on the hypothalamic and pituitary content of β-endorphin in ovariectomized female rats[21]. Surgical ovariectomy did not modify β-endorphin concentration in the hypothalamus of female rats. The administration of estradiol benzoate, norethisterone enanthate and progesterone in ovariectomized rats induced a significant increase of the peptide levels, while desogestrel and medroxyprogesterone acetate were inactive[22]. In the anterior pituitary, the ovariectomy induced a significant reduction in β-endorphin levels in comparison to fertile rats, while the administration of estradiol produced a restoration of β-endorphin content. When progesterone, norethisterone enanthate, or medroxyprogesterone acetate were given alone, they did not modify the concentrations of the peptide while the concentrations significantly increased after desogestrel administration. In ovariectomized rats the treatment with estradiol benzoate plus progestins reversed the effect induced by estradiol benzoate alone[21]. In the neurointermediate lobe, the ovariectomy in female fertile rats produced a decrease of β-endorphin content. Treatment with estradiol benzoate alone or with progesterone, desogestrel and medroxyprogesterone acetate induced an increase in β-endorphin levels to values similar to those of fertile controls, while norethisterone enanthate was not active in counteracting the effect of the ovariectomy. Progesterone and progestin treatment in association with estradiol benzoate did not modify the effect of estradiol benzoate alone[21]. Another neuropeptide modulated by gonadal steroids is neuropeptide Y. This peptide influences central behavior and neuroendocrine functions, by stimulating the pulsatile release of GnRH and gonadotropins. Experimental studies showed that estrogens are able to stimulate the synthesis and release of neuropeptide Y in the hypothalamus. In castrated female rats, gonadal steroid deficiency reduces neurosecretion of neuropeptide Y. Estrogens increase neuropeptide Y content in the median eminence and the synthesis of neuropeptide Y in arcuate nucleus, by inducing neuropeptide Y gene expression[23]. Indeed, recent findings have demonstrated several interactions between neuropeptide Y and β-endorphin neurons in the hypothalamus, therefore both estrogens and progestogens may indirectly exert modulatory effects on neuropeptide Y, inducing β-endorphin release[22].

A large number of studies have investigated the clinical effects of estro-progestin molecules on the CNS in postmenopausal women, with particular attention on the consequences of the neuroendocrine system modifications produced by withdrawal of gonadal hormones and on the effects of hormone replacement therapy (HRT).

A positive relationship has been demonstrated between circulating levels of estradiol and mood[24]. Studies regarding the effects of HRT on climacteric depression have shown a significant amelioration of mood in depressed postmenopausal women treated with estrogen[25,26–30], although other studies have not found a similar response to estrogen[29–31]. These different results may be due to a lower estrogen dosage or to the progestogen component of the combined preparations that were employed[32,33]. Generally, the doses of estrogens conventionally used do not improve mood in women with major depression but have a strong influence on mood and feeling of well-being in healthy non-depressed postmenopausal women[25,27–29,34–37]. The positive effects of estrogen on mood in postmenopausal women may relate to its effects on the adrenergic and serotoninergic tone. In fact, estrogen acts as a serotoninergic agonist by increasing serotonin synthesis and levels of its main metabolite 5-hydroxyindoleacetic acid.

Clinical studies have reported a frequent decrease in cognitive efficiency, including memory, in climacteric women[38]. Estrogen administration improves cognitive functions[33,39–42] by exerting a positive effect especially on memory and reaction time tests[40,42–45]. The employment of objective psychometric instruments to assess cognitive function has suggested that physiological levels of estrogen help in maintaining short- and long-term verbal memory, but have no effect on visual spatial memory. Although most studies on estrogen and cognition have found a positive effect of estrogen on memory processes, other studies have failed to demonstrate this effect[25,46,47]. The explanation for these discrepant findings is the difference in the selection of subjects and methodology. In particular, differences in the type and route of administration of hormonal preparations that are employed may account for some of the inconsistencies in the results. Different oral preparations are differentially absorbed and metabolized by the liver, whereas oral or transdermal administration of estrogen bypasses the initial hepatic metabolism. It is therefore reasonable to postulate that the method of administration and the different doses used explain some of the variance in the results. In addition, another important factor may be considered: in the postmenopausal period, estrogen administration enhances mood and subjective well-being. A depressed mood can have a negative impact on psychometric performance. Although several studies have demonstrated a secondary influence of estrogen on cognition through its effects on mood, others have not found a direct correlation[25,26,44,45,48]. Recent studies have demonstrated specific memory impairment, in surgically postmenopausal women[43,45], independent of the presence of affective disorders or other symptoms related to menopause. Estrogen may affect mood and cognition in an independent and direct manner.

Several studies focused the attention on the effect of estro-progestin compounds on the opioidergic system. In women, plasma β-endorphin levels change during the menstrual cycle and, in particular, the increase in circulating β-endorphin levels during the periovulatory phase seems to be related to ovulatory function[32]. This timing confirms the specific role of gonadal hormones in the modulation of the opioidergic system and shows that it is related to ovarian function. The increase in β-endorphin during the periovulatory phase seems to be related to the typical mid-cycle increase in plasma estradiol levels[49]. A decrease in plasma β-endorphin levels has been shown in postmenopausal women after surgical or spontaneous menopause[50]. The decrease in plasma β-endorphin has also been related to the pathogenesis of mood, behavior and nociceptive disturbances of the postmenopausal period. Estrogen treatment ameliorates the opiatergic activity and increases circulating β-endorphin levels to premenopausal values. Moreover, the administration of different progestogens does not modify the positive effect of estrogen on the opioidergic system[51]. Regarding the effects of progestins on neurovegetative symptoms and cognitive functions the few available data suggest that progestins do not modify the positive effects of estrogen[51].

ANDROGENS

Androgens are produced in women both by the ovaries and the adrenals, which synthesize androstenedione, testosterone and dehydroepiandrosterone (DHEA). Adrenals also produce DHEA sulfate (DHEAS). Testosterone is also obtained from the conversion of active precursors (androstenedione is the principal circulating precursor)[52]. In ovaries, androgens are secreted by the thecal cells under the control of LH. DHEA and its sulfate ester DHEAS are the major circulating adrenal cortex products[53–55]. DHEAS is synthesized from the conversion of free DHEA, which is secreted in large amounts (70–80%) by the adrenals. Twenty per cent of DHEA is produced by the ovaries. Both Δ5 androgens (DHEA and DHEAS) are peripherally converted into androstenedione, testosterone, dihydrotestosterone and estrogens. Commonly, less attention is focused on the activity of androgens in normal female physiology or on the consequences of their deficiency. Women with androgen deficiency may experience a variety of physical symptoms or psychological changes as a consequence of their endocrine state.

Several studies have investigated the effect of the climacteric and postmenopause on androgen synthesis and circulating levels. After menopause the principal source of circulating testosterone derives from the peripheral conversion of androstenedione and DHEAS. Circulating Δ5 androgen levels fall linearly with age, starting from the third decade of life, and are independent of the menopausal transition. The ratios of DHEA to testosterone and DHEAS to testosterone are not modified with age and it is logical that circulating testosterone levels should also decline with age as occurs for its main precursor. After the age of 70 years DHEAS levels are mantained at 20% or less of the maximum plasma concentrations, while cortisol levels remain unchanged[56].

Few studies have also focused attention on androgen replacement therapy and in particular on the symptomatology of the climacterium or of late postmenopause directly related to androgen deficiency, such as sexual disorders, loss of well-being and energy, mood disorders, neuroendocrine dysfunctions, metabolic and bone mass effects.

Androgens play a key role in female sexuality and libido. Androgen reduction contributes to the decline in sexual interest experienced by many women[57]. Little change in libido is described in women treated with estrogen replacement therapy[58,59]. Estrogen improves sexual satisfaction by ameliorating vaginal dryness or dyspareunia, but it does not seem to induce modification of libido in women without coital discomfort[60,61]. However, androgens remain only a small component in the management of the replacement therapy of menopause. Several studies showed the efficacy of parenteral testosterone administration[60-65]. Few data are available on long-term androgen replacement. To obtain a good response in terms of enhanced libido in postmenopausal androgen supplementation it seems that testosterone levels need to be restored to the physiological values found in young women[62].

Δ5 ANDROGENS AND THE BRAIN: BASIC RESEARCHES AND CLINICAL TRIALS

Several epidemiological, experimental and clinical trials have focused their attention on the actions of Δ5 androgens. Epidemiological studies have shown a relationship between the progressive decrease in circulating DHEA(S) levels and the increase in cardiovascular morbidity in men[66], breast cancer in women[67,68] and the decline of immune competence in both sexes[69].

Experimental studies in rodents showed a protective role of DHEA on the development of spontaneous carcinomas; an up-regulation of the immune system has also been reported[67,70,71]. Few studies have investigated the role of DHEA(S) on the CNS in humans. DHEA administration at 50 mg/day induced an

improvement in psychological and physical well-being in postmenopausal women[72], thus suggesting a specific role for DHEA supplementation on CNS functions (Figure 2). Recently, it has been shown that the oral administration of DHEA (50 mg/day) tends to determine an increase in well-being and mood only in women[73]. Moreover, another study described DHEA(S) as having antidepressant function (30–90 mg/day for 4 weeks) in middle-aged and elderly patients with major depression and low basal DHEA(S) levels[74].

On the other hand, DHEAS may directly affect the central nervous system. DHEA and DHEAS are also considered to be neurosteroids because they are produced in the CNS. The concentration of DHEA(S) in the CNS is 5–10 times greater with respect to plasma levels. Experimental studies indicate that the mammalian brain contains steroid precursors, such as cholesterol and lipid derivatives[75,76], but it is also able to metabolize other steroids coming from the peripheral circulation. The enzyme involved in the cleavage of cholesterol to pregnanolone and progesterone, localized in the mitochondria of glial cells, is cytochrome P450. This enzyme is encoded by the same P450 gene expressed in the adrenals and gonads and has been identified in rodents, cows and human brain. The origin of DHEA in the brain is unknown, since the adult rat brain does not have 17β-hydroxylase activity and cannot convert pregnanolone or progesterone to

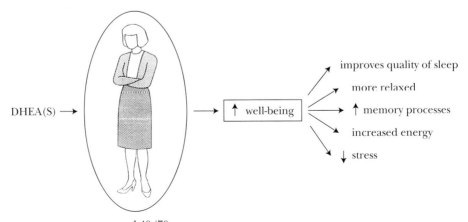

Figure 2 Effects of low-dose dehydroepiandrosterone(sulfate) DHEA(S) treatment in postmenopausal women

hydroxylated compounds, nor can it convert C21 or C19 steroids[77]. However, the concentrations of DHEA(S) in rat brain remain unchanged for a long time after the removal of gonads and adrenals. The synthesis of classical neurosteroids, including DHEA, probably proceeds through different pathways with respect to those of adrenals or gonads. In fact, glial cells contain additional steroid metabolizing enzymes that transform classical steroid hormones into a variety of compounds[75–77]. Experimental evidence suggests that the effects of DHEA and DHEAS on the CNS occur directly through a specific binding to the γ-aminobutyric acid$_A$ (GABA$_A$) receptor, thus blocking GABA-induced chloride transport or current in synaptoneurosomes and neurons in a dose-dependent manner, with an increase in neuronal excitability[78]. Moreover, a potentiating effect of DHEA on N-methyl-D-aspartate (NMDA) and sigma receptors has been reported in rat brain[77].

DHEA(S) AND NEUROENDOCRINE SYSTEMS

In order to clarify the effects of DHEA(S) on neuroendocrine functions, our group has recently investigated the effects of DHEA and DHEAS supplementation on the opiatergic tonus in postmenopausal women. In particular, the attention was focused on β-endorphin, the most important and biologically active endogenous opioid peptide, having behavioral, analgesic, thermoregulatory and neuroendocrine properties.

Clinical studies demonstrated that variations in circulating β-endorphin levels may be considered one of the markers of neuroendocrine function[78,79]. In postmenopausal women, the withdrawal of sex steroid hormones modifies neuroendocrine equilibrium by changing neuroactive transmitters. Regarding the opiatergic system, a decrease in plasma β-endorphin levels has been demonstrated postmenopause[80]. This reduction in circulating β-endorphin has been suggested to have a role in the mechanisms of hot flushes and sweats and in the pathogenesis of mood, behavior and nociceptive modifications[51]. Experimental and clinical studies have shown that β-endorphin synthesis and release is modulated by noradrenaline, dopamine, serotonin, acetylcholine, GABA and corticotropin-releasing factor[51]. In fertile subjects, a bolus injection of naloxone, an opioid receptor antagonist, and a bolus injection of clonidine, an α$_2$-presynaptic receptor agonist, increase β-endorphin levels. In postmenopause, a lack of β-endorphin response to clonidine and naloxone occurs and these findings suggest a postmenopausal impairment of adrenergic and opiatergic receptors in modulating β-endorphin release. HRT restores basal plasma β-endorphin levels to those present in fertile women as well as the β-endorphin response to clonidine and naloxone[51,81].

In a preliminary trial postmenopausal women ($n = 6$; age range 52–56 years; menopausal age > 3 years), having a normal body mass index (< 24 kg/m^2), received oral DHEA (100 mg/day) (Rottapharm, Milan, Italy) for 7 days. Women were submitted to a clonidine test (0.150 mg intravenously), before and after 7 days of treatment. Following 7 days of DHEA administration, a significant increase of plasma DHEA, DHEAS, androstenedione, testosterone, estrone and estradiol levels was found. On the contrary, basal plasma β-endorphin levels were not significantly modified after DHEA short-term administration. After the treatment a significant increase of plasma β-endorphin levels ($p < 0.01$, at 15 and 30 minutes) was observed in response to adrenergic activation with clonidine (Figure 3).

Further data have been obtained in postmenopausal women (menopausal age range 2–5 years; $n = 9$; age range 45–55 years), having a normal body mass index and basal plasma DHEA levels < 5 nmol/l. All women received DHEAS (50 mg by mouth/day) (Rottapharm, Milan, Italy). Subjects were observed monthly during the 3 months of therapy. Blood was drawn for the determination of basal plasma DHEA, DHEAS, androstenedione, 17-hydroxyprogesterone, testosterone, estrone, estradiol, sex hormone binding globulin, cortisol and β-endorphin levels. Before and after 3 months of therapy, β-endorphin levels were evaluated in response to three neuroendocrine tests: clonidine (0.150 mg), naloxone (4 mg intravenously) and fluoxetine (30 mg by mouth). DHEA and DHEAS levels significantly increased

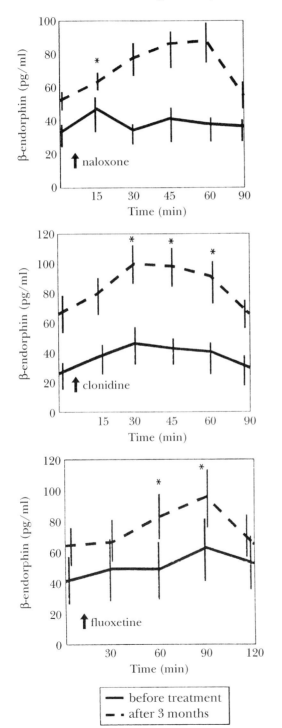

after the first month of DHEAS administration ($p < 0.05$). Androstenedione and testosterone levels showed a significant increase after each month of treatment ($p < 0.05$). Estradiol and estrone levels also increased significantly and progressively during the 3 months of treatment ($p < 0.05$). SHBG, cortisol, and 17 hydroxy-progesterone levels did not show significant variations. After the first month of therapy, a significant increase in basal plasma β-endorphin levels was observed ($p < 0.05$). The increase was confirmed after 2 and 3 months. While no response to the three tests was observed before treatment, a significant increase in plasma β-endorphin levels was shown after 3 months in response to clonidine naloxone tests.

According to the literature, both studies confirmed the significant increase in basal plasma levels of testosterone, and rostenedione, estrone and estradiol after DHEA(S) supplementation, indicating that the Δ5 androgen and its sulphate-conjugated ester may be converted into active steroids[72,82,83]. The increase in basal plasma β-endorphin levels after the first month of DHEAS therapy support an estrogen-like effect of the molecule on CNS. On the other hand, no similar findings were reported and this might be a consequence of the short-term DHEA administration. The treatment with DHEA(S) induces a restoration of the β-endorphin response to clonidine, naloxone and fluoxetine respectively. These findings suggest that DHEA(S) restores the neuroendocrine control of α^2-adrenergic, opioidergic and serotonin receptors on the anterior pituitary β-endorphin secretion. The modulation of neuroendocrine pathways after DHEAS supplementation may be mediated by a specific estrogenic action of DHEAS metabolites or, alternatively, by a similar receptorial specificity of DHEAS and estroprogestin compounds on opiatergic and adrenergic neurons. In

Figure 3 Mean ± SEM plasma β-endorphin response to clonidine, naloxone and fluoxetine test in postmenopausal women before and after dehydroepiandrosterone sulfate supplementation; β-endorphin levels in pg ml before treatment (solid lines) and after 3 months of treatment (broken lines),*$p < 0.05$ cf. time 0

conclusion, the present findings suggest that both the Δ5 androgens, and/or their metabolites, may be considered neuroendocrine correlates of the DHEA(S)-induced psychological and physical ameliorations.

CONCLUSION

These data support the idea that different estrogen, progestin and androgen molecules, used alone or in association, exert several effects on brain function. Gonadal hormones are of primary importance for the physiological brain function, acting both on the development and on the maintenance of the female behavior, cognition and reproductive function. However, at present, the knowledge concerning the implications of sex steroid hormones as control mechanisms of brain function is insufficient to be conclusive. Every year different kinds of molecules, numerous routes and regimens of administration are developed in HRT. Starting from this evidence, further studies are required to explain the specific role of endogenous and exogenous sex steroids on the CNS.

References

1. Genazzani AR, Petraglia F, Purdy RH. *The Brain: Source and Target for Sex Steroid Hormones.* Carnforth, UK: Parthenon Publishing Group, 1996
2. Speroff L, Glass RH, Kase NH. *Clinical Gynecological Endocrinology and Infertility*, 5th edn. Baltimore, MD: Williams and Wilkins, 1995
3. Alonso-Soleis R, Abreu P, Leopez-Coviella I, Hernandez G, Fajardo N. Gonadal steroid modulation of neuroendocrine transduction: a transynaptic view. *Cell Mol Neurobiol* 1996;3:357–82
4. Panay N, Sands RH, Studd JWW. Oestrogen and behaviour. In Genazzani AR, Petraglia F, Purdy RH, eds. *The Brain: Source and Target for Sex Steroid Hormones.* Carnforth, UK: Parthenon Publishing Group, 1996;257–76
5. Fuxe K, Gustafsson JA, Wetterberg L. *Steroid Hormone Regulation of the Brain.* Oxford: Pergamon, 1981;27–56
6. Karla SP. Gonadal steroid hormones promote interactive comunication. In Genazzani AR, Petraglia F, Purdy RH, eds. *The Brain: Source and Target for Sex Steroid Hormones.* Carnforth, UK: Parthenon Publishing Group, 1996;257–76
7. Matsumoto A. Synaptogenic action of sex steroids in developing and adult neuroendocrine brain. *Psychoneuroendocrinology* 1991;16:25–40
8. McEwen BS, Wooley CS. Estradiol and progesterone regulate neuronal structure and synaptic connectivity in adult as well as developing brain. *Exp Gerontol* 1994;29:431–6
9. Etgen AM, Karkanias GB. Estrogen regulation of noradrenergic signaling in the hypothalamus. *Psychoneuroendocrinology* 1994;19:603–10
10. Dickinson SL, Curzon G. 5-Hydroxytryptamine-mediated behavior in male and female rats. *Neuropharmacology* 1986;25:771–6
11. Biegon A, Bercovitz H, Samuel D. Serotonin receptor concentration during the estrous cycle of the rat. *Brain Res* 1980;187:221–5
12. Mendelson SD, McKittrick CR, McEwen BS. Autoradiographic analyses of the effects of estradiol benzoate on (^{3}H)-paroxetine binding the cerebral cortex and dorsal hippocampus of gonadectomized male and female rats. *Brain Res* 1993;601:299–301
13. Luine VN, McEwen BS. Effect of estradiol on turnover of Type A monoamine oxidase in the brain. *J Neurochem* 1977;28:1221–7
14. Panay N, Sands RH, Studd JWW. Estrogen and behaviour. In Genazzani AR, Petraglia F, Purdy RH, eds. *The Brain: Source and Target for Sex Steroid Hormones.* Carnforth, UK: Parthenon Publishing Group, 1996;257–76
15. Genazzani AR, Petraglia F, Silferi M, *et al.* Progestins modulate the action of estrogen on gonadotropin-releasing hormone, luteinizing hormone and prolactin in rat. *Gynecol Obstet Invest* 1990;29:197–202
16. Mishell DR, Klketzky OA, Brenner PF. The effect of contraceptive steroids on hypothalamic-pituitary function. *Am J Obstet Gynecol* 1977;128:60–6
17. Mann DR, Barraclough CA. Role of estrogen and progesterone in facilitating LH release in 4-day cyclic rats. *Endocrinology* 1973;93:694–7
18. Labrie F, Lagacè L, Drouin J. Direct and differential effects of sex steroids at the anterior pituitary

level on LH and FSH secretion. In Klopper A, Lerner AB, van der Molen HJ, Sciarra JJ, eds. *Research on Steroids*, Vol 8. London: Academic Press 1979;207

19. Panerai AE, Petraglia F, Sacerdote P, Genazzani AR. Mainly μ-opiate receptors are involved in luteinizing hormone and prolactin secretion. *Endocrinology* 1985;117:1096–9

20. Piva F, Limonta P, Dondi D, *et al.* Effects of steroids on the brain opioid system. *J Steroid Biochem Molec Biol* 1995:53,343–8

21. Genazzani AR, Petraglia F, Bergamaschi M, Genazzani AD, Facchinetti F, Volpe A. Progesterone and progestins modulate β-endorphin concentrations in the hypothalamus and in the pituitary of castrated female rats. *Gynecol Endocrinol* 1987;1:6–9

22. Genazzani AR, Petraglia F, Facchinetti F, *et al.* Steroid replacement increases beta-endorphin and beta-lipotropin plasma levels in postmenopausal women. *Gynecol Obstet Invest* 1988;26: 153–9

23. Fuxe K, Harfstrand A, Eneroth P, Zoli M, Agnati LF. Neuropeptide Y mechanisms in neuroendocrine regulation. In Genazzani AR, Montemagno U, Nappi C, Petraglia F, eds. *The Brain and Reproductive Function.* Carnforth, UK: Parthenon Publishing, 1988;45

24. Studd JWW, Smith RNJ. Estrogen and depression in women. *Menopause* 1994;1;33–7

25. Ditkoff EC, Crary WG, Cristo M, Lobo RA. Estrogen improves psychological function in asymptomatic postmenopausal women. *Obstet Gynecol* 1991;78:991–5

26. Daly E, Gray A, Barlow D, *et al.* Measuring the impact of menopausal symptoms on quality of life. *Br Med J* 1993;307:836–40

27. Limouzin-Lamothe M, Mairon N, LeGal J, *et al.* Quality of life after the menopause: influence of hormone replacement therapy. *Am J Obstet Gynecol* 1994;170:618–24

28. Montgomery JC, Brincat M, Tapp A, *et al.* Effect of oestrogen and testosterone implants on psychological disorder in the climacteric. *Lancet* 1987;i:297–9

29. Best N, Rees M, Barlow D, *et al.* Effect of estradiol implants on noradrenergic function and mood in menopausal patients. *Psychoneuroendocrinology* 1992;17:87–93

30. Klaiber EL, Broverman DM, Vogel W, *et al.* Estrogen replacement therapy for severe persistent depression in women. *Arch Gen Psych* 1979;36: 550–4

31. Coope J. Is oestrogen therapy effective in the treatment of menopausal depression? *J R Coll Gen Pract* 1981;31:134–40

32. Holst J, Backstrom T, Hammarback S, *et al.* Progestogen addition during oestrogen replacement therapy – effects on vasomotor

symptoms and mood. *Maturitas* 1989;11: 13–20.

33. Furuhjelm M, Feder-Freybergh P. The influence of estrogens on the psyche in climacteric and postmenopausal women. In van Keep PA, Albeaux M, Greenblatt R, eds. *Consensus on Menopause Research.* Baltimore: University Press, 1976;84–93

34. Palinkas LA, Barrett-Connor E. Estrogen use and depressive symptoms in postmenopausal women. *Obstet Gynecol* 1992;80:30–6

35. Michael C, Kantor H, Shore H. Further psychometric evaluation of older women – the effect of estrogen administration. *J Gerontol* 1970;25: 335–41

36. Ayward M. Estrogen and plasma tryptophan levels in perimenopausal patients. In Campbell S, ed. *The Management of the Menopause and Post-Menopausal Years.* Baltimore: University Park Press, 1976;135–47

37. Furuhjelm M, Carlstrom K. Treatment of climacteric and postmenopausal women with 17-beta-oestradiol and norethisterone acetate. *Acta Obstet Gynecol Scand* 1977;56:351–61

38. Halbreich U. Role of estrogen in postmenopausal depression. *Neurology* 1997;48(Suppl 7): S16–S20

39. Caldwell BM, Watson RI. Evaluation of psychological effects of sex hormone administration in aged women: results of therapy after 6 months. *J Gerontol* 1952;7:228–44

40. Hackman BW, Galbraith D. Six month study of oestrogen therapy with piperazine oestrone sulphate and its effect on memory. *Curr Med Res Opin* 1977;4(Suppl):21–7

41. Campbell S, Whitehead M. Oestrogen therapy and the menopausal syndrome. *Clin Obstet Gynecol* 1977;4:31–47

42. Fedor-Freybergh P. The influence of oestrogen on well being and mental performance in climacteric and postmenopausal women. *Acta Obstet Gynecol Scand* 1977;64(Suppl):5–69

43. Sherwin BB. Estrogen and/or androgen replacement therapy and cognitive functioning in surgically menopausal women. *Psychoneuroendocrinology* 1988;13:345–57

44. Sherwin BB, Phillips S. Estrogen and cognitive functioning in surgically menopausal women. *Ann NY Acad Sci* 1990;592:474–5

45. Phillips S, Sherwin BB. Effects of estrogen on memory function in surgically menopausal women. *Psychoneuroendocrinology* 1992;17:177–7

46. Rauramo L, Lagerspetz K, Engblom P, Punnonen R. The effect of castration and per-oral estrogen therapy on some psychological function. *Front Horm Res* 1975;13:94–104

47. Vanhulle R., Demol R. A double-blind study into the influence of estriol on a number of psychological tests in post-menopausal women. In van

Keep PA, Greenblatt RB, Albeaux-Fernet M, eds. *Consensus on Menopausal Research.* London: MTP Press, 1976;94–9

48. Kampen D, Sherwin BB. Estrogen use and verbal memory in healthy postmenopausal women. *Obstet Gynecol* 1994;83:979–83

49. Dennerstein L, Burrows GD, Hyman G, Sharpe K. Hormone therapy and effect. *Maturitas* 1979; 1:247–54

50. Sherwin B, Gelfand MM. A prospective one-year study of estrogen and progestin in post-menopausal women: effects on clinical symptoms and lipoprotein lipids. *Obstet Gynecol* 1989; 73:759–66

51. Stomati M, Bersi C, Rubino S, *et al*. Neuroendocrine effects of different oestradiol-progestin regimens in postmenopausal women. *Maturitas*, in press

52. Mc Loughin L, Grossman A, Tomlin S, *et al*. CRF-41 stimulates the release of beta-lipotropin and beta-endorphin in normal human subjects. *Neuroendocrinology* 1984;38:282–4

53. Judd HL, Bardin CW. Serum androstenedione and testosterone levels during the menstrual cycle. *J Clin Endocrinol Metab* 1973;36:475–81

54. Parker LN, Odell WD. Control of adrenal androgen secretion. *Endocr Rev* 1980;4:392–410

55. Yamaji T, Ibayashi H. Serum deydroepiandrosterone sulphate in normal and pathological conditions. *J Clin Endocrinol Metab* 1969;29:273–8

56. Hopper BR, Yen SSC. Circulating concentrations of dehydroepiandrosterone and dehydroepiandrosterone sulphate during puberty. *J Clin Endocrinol Metab* 1975;40:458–61

57. Davis SR, Burger HG. Androgens and the post-menopausal woman. *J Clin Endocrinol Metab* 1996;81:2759–63

58. Utian WH. The true clinical features of post-menopausal oophorectomy and their response to estrogen replacement therapy. *S Afr Med J* 1972;46:732–7

59. Campbell S, Whitehead M. Oestrogen therapy and the menopausal syndrome *Clin Obstet Gynecol* 1977;4:31–47

60. Studd JWW, Chakavarti S, Oram D. The climacteric. *Clin Obstet Gynecol* 1977;4:3–29

61. Studd JWW, Collins WP, Chakavarti S. Estradiol and testosterone implants in the treatment of psychosexual problems in postmenopausal women. *Br J Obstet Gynecol* 1988;84:314–15

62. Sherwin BB, Gelfand MM, Brender W. Androgen enhances sexual motivation in females: a prospective, crossover study of sex steroid administration in surgical menopause. *Psychosom Med* 1985;47:339–51

63. Burger HG, Hailes J, Menelaus M. The management of persistent symptoms with estradiol-testosterone implants: clinical, lipid and hormonal results. *Maturitas* 1984;6:351–8

64. Burger HG, Hailes J, Nelson J, Menelaus M. Effects of combined implants of estradiol and testosterone on libido in postmenopausal women. *Br Med J* 1987;294:936–7

65. Davis SR, McCloud P, Strauss BJC, Burger HG. Testosterone enhances estradiol's effects on postmenopausal bone density and sexuality. *Maturitas* 1995;21:227–36

66. Barret-Connor E, Khaw K, Yen SSC. A prospective study of DS mortality and cardiovascular disease. *N Engl J Med* 1986;315:1519–24

67. Helzlsouer KJ, Gordon GB, Alberg A, Bush TL, Comstock GW. Relationship of prediagnostic serum levels of DHEA and DS to the risk of developing premenopausal breast cancer. *Cancer Res* 1992;52:1–4

68. Bulbrook RD, Hayward JL, Spicer CC. Relation between urinary androgen and corticoid secretion excretion and subsequent breast cancer. *Lancet* 1975;2:395–8

69. Thoman ML, Weigle WO. The cellular and subcellular bases of immunosenescence. *Adv Immunol* 1989;46:221–61

70. Blauer KI, Rogers WM, Benton EW. Dehydroepiandrosterone antagonizes the suppressive effects of glucocorticoids on lymphocyte proliferation. Proceedings of the 71st Annual Meeting of the Endocrine Society, 1989

71. Rogers WM, Blauer KL, Bernton W. Dehydroepiandrosterone protection against dexamethasone induced thymic involution: flow cytometric and mechanism studies. Proceedings of the 71st Annual Meeting of The Endocrine Society, 1989

72. Morales AJ, Nolan JJ, Nelson JC, Yen SSC. Effects of replacement dose of dehydroepiandrosterone in men and women of advancing age. *J Clin Endocrinol Metab* 1994;78:1360–7

73. Wolf OT, Neumenn O, Helhammer DH, *et al*. Effects of a two-week physiological dehydroepiandrosterone substitution on cognitive performance and well-being in healthy elderly women and men. *J Clin Endocrinol Metab* 1997;82:2363–7

74. Wolkowitz OM, Reus VI, Roberts E, *et al*. Dehydroepiandrosterone (DHEA) treatment of depression. *Biol Psychiatr* 1997;41:311–18

75. Majewska MD. Neurosteroids: endogenous bimodal modulators of the GABA-A receptor. Mechanism of action and physiological significance. *Progr Neurobiol* 1992;38:379–95

76. Corpechot C, Young J, Calvel M, *et al*. Neurosteroids: 3α-hydroxy-5α-pregnan-20-one and its precursors in the brain, plasma, and steroidogenic glands of male and female rats. *Endocrinology* 1993;133:1003–9

77. Mellon SH. Neurosteroids: biochemistry, modes of action, and clinical relevance. *J Clin Endocrinol Metab* 1994;78:1003–8

78. Genazzani AR, Petraglia F, Mercuri N, *et al.* Effect of steroid hormones and antihormones on hypothalamic beta-endorphin concentrations in intact and castrated female rats. *J Endocrinol Invest* 1990;13:91–6

79. Petraglia F, Comitini G, Genazzani AR, *et al.* β-Endorphin in human reproduction. In Herz A, ed. *Opioids II.* Berlin: Springer-Verlag, 1993: 763–80

80. Schneider HPG, Genazzani AR. *A New Approach in the Treatment of Climacteric Disorders.* De Gruiter 1992:134–54

81. Majewska MD, Demirgoren S, Spivak CE, London ED. The neurosteroid DHEA is an allosteric antagonist of the GABA-A receptor. *Brain Res* 1990;526:143–6

82. Thijssen JHH, Nieuwenhuyse H. *DHEA: A Comprehensive Review.* Carnforth: The Parthenon Publishing Group, 1999

83. Mortola JF, Yen SSC. The effects of oral dehydroepiandrosterone on endocrine-metabolic parameters in postmenopausal women. *J Clin Endocrinol Metab* 1990;71:696–704

84. Berr C, Lafont S, Debuire B, Dartigues J-F, Baulieu EE. Relationship of dehydroepiandrosterone sulphate in the elderly functional and mental status, and short-term mortality: a French community-based study. *Proc Natl Acad Sci USA* 1996;93:13410–15

13

Depression, estrogen and neurotransmitters in the postmenopausal woman

J. S. Archer

INTRODUCTION

Mood changes and depression have been linked to hormonal changes in the menopausal woman. There are conflicting objective data that relate estrogen withdrawal to mood changes or depression. Estrogens can have a profound effect on the central nervous system (CNS). This review describes clinical depression, the effect of estrogen on CNS neurotransmitters and their biological activity, and clinical trials of estrogen on mood and/or depression in postmenopausal women.

DEPRESSION

As defined in the Diagnostic and Statistical Manual of Mental Disorders, Fourth Edition (DSM-IV), unipolar depressive diseases include major depressive disorder, dysthymia (a low-grade more tenacious depressed mood) and depressive disorder not otherwise specified (signs and symptoms of depression but not meeting criteria set for the other two disorders)[1]. Currently, depression is ranked as the world's fourth most devastating illness by the World Health Organisation[2]. There are projections that by the year 2020 depression will have climbed to second place behind heart disease[2]. The power of depression as an illness is underlined by the knowledge that only end-stage coronary heart disease causes more days of incapacity and only arthritis results in more chronic pain when compared to depression[1].

Approximately 15% of patients diagnosed with major depression will end their lives by suicide[3].

The prevalence of depressive disorders has been consistently higher in women than in men. These findings cross cultural, ethnic, socio-economic and geographical boundaries[4]. The National Comorbidity Survey reported lifetime prevalence rates of major depression at 21% in women compared to 13% in men, and dysthmia rates of 8% in women compared to 5% in men[4]. It has been suggested that not only do genetic and psychosocial factors account for this sexual disparity but also biological and thus neuro-endocrine factors, since this gender difference is seen only after the onset of puberty and persists until the age of 55[4].

DEPRESSION IN THE CLIMACTERIC

The fluctuating levels of sex hormones seen during a woman's menarchal life have been studied as a possible cause of a woman's increased susceptibility to dysphoria[5]. Some researchers have identified three life events that contain an increased risk of depression: premenstrual, postpartum and the climacteric[5].

However, controversy still exists with regard to whether there is an increased incidence of depression in the years surrounding menopause[6]. Involutional melancholia was included in the DSM-II published in 1968 but was removed from the successive editions as clinical studies failed to show a consistently higher rate of depression in postmenopausal women[7]. Earlier reports evaluated only women who attended menopause clinics and 65% were noted to be in the depressed range of the Zung self-rating depression scale[8]. This prevalence of dysphoric symptomatology was higher than that found in psychiatric clinics, indicating that this was a self-selected population and not a true representation of the average woman going through menopause[5,9]. Though several community-based studies have found no evidence of an increased rate of depressed mood and clinically defined depression at the time of menopause, other cross-sectional community-based studies disagree. These reports indicated prevalence rates of 16–20% during the climacteric, double the 9% point prevalence rate seen in the general female population[10,11].

Two prospective longitudinal studies that followed women as they went from the perimenopausal to menopausal stage found conflicting results. In both studies, menopausal status was determined by self-report of menstrual periods with no serum hormone measurements obtained[10,12]. Women were followed for 3 years in the Manitoba project[12]. The menopausal transition was not associated with depression except in the surgically menopausal group[12]. They did find a high rate of depression with 26% of all women being depressed during at least one of their interviews[12]. The Massachusetts Women's Health Study followed women for over 2 years with a transitory increase in depressed mood noted only in the women who remained perimenopausal during the study[10]. There was a common finding in both of these studies. Women who were experiencing a more pronounced rate of hormonal change were more likely to become depressed.

Several clinical studies have shown that women who have undergone a surgical menopause, thus experiencing a more precipitous drop in ovarian steroid serum levels, have more psychological symptomatology than those undergoing a natural menopause[12,13]. In fact, psychiatrists agree that hormone replacement therapy (HRT) is appropriate to prevent psychiatric sequelae in these women[13]. In addition,

those women with a long perimenopausal transition, and thus more likely to have fluctuating levels of estrogen, also suffer from a higher rate of depression[10,13]. In concordance with these findings, the absolute serum concentration of circulating hormonal levels does not distinguish between depressed and non-depressed women, indicating that the rate of change in hormonal levels is more indicative of psychological symptomatology[14].

Consequently, some researchers have concluded that if psychological symptomatology is present, it would be more likely to occur before and not after the cessation of menses[15]. In support of this hypothesis is one study that has shown that up to 80% of perimenopausal women, 48–53 years of age, develop mood disturbances[14,16]. Also, researchers have found a greater incidence of psychological symptoms in women aged 45–49 years with a peak suicide rate during this period[7]. There is no corresponding suicide peak in men at the same age[7].

If perimenopausal depression is related to fluctuating levels of hormones then women at risk for depression should include those women who have a prior history of depression related to hormonal changes. Such a situation has been identified in several studies. The Seattle Midlife Women's Health Study found that women with a history of premenstrual syndrome or postpartum depression were more likely to become depressed during the perimenopausal years[17]. The strongest predictor for depressed mood during the menopause was a history of premenstrual depression in another prospective longitudinal study[18]. Although the exact cause of premenstrual syndrome has not been elucidated, successful treatment of this disorder with 17β-estradiol appears to indicate a relative estrogen deficiency[5]. Depression is rare in the last trimester of pregnancy when hormonal levels are stable, but rates climb to 20% in the postpartum period, coinciding with a significant drop in estrogen levels[5]. The use of transdermal estradiol systems has been shown to be a successful treatment for postpartum depression[5]. The unifying characteristic of these three life stages that have been associated with depression in women appears to be low and/or fluctuating concentrations of serum estrogens[19].

The great majority of mood disorders are diagnosed and treated by the primary care provider such as an obstetrician/gynecologist[1]. Thus, it is imperative that physicians who treat women are not only able to recognize affective diseases but can treat them appropriately. In 1932 the first report of the antidepressant nature of estrogen in perimenopausal women was published[9]. Over 60 years later there remains no clear agreement as to the role of estrogen in the management of depression or depressed mood. If indeed low and fluctuating levels of estrogens are associated with depression in peri- and postmenopausal women, then the question must be answered as to the suitability of estrogen replacement therapy (ERT) for the treatment of depression in this group of women.

DEPRESSION AND STEROIDS

In the 1960s the role of neurotransmitters in the pathophysiology of depression was recognized. A biochemical deficiency in certain neurotransmitter systems was believed to result in affective disorders[1,20]. Initial work focused on the catecholamine system, with the earliest antidepressants known to affect the CNS concentrations of norepinephrine[1]. Neuroscience has now shown that the neurochemistry of the CNS is too detailed for just one neurotransmitter regulating mood and now multiple systems are known to play a role in the development of depression[1]. One prominent neurologist/psychiatrist, Mark George, refers to depression as 'depressions' to further delineate the numerous biological and pathophysiological bases and clinical appearances of this disease[21].

Recent advances in studies of brain function in humans have shown that the brain is a sexual organ and responds differently in males compared to females to a variety of stimuli[22]. Gonadal hormones not only exert 'organizational effects' during prenatal life to differentiate the brain according to gender but also 'activational effects' during adult life, which support this gender differentiation[23]. Gonadal

steroids are one of the most powerful peripherally generated biological signals in the CNS, affecting neurotransmitter synthesis, release, reuptake and receptor density number as well as enzymatic inactivation[7,24–26]. Gonadal steroids not only impact through the classical nuclear receptor and resultant protein synthesis (enzymes, neurotropic growth factors, neurotransmitters and neurotransmitter receptors) but also through direct membrane-mediated alterations[19,27]. Neurobiological changes in the CNS do result in psychiatric disorders such as depression[16] (Table 1).

Estrogen receptors have been found in areas of the brain that are involved in emotion, including the cerebral cortex, hypothalamus, hippocampus, amygdala and limbic forebrain[28]. Studies have shown that the limbic system, hypothalamus, γ-aminobutyric acid (GABA) receptors, dopamine, serotonin (5-hydroxytryptamine), cholinergic, glutaminergic and opiate systems are all sexually dimorphic[29]. All of these CNS neuroendrocrine functions have been implicated in the manifestation of the depressive state. Work done using positron emission tomography to image the brain during periods of self-induced sadness found that women and men both activated the limbic system[30]. The limbic area involved in the female subjects was eight times greater when compared to the male volunteers[21,30]. In addition it has been shown that areas of the brain that are lacking in classical estrogen receptors are still affected by this sex hormone, either by unrecognized estrogen receptors, membrane interactions, or via synaptic responses[31].

Table 1 Neurotransmitter involvement in depression and estrogen effects on central neurotransmitter levels

Depression	Estrogen
↓ Serotonin	↑ Serotonin
↓ Norepinephrine	↑ Norepinephrine
↓↑ Dopamine	↑↓ Dopamine
↑ Monoamine oxidase	↓ Monoamine oxidase
↓ γ-aminobutyric acid	↑ γ-aminobutyric acid
↓ Opioid	↑ Opioid
↑ β-adrenergic receptors	↓ β-adrenergic receptors

ESTROGEN AND SEROTONIN

The serotonergic system plays a substantial role in behaviors that are disturbed in affective disorders, including mood, sleep, sexual activity, appetite and cognitive ability[32]. Serotonin is a component in the development of depression, but whether this neurotransmitter is the key player is still being determined[32]. A new class of antidepressants are the selective serotonin-receptor uptake inhibitors (SSRI) which are extremely effective antidepressants despite their influence on just one neurotransmitter system[1].

Studies evaluating sexual behavior in animals have helped elucidate estrogen's role in the modulation of the serotonergic system. Basic animal investigations have found numerous effects of estrogen on serotonin synthesis, release, reuptake and catabolism, with most aspects of central monoamine metabolism being modulated by this sex hormone[33,34]. Estradiol administered to ovariectomized rats significantly increased the density of serotonin 2_A binding sites in the anterior frontal, anterior cingulate, olfactory tubercle, piriform cortex, nucleus accumbens and lateral dorsal raphe nucleus of the brain[35]. These areas in the CNS are involved in control of mood, emotion and behavior[35]. In addition, the serotonin 2_A receptors are involved in suicidal behavior[24]. This increase in serotonin 2_A receptor density would facilitate the propensity of neuronal cells to respond to a serotonin stimulus[24].

Imipramine, a tricyclic antidepressant, blocks the reuptake of serotonin in rats only when estrogen is present[36]. The reduction of serotonin 2_A receptor density by chronic treatment with imipramine does not occur unless estrogen is also available[37]. Estradiol administration to ovariectomized rats resulted in an acute reduction in serotonin 1 receptors with a later increase in serotonin receptor density in the hypothalamus, amygdala and preoptic area[38]. The expression of the gene coding for tryptophan hydroxylase, the rate limiting enzyme in serotonin synthesis, was significantly increased with the addition of estrogen in ovariectomized rhesus macaques[39].

In women of reproductive age, serotonin levels, platelet serotonin 2 receptor binding, serotonin uptake and 3H-imipramine binding all fluctuate according to the stage of the menstrual cycle and levels of ovarian hormones[40]. Platelet 3H-imipramine binding has been utilized as a biological index for depression as platelets are similar to binding sites in the brain and can modulate serotonin uptake[34,41]. Platelets concentrate serotonin through the serotonin transporter in a manner similar to that of serotonergic neurons in the CNS. Several studies have shown that a decrease in the number of platelet 3H-imipramine binding sites correlates with depressive symptomatology, indicating that decreased serotonin levels in platelets and therefore a correspondingly lower serotonin level in the CNS result in depression[34,41].

During the ovulatory period when estradiol levels are highest, a positive correlation was noted between estradiol levels and the density of 3H-imipramine binding sites on platelets and blood serotonin concentrations[14,42]. Thirty-one surgically menopausal women underwent a prospective double-blind cross-over study evaluating whether intramuscular estradiol treatment improved scores on the Beck Depression Inventory and the number of 3H-imipramine binding sites[14]. There was a positive correlation between mood, energy and number of 3H-imipramine binding sites on platelets with estradiol treatment which was reversed when the intramuscular placebo was begun[14].

Significantly lower blood concentrations of serotonin have been found in postmenopausal women when compared to premenopausal women[42]. Oral estradiol administered to these menopausal women increased serotonin blood levels to those compatible with the premenopausal state[42,43]. Estrogen also causes tryptophan, the precursor of serotonin, to be displaced from its binding sites to plasma albumin such that it increases the amount of free tryptophan available to the CNS[44].

There appears to be an age-associated decline in blood serotonin levels which would help explain why depression is more consistently seen with surgically menopausal women[42]. Younger women who undergo a surgical menopause have a more precipitous drop in both estrogen and serotonin levels, compared to older women undergoing natural menopause, and thus more psychological symptomatology.

Postmenopausal women with and without ERT were evaluated for their response to a serotonin agonist, meta-chlorophenylpiperazine (m-CPP), by measuring prolactin levels[40]. Women receiving ERT had an increased prolactin response with m-CPP compared to women not taking ERT, indicating that ERT had enhanced central serotonergic activity[40]. Other work which has supported a central increase in serotonin activity in women with estrogen treatment was done by Lippert and co-workers which showed a significant increase in urinary excretion of the serotonin metabolite, 5-hydroxyindole acetic acid after oral and transdermal administration of estradiol[26]. It has been found that an increase in serum estrogen levels within the physiological range will produce higher blood serotonin levels but supraphysiological doses of estrogens interrupt tryptophan metabolism, decrease serotonin uptake as well as down-regulate the estrogen receptor number and lead to depressive symptomatology[19,26,45].

ESTROGEN AND CATECHOLAMINES

In 1965, the catecholamine hypothesis of mood disorders was published by Schildkraut, suggesting that a deficiency in catecholamines, specifically norepinephrine, was associated with the depressive state[1]. Low levels of catecholamines, including norepinephrine, are considered to be important in precipitating a depressive event[7,46]. Several groups of antidepressants work by increasing levels of norepinephrine in the CNS, including tricyclic antidepressants, monoamine oxidase inhibitors, and serotonin-norepinephrine reuptake inhibitors[1].

Levels of norepinephrine were significantly increased after the administration of 17β-estradiol benzoate to cultures of hypothalamic tissue removed from female rats[47]. Estrogen appears to affect catecholaminergic synthesis, release, reuptake, metabolism and receptor function such that there is an overall stimulatory effect of estrogen on central norepinephrine activity and turnover[46]. A study evaluating women with 'postpartum blues' found significantly lower levels of norepinephrine on days when the self-rating mood scores were low[48].

Estrogen effects on the peripheral catecholamine system appear to be directly opposite to that found in the CNS. Several studies have shown that estrogen administration to postmenopausal women, who were then exposed to psychological stressors, had a decreased blood pressure response and attenuated increase in plasma norepinephrine, cortisol and glucocorticoid levels[49–51]. Due to advances in neuroscience and brain imaging it has been possible to demonstrate improved brain activation patterns and performance in postmenopausal women with regard to everyday memory tasks after ERT, most likely through increasing CNS acetylcholine concentrations[52,53]. Thus it is possible that the multiple positive effects of ERT on mood could also be related to improvement in daily function and response to stress in these women.

ESTROGEN AND DOPAMINE

Dopamine also plays a role in depression, with data suggesting that dopamine activity may be reduced in the depressive state with lower levels of dopamine found in depressed patients[54], though other work with depression has found increased dopamine activity with increased postsynaptic dopamine receptor binding[54]. Choreiform movement disorders have been seen during pregnancy and with the use of estrogen-containing oral contraceptives[55]. It has been postulated that elevated levels of estrogen cause a relative increase in dopamine neuronal function in the striatum with resultant chorea[55].

Dopaminergic neurons located within the substantia nigra have been separated into two classes, Type A and B[56]. Administration of 17-β estradiol to ovariectomized rats increased the activity of Type A and decreased the activity of Type B neurons[56]. Many antidepressants, including tricyclic antidepressants and monoamine oxidase inhibitors, induce subsensitivity of both dopamine Type A and B receptors, whereas estrogen acts in such a manner only on Type B receptors[56]. Estrogen also has an anti-depressant effect on the dopaminergic system by promoting a functional uncoupling of the D2 dopamine receptor in the anterior pituitary and decreasing dopamine receptors in the striatum[57,58].

Estrogen effects on the dopamine system though are not simple and unidirectional as some studies have shown an anti-dopaminergic effect of estrogen while others indicate that estrogen enhances dopamine function[56]. Ovariectomized rats had a significant increase in dopaminergic activity in the hippocampus and striatum which was reversed after chronic administration of estradiol benzoate[59], whereas other studies have shown that acute treatment with estradiol increases striatal dopamine metabolism and dopamine secretion from the hypothalamus[47,59].

ESTROGEN AND MONOAMINE OXIDASE

The monoamine oxidase inhibitors function as a class of antidepressants by inhibiting the monoamine oxidase enzyme which metabolizes the monoamine neurotransmitters such as norepinephrine, serotonin and dopamine[1]. Subcutaneous injections of estradiol to ovari-ectomized rats resulted in decreased activity of monoamine oxidase in the amygdala and hypo-thalamus[60]. This effect was blocked by concomi-tant administration of an estrogen antagonist[60]. In addition, the quantitative decrease in monoamine oxidase activity was related to the amount of estrogen given[60]. This effect of estro-gen was confirmed in two other studies utilizing ovariectomized rats. After injections with estradiol, monoamine oxidase activity was decreased only in areas of the brain known to have estrogen receptors, including the hypo-thalamus and locus coeruleus[61,62].

Monoamine oxidase activity increases after menopause, resulting in plasma monoamine oxidase activity in non-depressed premeno-pausal women that is 75% lower than levels found in non-depressed postmenopausal women, 600 c.p.m./ml and 2500 c.p.m./ml respectively[63]. Elevated levels of plasma mono-amine oxidase activity in depressed women have been shown to be significantly reduced, by approximately 60%, with the addition of ERT[63].

ESTROGEN AND GABA, OPIOID AND β-ADRENERGIC RECEPTORS

A decrease in the GABA system has also been associated with the depressive state. Cerebro-spinal fluid concentrations of GABA are low in depressed patients, GABA agonists repress depression and tricyclic antidepressants inhibit GABA uptake and stimulate its release[64]. Using rats, it has been shown that the postpartum period is associated with a significant decrease in the density of GABA-A receptors[64]. Also, administration of estradiol to ovariectomized rats resulted in the up-regulation of GABA receptors throughout the CNS with the anti-estrogen, tamoxifen, blocking this effect[65].

Postmenopausal women have lower opioid activity in the hypothalamus which is believed to be related to decreased serum estrogen levels[66]. After ERT, hypothalamic opioidergic activity is increased so that the elevated mood seen in treated postmenopausal women might be related to β-endorphin production[67,68].

Finally, increased β-adrenergic receptor density was found at post-mortem in brains of people who committed suicide[20]. In ovari-ectomized rats, a reduction in β-adrenergic receptors after chronic treatment with estradiol was noted[25,69]. This is the only result that is common to several forms of antidepressant therapy, including electroconvulsive shock, monoamine oxidase inhibitors, atypical anti-depressants and tricyclic antidepressants[25].

ESTROGEN TREATMENT IN WOMEN

For over 60 years the use of estrogen as an anti-depressant in peri- and postmenopausal women has been evaluated with no consensus reached as to its clinical effectiveness[9]. A meta-analysis of 111 articles published in 1995 on psychological symptoms of menopausal women receiving HRT concluded that there was no apparent positive correlation between HRT and psycho-logical improvement[70]. The authors also reported that few studies controlled for social stresses, vasomotor symptomatology, or placebo effect[70]. In addition, both standardized and non-standardized psychological tests were employed by these researchers[70]. In contrast, a meta-analysis performed 2 years later, of 26 published studies evaluating the use of HRT and ERT on depressed mood, found that ERT exerted a moderate to large effect on mood while the addition of progesterone dampened the positive impact of estrogen[71]. In addition, the authors point out that the antidepressant effect of estrogen may not be apparent until after 3 months of treatment[71]. Treatment strategies of less than 3 months duration might have contributed to the earlier studies showing no effect of ERT on mood.

Several of these studies were flawed by numerous confounding variables. The designation of peri- and postmenopausal status in these women was not consistent across the studies, with some researchers evaluating serum hormone levels and others determining patient status by history[71]. Plasma estrogen levels are variable from one woman to the next at the climacteric, with normal, low and even high estrogen levels found in these women, which further confounds the relationship between menopause and depression, such that the designation of a woman as peri- or postmenopausal does not ensure a hypoestrogenic state[34,72]. Work by Santoro and colleagues on perimenopausal serum steroid levels showed alternating hypergonadotropic hypoestrogenism as well as hyperestrogenism in these women[72]. In addition, there is a difference in diffusion rates across the blood–brain barrier for sex steroids, such that it is difficult to extrapolate serum estrogen levels to those present in the brain, and therefore it has been suggested that the patient can be used only as 'her own best bioassay'[19].

Researchers have used several psychological tests, including the Center for Epidemiologic Studies Depression Scale and Beck Depression Inventory, which might not be appropriate in peri- and postmenopausal women to measure depressed mood[12,71]. The Women's Health Questionnaire, which assesses mood and controls for somatic complaints, vasomotor symptoms and sleep disturbances, has been proposed as a more applicable test[73]. The 'domino effect' of depression in postmenopausal women suggests that estrogen deficiency results in vasomotor symptomatology and sleep disturbances which then can lead to psychological symptoms of depression[74]. If vasomotor symptoms are controlled for, then the antidepressant effect of estrogen alone can be evaluated.

One study divided a group of healthy perimenopausal women with moderate vasomotor symptoms into treatment protocols which used two different dosages of conjugated equine estrogens with or without medroxyprogesterone acetate[75]. All groups had similar control of their hot flushes and felt a subjective improvement in mood but the group receiving the higher dose of conjugated equine estrogens reported a greater sense of well-being, while the addition of medroxyprogesterone acetate dampened this positive mood[75]. In additional work by Ditkoff and associates, surgically menopausal women with no vasomotor symptomatology showed improvement in depression scores while on conjugated equine estrogens[76].

Another hypothesis for ERT is that estrogen has a 'mental tonic' effect which improves mood but does not treat clinical depression[53,76]. There are only a few case reports in the literature that describe a clinical antidepressant effect of estrogen. A case study of high dose conjugated equine estrogens (15–25 mg doses) reported its use as an effective antidepressant in a group of 23 severely depressed pre- and postmenopausal women[63]. Another case report of a 35-year-old woman who had a 24-year history of numerous depressive and manic episodes, previously treated with several psychotropic agents and hospitalized four times, had significant improvement in her mood, cognition, libido and energy level when placed on a combination oral contraceptive pill[77].

The mental tonic effect of ERT has been supported by several studies, including one that reported decreased depression scores, increased hypomanic scores and a decrease in a schizophrenia scale in women taking conjugated equine estrogens[76]. A well-designed prospective cross-over study by Barbara Sherwin evaluated healthy non-depressed premeno-pausal women who had undergone psycho-logical testing prior to total abdominal hyster-ectomy and bilateral salpingo-oophorectomy for benign disease[28]. They were then placed on monthly intramuscular injections of either estrogen, androgen, estrogen–androgen, or placebo for 3 months[28]. During the fourth month all participants received placebo before crossing over to a new treatment[28]. For both treatment stages, women who received placebo had higher depression scores when compared to the women receiving any of the hormone preparations[28].

It must be emphasized that all the clinical trials used different HRT strategies, including various forms of estrogens, androgens and progestins with varying routes of administra-tion. Androgens have been shown to enhance mood, possibly by their 'energizing properties' and by aromatization to estrogen in the CNS[78]. It has been noted that progestins have a negative effect on mood, resulting in increased depres-sion scores[67,75,79]. The mechanism of progestin effect could be related to the sedative and anesthetic effects of progesterone on CNS neurotransmitters but it could also be due to estrogen receptor depletion and increasing monoamine oxidase activity[19]. In rats, chronic estrogen treatment caused an increase in the number of cortical serotonin 2 receptors but when progesterone was given in combination with estrogen there was no increase noted in serotonin 2 receptor binding[25]. Not all progestins are equal as each has its own variable effect on mood[80].

Cyclic mood and behavioral symptoms have been associated with sequential HRT and may improve with a switch to continuous combined estrogen plus progestin therapy[6]. Continuous HRT in low dosages has been shown to have fewer psychological side-effects[6,80]. Uriel Halbreich has successfully used cyclic adminis-tration of ERT with no progestins, but practi-tioners must use caution with this clinical regimen[80].

Several studies have concluded that the administration of transdermal estrogen, rather than an oral route, has a more positive effect on psychological symptomatology because serotonin is more effectively induced by the con-sistent and continuous delivery of estrogen[49]. Supraphysiological levels of estrogen may actu-ally down-regulate estrogen receptor activity and have a negative impact on mood[19]. So the addition of ERT to women who might be hyperestrogenic despite their peri- and post-menopausal status might result in an increase in negative mood. Finally, the use of other estrogens rarely used in ERT, such as 17β-hydroxyestradiol, ethinylestradiol and estriol, have a positive impact on blood serotonin levels and mood in postmenopausal women[7,42].

There are several published articles which support the antidepressant nature of estrogen. Four women, with no prior psychiatric illnesses, developed panic disorder and/or major depres-sion with and without psychotic features while on gonadotropin-releasing hormone (GnRH) agonists for treatment of endometriosis[81]. Three of the four responded with administra-tion of an SSRI, sertraline (Zoloft)[81]. Rapid mood cycling has been acknowledged as a com-plication of antidepressant medications and has been found to occur with estrogen as well[82]. A postmenopausal woman with severe depression developed rapid cycles of euthymia, hypomania and depression when started on conjugated equine estrogens and had an abrupt cessation of the mood cycling when her ERT was stopped[82].

Another case study involved a group of women with major depression who had a history of a good response with antidepressants, who subsequently failed treatment for their recur-rent depression after they had been placed on tamoxifen, an antiestrogen[83]. Work done by Schneider and colleagues with clinically depressed women over the age of 60 revealed a possible synergistic effect between estrogen and the SSRI, fluoxetine (Prozac) such that lower doses of antidepressants might be efficacious in women already on ERT[74,82]. This correlates with other work that has shown a decreased dosage of antidepressants required during the follicular phase of the menstrual cycle in young cycling women[7]. A community-based sample of post-menopausal women found a decreased risk of depressed mood in women over the age of 60 if they were on ERT[11]. It is possible that ERT might prevent the development of depression in this older age group[11].

If decreasing levels of estrogen in the CNS account for the increased likelihood of depression in women, then this could explain why men are at a reduced risk for affective disorders. Plasma testosterone levels in men are nearly 1000 times greater than estradiol concentrations in women[35]. Aromatization of testosterone into 17β-estradiol in the CNS could result in brain levels of this estrogen just as high as those seen in women[35]. But aging men do not have the abrupt drop in plasma sex hormone levels that are seen in women going through the menopause[35].

CONCLUSION

Currently two out of three depressed patients are female with clinical depression considered an 'endemic part of the female experience'[2,74]. Several researchers have concluded that the question is not whether mood is associated with levels of sex steroids, but instead to determine which women are affected by these changes and the appropriate treatment for them[2]. Antidepressants are not a panacea as 30% of patients do not respond to these medications, while others react only partially or cannot tolerate the numerous side-effects[21,84]. The use of ERT with its concomitant benefits to the cardiovascular, musculoskeletal, genitourinary and neurological systems might be a reasonable first step in the treatment of mild to moderate depression in the peri- and postmenopausal woman. The potential synergistic effect of estrogen with antidepressants might allow a lower dosage of antidepressants to be used and help those patients whose symptoms are refractory to conventional psychopharmacology. Alternative HRT strategies can be employed in women who do not have elevation of their mood with their initial HRT. The multiple and complex effects of estrogen on CNS neurotransmitters are still being investigated, not only with regard to mood disorders but also in terms of cognitive function in the peri- and postmenopausal woman.

References

1. Barbieri RL, Cohen LS, Ling FW, *et al.* Depressive disorders in women: diagnosis, treatment and monitoring. *APGO Educational Series on Women's Health Issues* 1997.
2. Foote D, Seibert S. The age of anxiety. *Newsweek* Spring/Summer 1999:68–75
3. Blumenthal SJ. Women and depression. *J Women's Health* 1994;3:467–79
4. Pearlstein T, Rosen K, Stone AB. Mood disorders and menopause. *Endocrinol Metab Clin North Am.* 1997;26:279–94
5. Studd JWW, Smith RNJ. Estrogens and depression in women. *Menopause* 1994;3:467–79
6. Schmidt PJ, Rubinow DR. Menopause-related affective disorders: a justification for further study. *Am J Psychiatr* 1991;148:844–52
7. Vliet EL, Davis VLH. New perspectives on the relationship of hormone changes to affective disorders in the perimenopause. *NAACOGS Clin Issu Perinat Women's Health Nurs* 1991;2:453–71
8. Anderson E, Hamburger S, Liu JH, *et al.* Characteristics of menopausal women seeking assistance. *Am J Obstet Gynecol* 1987;156:428–33
9. Smith RNJ, Studd JWW. Estrogens and depression in women. In Lobo RA, ed. *Treatment of the Postmenopausal Woman: Basic and Clinical Aspects.* New York: Raven Press, 1994;119–27
10. Avis NE, McKinlay SM. The Massachusetts women's health study: an epidemiologic investigation of the menopause. *JAMWA* 1995;50:45–63
11. Palinkas LA, Barrett-Connor E. Estrogen use and depressive symptoms in postmenopausal women. *Obstet Gynecol* 1992;80:30–6
12. Kaufert PA, Gilbert P, Tate R. The Manitoba Project: a re-examination of the link between menopause and depression. *Maturitas* 1992;14:143–55
13. Khastgir G, Studd J. Hysterectomy, ovarian failure, and depression. *Menopause* 1998;5:113–22
14. Sherwin BB, Suranyi-Cadotte BE. Up-regulatory effect of estrogen on platelet 3H-imipramine

binding sites in surgically menopausal women. *Biol Psychiatr* 1990;28:339–48

15. Pearlstein TB. Hormones and depression: what are the facts about premenstrual syndrome, menopause and hormone replacement therapy? *Am J Obstet Gynecol* 1995;173:646–53

16. Plotsky PM, Owens MJ, Nemeroff CB. Psychoneuroendocrinology of depression. Hypothalamic–pituitary–adrenal axis. *Psychiatr Clin North Am* 1998;21:293–307

17. Woods NF, Mitchell ES. Patterns of depressed mood in midlife women: observations from the Seattle Midlife Women's Health Study. *Res Nurs Health* 1996;19:111–23

18. Hunter MS. Somatic experience of the menopause: a prospective study. *Psychosom Med* 1990; 52:357–67

19. Arpels JC. The female brain hypoestrogenic continuum from the premenstrual syndrome to menopause. A hypothesis and review of supporting data. *J Reprod Med* 1996;41:633–9

20. Nemeroff CB, Musselman DL, Nathan KI, *et al.* Pathophysiological basis of psychiatric disorders: Focus on mood disorders and schizophrenia. *Psychiatry Volume 2.* Philadelphia, USA: WB Saunders Company, 1997:258–72

21. Schrof JM, Schultz S. Melancholy nation. *U.S. News & World Report* March 8, 1999:56–63

22. Stahl SM. Estrogen makes the brain a sex organ. *J Clin Psychiatr* 1997;58:421–2

23. Fillit H. Future therapeutic developments of estrogen use. *J Clin Pharmacol* 1995;35:25S–28S

24. Sumner BEH, Fink G. Estrogen increases the density of 5-hydroxytryptamine 2A receptors in cerebral cortex and nucleus accumbens in the female rat. *J Steroid Biochem Molec Biol* 1995;54: 15–20

25. Biegon A, Reches A, Snyder L, *et al.* Serotonergic and noradrenergic receptors in the rat brain: modulation by chronic exposure to ovarian hormones. *Life Sci* 1983;32:2015–21

26. Lippert TH, Filshie M, Muck AO, *et al.* Serotonin metabolite excretion after postmenopausal estradiol therapy. *Maturitas* 1996;24:37–41

27. Ffrench-Mullen JMH, Spence KT. Neurosteroids block Ca+2 channel current in freshly isolated hippocampal CA1 neurons. *Eur J Pharmacol* 1991; 202:269–72

28. Sherwin BB. Impact of the changing hormonal milieu on psychological functioning. In Lobo RA, ed. *Treatment of the Postmenopausal Woman: Basic and Clinical Aspects.* New York: Raven Press, 1994;119–27

29. Majewska MD. Sex differences in brain morphology and pharmacodynamics. In Jensvold MF, Halbreich U, Hamilton JA, eds. *Psychopharmacology and Women: Sex, Gender and Hormones.* Washington DC: American Psychiatric Press, 1996;73–83

30. George MS, Ketter TA, Parekh PI, *et al.* Gender differences in regional cerebral blood flow during transient self-induced sadness or happiness. *Biol Psychiatr* 1996;40:859–71

31. McEwen BS, Alves SE, Bulloch K, *et al.* Ovarian steroids and the brain: implications for cognition and aging. *Neurology* 1997;48:S8–S15

32. Meltzer HY. Role of serotonin in depression. *Ann N Y Acad Sci* 1990;600:486–95

33. Maswood S, Stewart G, Uphouse L. Gender and estrous cycle effects on the 5-HT1A agonist, 8-OH-DPAT, on hypothalamic serotonin. *Pharmacol Biochem Behav* 1995;51:807–13

34. Guicheny P, Leger D, Barraat J, *et al.* Platelet serotonin content and plasma tryptophan in peri- and postmenopausal women: variations with plasma oestrogen levels and depressive symptoms. *Eur J Clin Invest* 1988;18:297–304

35. Fink G, Sumner BEH, Rosie R, *et al.* Estrogen control of central neurotransmission: effect on mood, mental state, and memory. *Cell Mol Neurobiol* 1996;16:325–44

36. Fludder JM, Tonge SR, Leonard BE. Modification by ethinyloestradiol and progesterone of the effects of imipramine on 5-hydroxytryptamine metabolism in discrete areas of rat brain. *Br J Pharmacol* 1997;60:309P–10P

37. Kendall DA, Stancel GM, Enna SJ. Imipramine: effect of ovarian steroids on modifications in serotonin receptor binding. *Science* 1981;211: 1183–5

38. Biegon A, McEwen BS. Modulation by estradiol of serotonin 1 receptors in brain. *J Neurosci* 1982;2:199–205

39. Pecins-Thompson M, Brown NA, Kohama SG, *et al.* Ovarian steroid regulation of tryptophan hydroxylase mRNA expression in rhesus macaques. *J Neurosci* 1996;16:7021–9

40. Halbreich U, Rojansky N, Palter S, *et al.* Estrogen augments serotonergic activity in postmenopausal women. *Biol Psychiatr* 1995;37:434–41

41. Roy A, Everett D, Pickar D, *et al.* Platelet tritiated imipramine binding and serotonin uptake in depressed patients and controls. *Arch Gen Psychiatr* 1987;44:320–7

42. Gonzales GF. Blood levels of 5-hydroxytryptamine in human beings under several physiological situations. *Life Sci* 1980;27: 647–50

43. Gonzales GF, Carrillo C. Blood serotonin levels in postmenopausal women: effects of age and serum oestradiol levels. *Maturitas* 1993;17:23–9

44. Sherwin BB. Menopause, early aging and elderly women. In Jensvold MF, Halbreich U, Hamilton JA, eds. *Psychopharmacology and Women: Sex, Gender and Hormones.* Washington DC: American Psychiatric Press, 1996;225–37

45. Rehavi M, Sepcuti H, Weizman A. Upregulation of imipramine binding and serotonin uptake by

estradiol in female rat brain. *Brain Res* 1987;410: 135–9

46. Janowsky DS, Halbreich U, Rausch J. Association among ovarian hormones, other hormones, emotional disorders and neurotransmitters. In Jensvold MF, Halbreich U, Hamilton JA, eds. *Psychopharmacology and Women: Sex, Gender and Hormones.* Washington DC: American Psychiatric Press, 1996;85–106

47. Paul SM, Axelrod J, Saavedra JM, *et al.* Estrogen-induced efflux of endogenous catecholamines from the hypothalamus in vitro. *Brain Res* 1979; 178:499–505

48. Kuevi V, Causon R, Dixson AF, *et al.* Plasma amine and hormone changes in 'post-partum blues'. *Clin Endocrinol* 1983;19:39–46

49. Lindheim SR, Legro RS, Bernstein L, *et al.* Behavioral stress responses in premenopausal and postmenopausal women and the effects of estrogen. *Am J Obstet Gynecol* 1992;167:1831–6

50. Owens JF, Stoney CM, Matthews KA. Menopausal status influences ambulatory blood pressure levels and blood pressure changes during mental stress. *Circulation* 1993;88:2794–802

51. Komesaroff PA, Esler MD, Sudhir K. Estrogen supplementation attenuates glucocorticoid and catecholamine responses to mental stress in perimenopausal women. *J Clin Endocrinol Metab* 1999;84:606–10

52. Shaywitz SE, Shaywitz BA, Pugh KR, *et al.* Effect of estrogen on brain activity patterns in postmenopausal women during working memory tasks. *JAMA* 1999;281:1197–202

53. Sherwin BB. Hormones, mood, and cognitive function in postmenopausal women. *Obstet Gynecol* 1996;87:20S–6S

54. Thase ME, Howland RH. Biological processes in depression: an updated review and integration. In Beckham EE, Leber WR, eds. *Handbook of Depression. Second Edition.* New York: The Guilford Press, 1995;213–79

55. Hruska RE, Ludmer LM, Pitman KT, *et al.* Effects of estrogen on striatal dopamine receptor function in male and female rats. *Pharmacol Biochem Behav* 1982;16:285–91

56. Chiodo LA, Caggiula AR. Substantia nigra dopamine neurons: alterations in basal discharge rates and autoreceptor sensitivity induced by estrogen. *Neuropharmacology* 1983;22: 593–9

57. Becker JB. Estrogen rapidly potentiates amphetamine-induced striatal dopamine release and rotational behavior during microdialysis. *Neurosci Lett* 1990;118:169–71

58. Munemura M, Agui T, Sibley DR. Chronic estrogen treatment promotes a functional uncoupling of the D2 dopamine receptor in rat anterior pituitary gland. *Endocrinology* 1989;124: 346–55

59. Bitar MS, Ota M, Linnoila M, *et al.* Modification of gonadectomy-induced increases in brain monoamine metabolism by steroid hormones in male and female rats. *Psychoneuroendocrinology* 1991;16:547–57

60. Luine VN, Khylchevskaya RI, McEwen BS. Effect of gonadal steroids on activities of monoamine oxidase and choline acetylase in rat brain. *Brain Res* 1975;86:293–306

61. Chevillard C, Barden N, Saavedra JM. Estradiol treatment decreases type A and increases type B monoamine oxidase in specific brain stem areas and cerebellum of ovariectomized rats. *Brain Res* 1981;222:177–81

62. Luine VN, Rhodes JC. Gonadal hormone regulation of MAO and other enzymes in hypothalamic areas. *Neuroendocrinology* 1983;36:235–41

63. Klaiber EL, Broverman DM, Vogel W, *et al.* Estrogen therapy for severe persistent depressions in women. *Arch Gen Psychiatr* 1979;36:550–4

64. Majewska MD. Neurosteroids: endogenous bimodal modulators of the GABA$_A$ receptor. Mechanism of action and physiological significance. *Prog Neurobiol* 1992;38:379–95

65. Maggi A, Perez J. Estrogen-induced up-regulation of γ-aminobutyric receptors in the CNS of rodents. *J Neurochem* 1986;47:1793–7

66. Schurz B, Wimmer-Greinecker G, Metka M, *et al.* β-endorphin levels during the climacteric period. *Maturitas* 1988;10:45–50

67. Blum I, Vered Y, Lifshitz A, *et al.* The effect of estrogen replacement therapy on plasma serotonin and catecholamines of postmenopausal women. *Isr J Med Sci* 1996;32:1158–62

68. D'Amico JF, Greendale GA, Lu JKH, *et al.* Induction of hypothalamic opioid activity with transdermal estradiol administration in postmenopausal women. *Fertil Steril* 1991;55:754–8

69. Wagner HR, Crutcher KA, Davis JN. Chronic estrogen treatment decreases β-adrenergic responses in rat cerebral cortex. *Brain Res* 1979;171:147–51

70. Pearce J, Hawton K, Blake F. Psychological and sexual symptoms associated with the menopause and the effects of hormone replacement therapy. *Br J Psychiatr* 1995;167:163–73

71. Zweifel JE, O'Brien WH. A meta-analysis of the effect of hormone replacement therapy upon depressed mood. *Psychoneuroendocrinology* 1997; 22:189–212

72. Santoro N, Brown JR, Adel T, *et al.* Characterization of reproductive hormonal dynamics in the perimenopause. *J Clin Endocrinol Metab* 1996;81: 1495–501

73. Gillis S, Waltrous M, Mik J. Quality of life in peri- and postmenopause: a multi-country analysis using the women's health questionnaire. Poster presented at The North American Menopause Society, September 1997.

74. Landau C, Milan FB. Assessment and treatment of depression during the menopause: a preliminary report. *Menopause* 1996;3:201–7

75. Sherwin BB, Gelfand MM. A prospective one-year study of estrogen and progestin in postmenopausal women: effects on clinical symptoms and lipoprotein lipids. *Obstet Gynecol* 1989;73:759–766

76. Ditkoff EC, Crary WG, Cristo M, *et al.* Estrogen improves psychological function in asymptomatic postmenopausal women. *Obstet Gynecol* 1991;78:991–5

77. Price WA, Giannini AJ. Antidepressant effects of estrogen. *J Clin Psychiatr* 1985;46:506

78. Sherwin BB. Affective changes with estrogen and androgen replacement therapy in surgically menopausal women. *J Affect Disord* 1988;14:177–87

79. Holst J, Backstrom T, Hammarback S, *et al.* Progestogen addition during oestrogen replacement therapy – effects on vasomotor symptoms and mood. *Maturitas* 1989;11:13–20

80. Halbreich U. Role of estrogen in postmenopausal depression. *Neurology* 1997;48:S16–S20

81. Warnock JK, Bundren JC. Anxiety and mood disorders associated with gonadotropin-releasing hormone agonist therapy. *Psychopharm Bull* 1997;33:31–16

82. Oppenheim G. A case of rapid mood cycling with estrogen: implications for therapy. *J Clin Psychiatr* 1984;45:34–5

83. Halbreich U. Gonadal hormones and anti-hormones, serotonin and mood. *Psychopharm Bull* 1990;26:291–5

84. McElroy SL, Keck PE, Friedman LM. Practical management of antidepressant side effects: an update. In Hales RE, Yudofsky SC, eds. *Practical Clinical Strategies in Treating Depression and Anxiety Disorders in a Managed Care Environment.* Washington DC: American Psychiatric Association, 1996;39–48

14

Hormones and hemostasis

A. Cano

THE HEMOSTATIC SYSTEM

Hemostasis is a physiological mechanism that maintains blood fluidity within the vascular tree. The privation of that function leads to disorders such as acute coronary heart syndrome, increasingly recognized as a primary consequence of a local imbalance of the hemostatic mechanism[1-3]. Also, hemostasis prevents the loss of blood through breach disruptions in the normal vasculature. Such crucial functions cannot be left under the control of a simple, brittle system. Hemostasis is, in fact, a complex mechanism resulting from the dynamic equilibrium between pro-coagulant and anticoagulant checks and balances, together with pro- and antifibrinolytic activities.

In the normal state, the system works to prevent the local accumulation of activated blood-clotting enzymes and complexes. In the case of a vascular injury, circulating platelets are exposed to the subendothelial layers and, subsequently, attach to the injured surface, and become highly adherent. The bound platelets degranulate and provide receptors for the assembly of blood-clotting enzyme complexes[4-6]. Together with the activation of platelets, the exposure to non-vascular cell-bound tissue factor in the subendothelial space activates the extrinsic pathway of blood coagulation. Figure 1 is a simplified summary depicting the cascade of proteolytic reactions involved in the extrinsic pathway, whose final step is the generation of fibrin monomers as a result of the cleavage of fibrinogen by thrombin. These monomers polymerize and link to one

another to form a chemically stable clot. Thus, the coagulation cascade shows the remarkable ability to amplify the signal generated by a small initiating stimulus into a potentially explosive chain reaction. This is accomplished by a well-orchestrated participation of distinct procoagulant factors, which are zymogens providing a reservoir ready to transform into active proteases, then receiving the suffix 'a'. As shown in Figure 1, activation of factor X to Xa links the intrinsic and extrinsic pathways of the coagulation cascade. Factor XII initiates the extrinsic pathway, but its importance for the formation of the thrombus is dubious, since patients with hereditary factor XII deficiency do not suffer from bleeding diathesis.

The limiting factor of that potentially uncontrolled reaction is provided by the natural anticoagulant mechanisms. Antithrombin III and protein C, with the concurrent participation of its co-factor protein S, are the main actors of this system. The activity of antithrombin III is potentiated by the presence of endogenous heparan sulfate, whereas protein C is activated by thrombin, when in presence of thrombomodulin, a protein bound to endothelial cells. The antithrombin III pathway inhibits several activated coagulation enzymes by forming complexes, like the thrombin–antithrombin III complexes (TAT), which are rapidly cleared from the circulation by the reticuloendothelial system. The thrombomodulin-activated protein C (APC) inhibits coagulation by proteolytic cleavage of

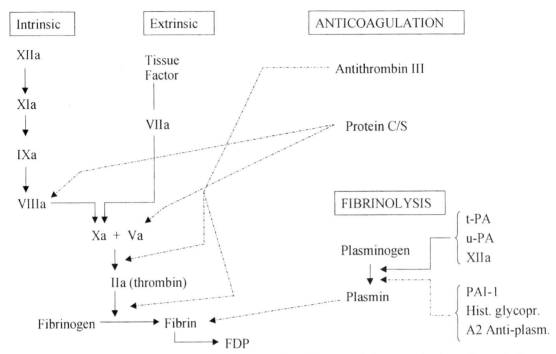

COAGULATION CASCADE

Figure 1 This figure includes a schematic representation of the coagulation cascade, the anticoagulation system, and fibrinolysis, the three mechanisms which regulate the hemostatic system. On the left, the coagulation cascade is represented by both the intrinsic and the extrinsic arms, described through only the activated form of the distinct enzymes. Coagulation initiates by interaction of tissue factor bound to the cell membranes with factor VIIa. Activation of factor X links the extrinsic and intrinsic pathways, although factor VIIa also activates factor IX (not shown in the figure). Factor Xa converts prothrombin to thrombin in a reaction activated by factor Va. Anticoagulation is carried into effect by the antithrombin III and the protein C/S pathways. Antithrombin III neutralizes thrombin instantly, and also inhibits other enzymes of the cascade, such as XIa, IXa, and Xa. The protein C/S pathway interacts with thrombomodulin (not shown in the figure) to inactivate factors Va and VIIIa. The fibrinolytic activity resides in the conversion of plasminogen to plasmin, a protease which degrades fibrin to fibrin degradation products (FDP). Plasminogen is activated by tissue plasminogen activator (t-PA), urokinase plasminogen activator (u-PA) and factor XIIa, whereas plasminogen activator inhibitor type 1 (PAI-1) exerts an anti-fibrinolytic effect together with histidine glycoprotein and α2 anti-plasmin. Links are represented by solid (when stimulatory) or dashed (when inhibitory) arrows

activated factors VIII and V; the R506Q mutation in factor V, also known as factor V Leiden, is therefore a major cause of resistance to APC[7].

Fibrinolysis is, finally, a mechanism of the hemostatic system which regulates fibrin formation through a controlled degradation of fibrin by plasmin. Plasmin is a powerful protease which derives from plasminogen, a zymogen whose activation is regulated by a system of activators and inhibitors. Among them, tissue plasminogen activator (t-PA) is produced in the endothelium and, in the presence of fibrin, activates plasminogen to produce plasmin. Plasminogen activator inhibitor type 1 (PAI-1) is produced in endothelial and hepatic cells and, in balance with t-PA, constitutes the major ruler of fibrinolysis[8]. Other minor regulators of fibrinolysis are factor XIIa and urokinase plasminogen activator (u-PA) among the activators, and histidine glycoprotein and α2-antiplasmin, among the inhibitors[8].

It is important to note that, together with the self limitation of the activation of the cascade, as determined by the interplay between the prothrombotic and the anticoagulant mechanisms, the clot is a focal lesion. This characteristic may be understandable in the context of the local endothelial disruption that generates an imbalance of the system, as described above, but may be puzzling in cases of systemic alterations in the hemostatic system, which also originate thrombotic lesions in discrete areas of the vascular tree. The correct understanding of the particulars which condition the focality of the thrombotic lesion is becoming a crucial point in the clarification of the mechanisms of hemostasis.

FACTORS UNDERLINING THE FOCALITY OF THE THROMBOTIC LESIONS

There is actually little doubt that, in keeping with the triad of Virchow, the three mechanisms that condition the thrombotic phenotype are the two already mentioned, local injury to the vessel wall and procoagulant activation of the hemostatic equilibrium, and third, the decrease in blood flow. The relative implication of each of those three determinants in the formation of a clot at a certain site of the vascular tree is as yet unknown.

The weight of the vessel wall factor is probably of particular relevance when considering the hemostatic actions of the ovarian steroids, where there seems to be a trend favoring venous thrombosis, whereas the opposite holds for the arterial tree. In addition to this general segregation into either the venous or the arterial vessels, there may also be thrombotic lesions specifically linked to a more concrete vascular place. The frequent location at the portal, hepatic, and mesenteric veins in cases of paroxysmal nocturnal hemoglobinuria[9,10] is a clear example. Other clinical observations, like the predisposition to cause thrombosis in the retina or placenta vessels in patients with the antiphospholipid–antibody syndrome, additionally illustrate this characteristic action of the hemostatic system.

There is also a certain association between the nature of hemostatic imbalance and the phenotype of the lesion in some cases. For example, congenital deficiencies of antithrombin III, protein C and protein S are preferentially associated with a higher risk of deep venous, but not arterial, thrombosis[11,12]. However, mutations in the factor V gene (factor V Leiden), and in the prothrombin gene, determine a higher risk for not only deep venous thrombosis of the legs and brain[13,14] but also arterial thrombosis of the coronary tree in women who smoke[13,15].

To complicate things further, it appears that the conjunction of distinct combinations of the three Virchow's mechanisms may also create specific phenotypes, as is the case of the higher perioperative risk of venous thrombotic episodes resulting from the decreased flow, focal disruption of the vessel wall, and deficiencies in the anticoagulant system[16].

Given the complexity of this scenario, clarifying the effects of the ovarian steroids is a rather intricate task. A rational approach might be, perhaps, to contrast the clinical observations with the biological data, since this might help to raise hypotheses on the already dark areas of the hormonal action. This should be done while keeping in mind that the net effect on clotting and fibrinolysis and the potential clinical implications of hormone replacement therapy (HRT), are still unclear; existing data derive from population-based studies or small trials assessing biological intermediates of hemostasis, whose variability and definitive clinical relevance is not completely confirmed.

CLINICALLY OBSERVABLE EFFECTS OF HORMONES ON THE HEMOSTATIC SYSTEM

One principal lesson of the numerous studies on the thrombogenic role of ovarian steroids has been that this is a dose-dependent phenomenon, mainly linked to estrogens[17]. The coronary heart disease events detected in women who were using the old oral contraceptives were drastically reduced when the estrogenic component was diminished. The more recent data provided by studies on women using the modern preparations with either 30 or 20 µg of ethinyl estradiol have shown neutral effects on coronary heart disease[18]. The relative risk for venous thrombosis, on the contrary, seems still increased, although the absolute risk is as low as 4.6 cases per 10 000 exposed woman years[19].

The distinct formulations employed in HRT almost universally include natural estrogens. Their lower potency is clearly reflected in their markedly diminished effect on hemostasis, the effect on thrombin generation being virtually immeasurable[20]. The perception exists that, within the estrogenic dose range accomplished by HRT, the improvement in fibrinolytic capacity may exceed the activation of baseline coagulation, as suggested by the preservation of a marked reduction in PAI-I in the presence of undetectable activation of coagulation[21,22]. In fact, there is general agreement on the protective effect of HRT on arterial thrombogenesis. Nonetheless, four distinct retrospective studies[23–26] have presented concordant data on an association between the use of HRT and a mean relative risk of deep venous thrombosis oscillating between 2.1 and 3.6. Together with the variables at work in this different behavior of the arterial and venous trees, the fact that the lower estrogen–progestin dosages used in HRT maintain the venous thrombotic risk of oral contraceptives may possibly be influenced by the implication of risk factors other than the induction of a hemostatic imbalance.

The clinical effects of progestins seem of less importance. As for estrogens, part of the information on the progestin action has been gathered from studies in the field of contraception, with the use of progestin-only pills. Although the data are scarce, most authors agree that there is no consistent pattern of clinical effects on hemostasis[17]. There has been recent controversy, however, on the risk of venous thromboembolism among users of gestodene and desogestrel, two third-generation progestins, versus levonorgestrel-containing combined oral contraceptives. The retrospective nature of the original studies, together with the possible influence of distinct types of bias[19,27], have deactivated the original prevention. Moreover, as confirmed in a recent review, an analysis of the 17 comparative studies showed

no difference between the desogestrel- and gestodene-containing and the levonorgestrel-containing oral contraceptives[28].

In short, the inconsistencies linked to the eventual role of progestins on thrombogenesis leave estrogen as the main actor in this scenario. The following sections will be dedicated, therefore, to reviewing the biological data about the action of estrogens on two factors of the Virchow's triad, the balance between the procoagulant, anticoagulant and fibrinolytic factors, and the endothelium. There is less wealth of data concerning eventual modifications of the blood flow in venous territories.

THE BIOLOGICAL EFFECT OF ESTROGENS ON THE HEMOSTATIC BALANCE

As mentioned above, the procoagulant factors are inactive zymogens which require activation to develop their potential functionality. It is important to note that the coagulant factors are present in concentrations far in excess of the physiological need. Accordingly, changes in the plasma level of inactive zymogens, as it occurs after use of estrogens in HRT, may have little impact. Some procoagulant factors have been ascribed estrogen regulation of their genes, such as factor XII[29], factor VII[30], factors VIII and IX[20] and fibrinogen[30–32]

It seems therefore, and this is an important conclusion when trying to measure clinically any activation of coagulation, that functional measurements should be preferable to the assessment of protein concentrations of zymogens[33]. The TAT complexes, for example, may give a better idea of the amount of thrombin that has been produced. Fibrinopeptide A (FPA), a peptide which is released from fibrinogen by the action of thrombin, may be taken to gain information on thrombin activity. However, both the TAT complexes and the FPA may be artificially increased by venepuncture and have a short half-life, two facts which make their reliable measurement difficult. The fragment 1+2 (F1+2) constitutes the amino terminus of the prothrombin which is split during prothrombin activation, and has a long half-life;

F1+2 is therefore a reliable marker of the generation of thrombin. The degradation products of fibrin (FDP) may be taken, for similar reasons, as an indicator of fibrinolytic activity, since the activity of plasmin cannot be measured directly due to the short half-life of the enzyme. The use of estrogens in oral contraception, and at a lower level in replacement therapy after menopause, has been suggested to slightly increase markers of thrombin generation and activity such as the prothrombin F1+2, TAT complexes and FPA[34], although this issue remains debatable in the literature.

The activators of the anticoagulant system reside mainly on the endothelium, as is the case of thrombomodulin (protein C) and heparin-like glycoproteins (AT-III). Other modulators of the protein C/S pathway are factor V, which acts as a cofactor, and the C4b-binding protein, an inhibitor of the complement pathway that forms a complex with protein S. A decrease in C4b-binding globulin, as induced by estrogens in one study[35], elevates the amount of free protein S, thus increasing its activity. Both protein S and AT-III exhibit a very wide range of normality, an important point that invalidates any conclusion obtained from small modifications in their circulating levels, as has been described for estrogens[36] (Figure 2). The level at which AT-III would significantly increase the risk of thrombosis is unknown, but studies in families, with congenital AT-III deficiency suggest that it would have to be reduced to about 50% of its normal activity. The prevalence of congenital deficiencies of any of the three components of the anticoagulant system is, however, rare. This is at variance with the prevalence of APC resistance due to factor V Leiden, which varies from 2% to 15% in a White population[37].

The increased susceptibility of the population with genetic deficiencies in the anticoagulant system may influence the higher relative risk of venous thromboembolism ascribed to estrogens. This association has been clearly observed for oral contraceptives[38,39]. In fact, the continuous activation of the coagulation cascade in vivo seems confirmed by the detection of low, but measurable, plasma levels of reaction products of coagulation and fibrinolysis in the normal population. This tonic low-grade activation of coagulation requires a continuous activity of the anticoagulant and the fibrinolytic systems. The reduction in the 'safety margin' determined by a genetic deficiency in any of the components of the anticoagulant system may condition a higher thrombotic risk, which is increased by estrogens[35,37–39]. This effect, nonetheless, must be small in HRT users where, as mentioned above, the lower estrogenic dose leaves the hemostatic balance very close to neutrality, if not displaced towards the antithrombotic side (see below). Therefore, the extremely low, but still detectable, increased risk of venous thrombosis with HRT may be influenced by alternative variables. The older age of women receiving HRT may possibly exert an influence, since age is a demonstrated risk factor for venous thrombosis[40]. A hypothetical influence of variables distinct to the activation of procoagulants, such as the reduction in the venous blood flow, the third mechanism of the Virchow's triad, may also be operative. This is actually the likely mechanism operating in the prothrombotic effect of immobilization or, more clearly, venous occlusion.

THE SIGNIFICANCE OF PARTICULAR RISK MARKERS

The scant consideration received by the changes induced by estrogens on the levels of circulating procoagulant zymogens or members of the anticoagulant system contrasts with the attention paid to factors whose concentration

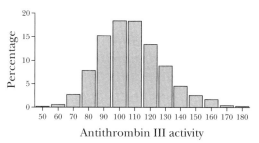

Figure 2 Distribution of plasma antithrombin III levels among 6737 women, aged 45–64 years, who participated in the Atherosclerosis Risk in Communities Study (from ref. 36 with permission)

has been considered clinically relevant. There is general agreement on the value of these factors, despite the awareness of the fact that much of the evidence supporting their relevance comes from retrospective studies and, as a consequence, suffers from methodological insufficiencies. As shown by clinical observations, there may be preferential identification of particular markers with either venous or arterial thrombosis.

Making an abstraction of an eventual implication of the other two components of the Virchow' triad, there is evidence favoring the concept of hypercoagulability as a main determinant of venous thrombosis. This conclusion is obtained from: the observation of a high prevalence of APC resistance or other anticoagulant deficiencies[14,39,41] among patients with venous thrombosis, and the association of recognized triggers of venous thrombosis, such as immobilization, trauma, or venous occlusion, with increased coagulant activity as depicted by raised F1+2 and FDPs[33].

In the arterial tree, an increase in either the level of fibrinogen or the activity of factor VII has been associated with higher risk of myocardial infarction, possibly the most severe complication of arterial thrombosis[42–46]. The hypofunctional status of the fibrinolytic system may be also relevant, as suggested by the rise in PAI-1 detected in coronary heart disease, and the poor prognosis linked to that increase[46–55]. Elevated levels of lipoprotein(a) (Lp(a)) have been shown to behave as an independent risk factor for cardiovascular disease, an observation that possibly may be also ascribed to hypofunctional fibrinolysis, since several studies have found that Lp(a) interferes with the fibrinolytic system because of its structural similarity to plasminogen[56]. In this connection, the generation of plasmin has been shown to be inhibited in postmenopausal women with high Lp(a) levels[57]. However, Lp(a)'s role as an independent risk factor is not completely clear[58], and there are no clinical data demonstrating that lowering Lp(a) results in reduced coronary heart disease risk. The same criticism may be applied to factor VII and fibrinogen.

THE EFFECT OF HRT

Some reports suggest that HRT increases the concentration of factor VII[22,59–61], although this was not confirmed in other studies, where factor VII remained unchanged[45,63,64], or even decreased[30,62,65]. An interesting observation supporting the inductive effects of estrogens comes from the finding of a close interrelationship of factor VII and triglyceride[66], since estrogens, particularly through the oral route, are known to increase triglyceride levels. Reduction in the level of circulating fibrinogen during HRT has been detected in most[30–32,61,65.67,68] but not all[45] studies, with no difference between estrogen and combined HRT.

Fibrinolysis seems enhanced by HRT in most studies. A prospective study on 75 postmenopausal women demonstrated a reduction in PAI-1 and an increase in t-PA in women under HRT, both effects remaining after 1 year of treatment. The reduction of PAI-1 was observed in women receiving oral, but not transdermal, estrogens. In a cohort of 749 women from the Framingham Offspring Study it was shown that high estrogen status was associated with greater fibrinolytic potential (lower PAI-1 levels)[69]. Similar profibrinolytic changes were observed in other studies with distinct HRT regimens[22,61,68,70]. A recent study has clarified some molecular aspects of the estrogenic action on the circulating levels of PAI-1[71]. The 4/5 guanosine (4G/5G) polymorphism in the promoter region of the PAI-1 gene has been shown to be associated with higher levels of plasma PAI-1 activity. The 4G allele has higher activity than the 5G allele because the 5G allele contains an additional binding site for a DNA-binding protein that could be a transcriptional repressor[72,73]. In a group of postmenopausal women with coronary heart disease (CHD), the levels of PAI-1 correlated with the 4G allele dosage (Figure 3)[71]. Also the HRT-induced decrease in PAI-1 correlated with the 4G allele dosage (Figure 4)[71].

Additional effects on fibrinolysis may be brought about by changes in the circulating concentration of Lp(a). Increases in the concentration of Lp(a) were detected under the hypoestrogenic status of menopause, either

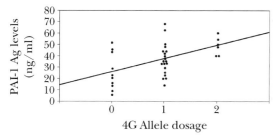

Figure 3 Correlation between plasminogen activator inhibitor type 1 (PAI-1) antigen levels and 4G allele dosage in a group of women with coronary heart disease. The 4G/4G genotype, ascribed to the 2 category at the *x* axis, is associated with the highest PAI-1 levels (from ref. 71, with permission)

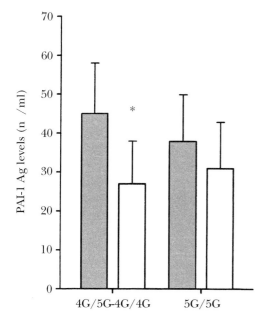

Figure 4 Influence of the plasminogen activator inhibitor type 1 (PAI-1) promoter 4G/5G genotype on the variation in PAI-1 antigen levels under hormone replacement therapy (HRT). The presence of the 4G allele (4G/5G or 4G/4G genotype) determined susceptibility to HRT, as shown by the bars on the left, where the levels of antigenic PAI-1 significantly decreased. In contrast, PAI levels remained unchanged in cases with the 5G/5G genotype, as shown by the bars on the right. Values are mean ± SEM; tinted bars, PAI-1 levels before HRT; open bars, PAI-1 levels after 3–4 months HRT; *$p < 0.05$ (from ref 71, with permission)

natural[74] or surgical[75]. The administration of estrogens, accordingly, is followed by a reduction in the Lp(a) levels[61,74,76,77], an effect which is not down-regulated by progestins[74]. Interest-ingly, the decrease in Lp(a) levels by HRT is particularly evident in women undergoing higher Lp(a) increases with menopause, and after oral estrogens, with or without progestins[57]. Also of interest, the apolipoprotein (a) component of Lp(a) shows a size polymorphism, with individual isoforms ranging in apparent molecular weights from about 250–800 kD[78,79]. The low molecular weight apo (a) isoforms show higher plasmin inhibition than high molecular weight apo (a) isoforms, and tend to accumulate in women suffering higher Lp(a) increases with menopause, the most estrogen-sensitive population sample[57].

In sum, most of the observed actions of HRT on relevant risk factors in hemostatic balance seem to promote a beneficial effect. The available clinical observations, despite the methodological limitation of the studies, seem unanimous in suggesting a very low but detectable risk of venous thrombosis. Therefore, one may speculate on the possible influence of alternative variables, where the effect of HRT on either the vessel wall or the blood flow operate as possible factors.

BIOLOGICAL EFFECTS OF ESTROGENS ON THE VESSEL WALL

In addition to the effects of estrogens on the distinct factors involved in the hemostatic balance, the implication of the vascular wall in the mechanisms of thrombogenesis requires analysis of the eventual effect of estrogens at that level.

The role of endothelium in the hemostatic control

The vascular wall is subjected to a continuous remodelling process, where the three main cellular components, endothelium, smooth myocytes and fibroblasts establish complex paracrine and autocrine interactions[80]. The endothelium holds a principal position, in part due to its location, in the interplay between the external stimuli and the rest of the structures of the vessel wall.

In addition to its role as the main sensor, the endothelium generates an ample range of mediators able to act on its own cells and on the neighborhood[81]. The endothelial products are qualified to regulate immune responses, vascular tone and hemostasis. Vasodilators, such as nitric oxide and prostacyclin, and vasoconstrictors, such as endothelin-1 and platelet-activating factor (PAF)[82], are principal pieces of that machinery. The aggregation of platelets is prevented by the combined influence of prostacyclin and nitric oxide, together with ADPase, an enzyme detected in the endothelial surface, which degrades ADP from activated platelets, thus preventing their activation[83,84].

The healthy endothelium prevents thrombosis by instruments other than its antiaggregatory properties on platelets. Thrombomodulin is an endothelial surface protein that binds thrombin, making it incapable of activating platelets or cleaving fibrinogen. The resulting complex activates protein C. Endothelial cells also synthesize t-PA. Finally, the intact endothelium is a surface anticoagulant. The endothelial cell membranes are covered by glycoproteins and proteoglycans like heparan sulfate, the cofactor to antithrombin III. The glycoproteins condition a negatively charged environment that impairs the adhesion of platelets and the initiation of the intrinsic pathway of coagulation[85].

Endothelial dysfunction is followed by an impaired ability to release vasodilator and antiaggregatory factors, and by the promoted release of vasoconstrictor and proaggregatory substances. Among the latter, the Von Willebrand factor (vWF) is an adhesive protein found in plasma, endothelial cells and the storage granules of platelets. This factor mediates platelet adhesion to vascular subendothelium[86,87]. PAF, also produced by adequately stimulated endothelial cells, is a lipid inflammatory mediator which induces platelet aggregation through binding to a surface receptor present in the platelet membrane[88]. Endothelial dysfunction may result from several diseases, including atherosclerosis, diabetes mellitus, hypertension, or hypercholesterolemia. Also, some level of dysfunction has been linked to the hypoestrogenic state of menopause.

In conclusion, it seems that the endothelium is a crucial element among the components of the vascular wall with a regulatory potential on hemostasis. A healthy endothelium warrants protection against the activation of platelets and the intrinsic pathway of coagulation, two principal factors in the constitution of a clot. The fact that the hemostatic imbalances favoring thrombosis do not promote a diffuse thrombotic diathesis but, on the contrary, a focal lesion, is undoubtedly influenced by circumstances related to the endothelium, perhaps even to regional differences within the vascular tree[89].

The action of estrogens

Thanks to the intervention of an ample range of mediators, the endothelial cells establish a complex system of reciprocal relationships with their microenvironment. As a result, the profile of the endothelial function may differ with the signals received from the neighborhood. The development of atherosclerosis within the arterial tree clearly defines an important difference between the venous and the arterial walls. The inflammatory milieu defined by atherosclerosis is associated with an array of functional derangements in endothelial cells[88,90]. Thus, the balance between endothelial mediators with vasodilator/antiaggregatory and vasoconctrictor/aggregatory effects is disrupted in favor of the latter. The production of nitric oxide and prostacyclin is diminished, while the disruption of the endothelial lining of blood vessels exposes the subendothelial matrix, which contains vWF and fibrinogen[88]. A well-organized system of distinct adhesion molecules[87,91,92] operates to determine platelet aggregation, a first step to form a hemostatic plug or a thrombus[4–6]. There is a concomitant stimulation in the expression of P-selectin, an adhesion molecule also found in activated platelets, which mediates the deceleration of platelets prior to their aggregation. Additionally, the initiation and progression of atherosclerosis has been associated with oxidation of low-density lipoproteins (LDL), which may therefore act as an indirect promoter of thrombogenesis[93].

Estrogens are known to protect the endothelium from most of those dysfunctions in atherosclerotic vessels, and therefore to act as antithrombotic factors in that context. Estrogens display a multitude of functions which protect the vessel wall from atherosclerosis, thus determining an antithrombotic effect on the arteries. Among the protective actions, estrogens diminish the vasomotor tone through both short-term and long-term effects on the vasculature[94,95], an effect that seems to be obtained through both non-genomic and genomic mechanisms[94], and that has been recognized as relevant in the initiation and progression of atherosclerosis[90]. The promotion of vasodilator/antiaggregatory substances, such as nitric oxide and prostacyclin[95–97], together with the diminution of vasoconstrictors/proaggregatory substances, such as endothelin-1[98,99], are only examples of distinct mechanisms involved in that effect. In this connection, data from animal models show that estrogens inhibit platelet aggregation[100]. Also, 17β-estradiol has antioxidant effects *in vitro*, which seems to be confirmed *in vivo* by the observation of an increase in the lag-time for oxidation of the LDL obtained from postmenopausal women treated with 17β-estradiol at a physiological dose[101]. Additionally, estrogens have trophic effects on endothelium, as demonstrated by their ability to promote cell growth *in vitro*[102] and *in vivo*[103], and by their confirmed inhibition of the apoptosis of cultured endothelial cells[104]. To add more protection, there are data supporting an inhibiting effect of estrogens on the expression of adhesion molecules by vascular cells[105]. These protective effects of estrogens have been confirmed in postmenopausal women by the modification of the circulating levels of markers of endothelial function, such as soluble P-selectin, vWF, soluble thrombomodulin, and t-PA, to the premenopausal state[106].

As a conclusion, there are distinct experimental lines of evidence suggesting that at the vascular wall, one of the three elements of the Virchow's triad, the action of estrogens, may be antithrombotic. This action may be conducted through morphological and functional restoration of the endothelial function, and therefore, may be particularly operative at the arterial level, where atherosclerosis acts as a disturbing endothelial element. This hypothesis may also explain in part the contrasting effect on the venous tree, where in the setting of an already functional endothelium, estrogens seem to slightly increase the thrombotic risk. Most probably, however, the level of complexity of the mechanisms conditioning the induction of, or protection from, the generation of a hemostatic plug in either veins or arteries is much higher. The fact that the amelioration of the endothelial function in arteries determines a hemostatic balance leaning to the opposite of that found in veins, where the endothelial function seems preserved, calls for a role of distinct local factors. Research at that level may shed light on many of the paradoxical hemostatic effects of estrogens on arteries and veins.

ACKNOWLEDGEMENT

This paper was supported by grant 1FD97–1035–C02–01 from the Spanish Ministry for Education and Culture.

References

1. Fuster V, Badimon L, Badimon JJ, *et al.* The pathogenesis of coronary artery disease and the acute coronary syndromes. *N Engl J Med* 1992; 326:242–50
2. Fuster V, Badimon L, Badimon JJ, *et al.* The pathogenesis of coronary artery disease and the acute coronary syndromes. *N Engl J Med* 1992; 326:310–18
3. Badimon L, Bayés-Genís A. Effects of progestogens on thrombosis and atherosclerosis. *Hum Reprod Update* 1999;5:191–9

4. Kroll MH, Harris TS, Moake JL, *et al.* von Willebrand factor binding to platelet GpIb initiates signals for platelet activation. *J Clin Invest* 1991;88:1568–73

5. Harker LA. Platelets and vascular thrombosis. *N Engl J Med* 1994;330:1006–7

6. Lefkovits J, Plow EF, Topol EJ. Platelet glycoprotein IIb/IIIa receptors in cardiovascular medicine. *N Engl J Med* 1995;332:1553–9

7. Bertina RM, Koeleman BPC, Koster T, *et al.* Mutation in blood coagulation factor V associated with resistance to activated protein C. *Nature* 1994;369:64–7

8. Notelovitz M. Hormone therapy and hemostasis. In Lobo RA, ed. *Treatment of the Postmenopausal Woman. Basic and Clinical Aspects.* New York: Raven Press, 1994;271–81

9. Hillmen P, Lewis SM, Bessler M, *et al.* Natural history of paroxysmal nocturnal hemoglobinuria. *N Engl J Med* 1995;333:1253–8

10. Socie G, Mary JY, de Gramont A, *et al.* Paroxysmal nocturnal haemoglobinuria: long-term follow-up and prognostic factors. *Lancet* 1996; 348:573–7

11. De Stefano V, Finazzi G, Mannucci PM. Inherited thrombophilia: pathogenesis, clinical syndromes, and management. *Blood* 1996;87: 3531–44

12. Thomas DP, Roberts HR. Hypercoagulability in venous and arterial thrombosis. *Ann Intern Med* 1997;126:638–44

13. Price DT, Ridker PM. Factor V Leiden mutation and the risks for thromboembolic disease: a clinical perspective. *Ann Intern Med* 1997;127: 895–903

14. Martinelli I, Sacchi E, Landi G, *et al.* High risk of cerebral-vein thrombosis in carriers of a prothrombin-gene mutation and in users of oral contraceptives. *N Engl J Med* 1998;338: 1793–7

15. Rosendaal FR, Siscovick DS, Schwartz SM, *et al.* Factor V Leiden (resistance to activated protein C) increases the risk of myocardial infarction in young women. *Blood* 1997;89:2817–21

16. Pabinger I, Schneider B. Thrombotic risk in hereditary antithrombin III, protein C, or protein S deficiency: a cooperative, retrospective study. *Arterioscler Thromb Vasc Biol* 1996;16:742–8

17. Winkler UH. Effects of progestins on cardiovascular diseases: the haemostatic system. *Hum Reprod Update* 1999;5:200–4

18. Acute myocardial infarction and combined oral contraceptives: results of an international multicentre case–control study. WHO Collaborative Study of Cardiovascular Disease and Steroid Hormone Contraception. *Lancet* 1997; 349:1202–9

19. Todd JC, Lawrenson R, Farmer RDT, *et al.* Venous thromboembolism disease and combined oral contraceptives: a re-analysis of the MediPlus database. *Hum Reprod* 1999;14:1500–5

20. Lowe GDO, Rumley A, Woodward M, *et al.* Epidemiology of coagulation factors, inhibitors and activation markers: The Third Glasgow MONICA Survey I. Illustrative reference ranges by age, sex and hormone use. *Br J Haematol* 1997;97:775–84

21. Winkler UH. Menopause, hormone replacement therapy and cardiovascular disease: a review of haemostaseological findings. *Fibrinolysis* 1992;6:5–10

22. Kroon UB, Silfverstolpe G, Tengborn L. The effects of transdermal estradiol and oral conjugated estrogens on haemostasis variables. *Thromb Haemost* 1994;71:420–3

23. Daly E, Vessey MP, Hawkins MM, *et al.* Risk of venous thromboembolism in users of hormone replacement therapy. *Lancet* 1996;348:977–80

24. Jick H, Derby LE, Myers MW, *et al.* Risk of hospital admission for idiopathic venous thromboembolism among users of postmenopausal oestrogens. *Lancet* 1996;348:981–3

25. Grodstein F, Stampfer MJ, Goldhaber SZ, *et al.* Prospective study of exogenous hormones and risk of pulmonary embolism in women. *Lancet* 1996;348:983–7

26. Gutthan SP, Rodriguez LAG, Castellsague J, *et al.* Hormone replacement therapy and risk of venous thromboembolism: population based case-control study. *Br Med J* 1997;314:796–800

27. Balasch J. The 'pill scare II' two years later. *Eur J Contracep Health Care* 1997;2:149–59

28. Winkler UH. Effects on hemostatic variables of desogestrel- and gestodene-containing oral contraceptives in comparison with levonorgestrel-containing oral contraceptives: a review. *Am J Obstet Gynecol* 1998;179:S51–6

29. Farsetti A, Miniti S, Citarella F, *et al.* Molecular basis of estrogen regulation of Hageman factor XII gene expression. *Endocrinology* 1995;136: 5076–83

30. Kroon UB, Tengborn L, Rita H, *et al.* The effects of transdermal oestradiol and oral progestogens on haemostasis variables. *Br J Obstet Gynaecol* 1997;104 (Suppl. 16):32–7

31. Frohlich M, Schunkert H, Hense HW, *et al.* Effects of hormone replacement therapies on fibrinogen and plasma viscosity in postmenopausal women. *Br J Haematol* 1998;100:577–81

32. Conard J, Gompel A, Pelissier C, *et al.* Fibrinogen and plasminogen modifications during oral estradiol replacement therapy. *Fertil Steril* 1997;68:49–53

33. Winkler UH. Hormone replacement therapy and hemostasis: principles of a complex interaction. *Maturitas* 1996;24:131–45

34. Chae CU, Ridker PM, Manson JE. Postmenopausal hormone replacement therapy and

cardiovascular disease. *Thromb Haemost* 1997; 77:770–80

35. Kessler CM, Szymanski LM, Shamsipour Z, *et al.* Estrogen replacement therapy and coagulation: relationship to lipid and lipoprotein changes. *Obstet Gynecol* 1997;89:326–31

36. Conlan MG, Folsom AR, Finch A, *et al.* Antithrombin III: associations with age, race, sex and cardiovascular disease risk factors. *Thromb Haemost* 1994;72:551–6

37. Bertina RM, Rosendaal FR. Venous thrombosis. The interaction of genes and environment. *N Engl J Med* 1998;338:1840–1

38. Vandenbroucke JP, Koster T, Briët E, *et al.* Increased risk of venous thrombosis in oral-contraceptive users who are carriers of factor V Leiden mutation. *Lancet* 1994;344:1453–7

39. Martinelli I, Landi G, Merati G, *et al.* Factor V gene mutation is a risk factor for cerebral venous thrombosis. *Thromb Haemost* 1996;75: 393–4

40. Anderson FA, Wheeler HB, Goldberg RJ, *et al.* A population-based perspective of the hospital incidence and case-fatality rates of deep vein thrombosis and pulmonary embolism. The Worcester DVT Study. *Archiv Intern Med* 1991; 151:933–8

41. Zivelin A, Griffin JH, Xu X, *et al.* A single genetic origin for a common Caucasian risk factor for venous thrombosis. *Blood* 1997;89: 397–402

42. Lee AJ, Smith WCS, Lowe GDO, *et al.* Plasma fibrinogen and coronary risk factors: the Scottish Heart Health Study. *J Clin Epidemiol* 1990;43:913–19

43. Wilhelmsen L, Svärdsudd K, Korsan-Bengtsen K, *et al.* Fibrinogen as a risk factor for stroke and myocardial infarction. *N Engl J Med* 1984;311: 501–5

44. Meade TW, Mellows S, Brozovic M, *et al.* Haemostatic function and ischaemic heart disease: principal results of the Northwick Park Heart Study. *Lancet* 1986;ii:533–7

45. Scarabin PY, Alhenc-Gelas M, Plu-Bureau G, *et al.* Effects of oral and transdermal estrogen/progesterone regimens on blood coagulation and fibrinolysis in postmenopausal women. A randomized controlled trial. *Arterioscler Thromb Vasc Biol* 1997;17:3071–8

46. Scarabin PY, Aillaud MF, Amouyel P, *et al.* Associations of fibrinogen, factor VII and PAI-1 with baseline findings among 10,500 male participants in a prospective study of myocardial infarction – the PRIME Study. Prospective epidemiological study of myocardial infarction. *Thromb Haemost* 1998;80:749–56

47. Aznar J, Estellés A, Tormo G, *et al.* Plasminogen activator inhibitor activity and other fibrinolytic

variables in patients with coronary artery disease. *Br Heart J* 1988;59:535–41

48. Páramo JA, Colucci M, Collen D. Plasminogen activator inhibitor in the blood of patients with coronary artery disease. *Br Med J* 1985;291: 573–4

49. Hamsten A, Wiman B, De Faire U, *et al.* Increased plasma levels of a rapid inhibitor of tissue plasminogen activator in young survivors of myocardial infarction. *N Engl J Med* 1985;313: 1557–63

50. Estellés A, Tormo G, Aznar J, *et al.* Reduced fibrinolytic activity in coronary heart disease in basal conditions and after exercise. *Thromb Res* 1985;40:373–83

51. Hamsten A, De Faire U, Walldius G, *et al.* Plasminogen activator inhibitor in plasma: risk factor for recurrent myocardial infarction. *Lancet* 1987;ii:3–9

52. Thogersen AM, Jansson JH, Boman K, *et al.* High plasminogen activator inhibitor and tissue plasminogen activator levels in plasma precede a first acute myocardial infarction in both men and women: evidence for the fibrinolytic system as an independent primary risk factor. *Circulation* 1998;98:2241–7

53. Gottsauner-Wolf M, Sochor H, Hornykewycz S, *et al.* Predictive value of PAI-1 plasma activity and thallium perfusion imaging for restenosis after percutaneous transluminal angioplasty in clinically asymptomatic patients. *Thromb Haemost* 1999;81:522–6

54. Cesari M, Rossi GP. Plasminogen activator inhibitor type 1 in ischemic cardiomyopathy. *Arterioscler Thromb Vasc Biol* 1999;19:1378–86

55. Wiman B. Predictive value of fibrinolytic factors in coronary heart disease. *Scand J Clin Lab Invest Suppl* 1999;230:23–31

56. Edelberg JM, Pizzo SV. Lipoprotein (a): the link between impaired fibrinolysis and atherosclerosis. *Fibrinolysis* 1991;5:135–43

57. Estellés A, Cano A, Falcó C, *et al.* Lipoprotein (a) levels and isoforms and fibrinolytic activity in postmenopause – influence of hormone replacement therapy. *Thromb Haemost* 1999;81: 104–10

58. Ridker PM. An epidemiologic reassessment of lipoprotein(a) and atherothrombotic risk. *Trends Cardiovasc Med* 1995;5:225–9

59. Boschetti C, Cortellaro M, Nencioni T, *et al.* Short- and long-term effects of hormone replacement therapy (transdermal estradiol vs oral conjugated equine estrogens, combined with medroxyprogesterone acetate) on blood coagulation factors in postmenopausal women. *Thromb Res* 1991;62:1–8

60. Habiba M, Andrea A, Philipps B, *et al.* Thrombophilia and lipid profile in post-menopausal women using a new transdermal

oestradiol patch. *Eur J Obstet Gynecol Reprod Biol* 1996;66:165–8

61. Andersen LF, Gram J, Skouby SO, *et al.* Effects of hormone replacement therapy on hemostatic cardiovascular risk factors. *Am J Obstet Gynecol* 1999;180:283–9

62. Scarabin PY, Plu-Bureau G, Bara L, *et al.* Haemostatic variables and menopausal status: influence of hormone replacement therapy. *Thromb Haemost* 1993;70:584–7

63. Saleh AA, Dorey LG, Dombrowski MP, *et al.* Thrombosis and hormone replacement therapy in postmenopausal women. *Am J Obstet Gynecol* 1993;6:1554–7

64. Nabulsi AA, Folsom AR, White A, *et al.* Association of hormone-replacement therapy with various cardiovascular risk factors in postmenopausal women. *N Engl J Med* 1993;328:1069–75

65. Lindoff C, Peterson F, Lecander I, *et al.* Transdermal estrogen replacement therapy: beneficial effects on hemostatic risk factors for cardiovascular disease. *Maturitas* 1996;24:43–50

66. Skartlien AH, Lyberg-Beckmann S, Holme I, *et al.* Effect of alteration in triglyceride levels on factor VII-phospholipid complexes in plasma. *Arteriosclerosis* 1989;9:798–801

67. PEPI Trial Writing Group. Effects of estrogen/progestin on heart disease risk factors in postmenopausal women. *JAMA* 1995;273:199–208

68. Meilahn EN, Cauley JA, Tracy RP, *et al.* Association of sex hormones and adiposity with plasma levels of fibrinogen and PAI-1 in postmenopausal women. *Am J Epidemiol* 1996;143:159–66

69. Gebara OCE, Mittleman MA, Sutherland P, *et al.* Association between increased estrogen status and increased fibrinolytic potential in the Framingham Offspring Study. *Circulation* 1995;91:1952–8

70. Notelovitz M. Progestogens and coagulation. *Int Proc J* 1989;1:229–34

71. Grancha S, Estellés A, Tormo G, *et al.* Plasminogen activator inhibitor-1 (PAI-1) promoter 4G/5G genotype and increased PAI-1 circulating levels in postmenopausal women with coronary artery disease. *Thromb Haemost* 1999;81:516–21

72. Dawson S, Wiman B, Hamsten A, *et al.* The two allele sequences of a common polymorphism in the promoter of the plasminogen activator inhibitor (PAI-1) gene respond differently to interleukin-1 in hepG2 cells. *J Biol Chem* 1993;268:10739–45

73. Eriksson P, Kallin B, van't Hooft FM, *et al.* Allele-specific increase in basal transcription of the plasminogen-activator inhibitor 1 gene is associated with myocardial infarction. *Proc Natl Acad Sci USA* 1995;92:1851–5

74. Gilabert J, Estellés A, Cano A, *et al.* The effect of estrogen replacement therapy with or without progestogen on the fibrinolytic system and coagulation inhibitors in postmenopausal status. *Am J Obstet Gynecol* 1995;173:1849–54

75. Kim CJ, Ryu WS, Kwak JW, *et al.* Changes in Lp(a) lipoprotein and lipid levels after cessation of female sex hormone production and estrogen replacement therapy. *Arch Intern Med* 1996;156:500–4

76. Haines CJ, Chung TK, Masarei JR, *et al.* An examination of the effect of combined cyclical hormone replacement therapy on lipoprotein(a) and other lipoproteins. *Atherosclerosis* 1996;119:215–22

77. Honggi W, Lippuner K, Riesen W, *et al.* Long-term influence of the different postmenopausal hormone replacement regimens on serum lipids and lipoprotein(a): a randomised study. *Br J Obstet Gynecol* 1997;104:708–17

78. Uttermann G, Kraft HG, Menzel HJ, *et al.* Genetics of the quantitative Lp(a) lipoprotein trait. I. Relation of Lp(a) glycoprotein phenotypes to Lp(a) lipoprotein concentrations in plasma. *Hum Genet* 1988;78:41–6

79. Kamboh MI, Ferrel RE, Kottke BA. Expressed hypervariable polymorphism of apolipoprotein(a). *Am J Hum Genet* 1991;49:1063–74

80. Gibbons GH, Dzau VJ. The emerging concept of vascular remodelling. *N Engl J Med* 1994;330:1431–8

81. Änggard EE. The endothelium – the body's largest endocrine gland? *J Endocrinol* 1990;127:371–5

82. Vane JR, Änggard EE, Botting RM. Regularity functions of the vascular endothelium. *N Engl J Med* 1990;323:27–36

83. Marcus AJ, Safier LB, Broekman MJ, *et al.* Thrombosis and inflammation as multicellular processes: significance of cell–cell interactions. *Thromb Haemost* 1995;74:213–17

84. Marcus AJ, Broekman MJ, Drosopoulos JH, *et al.* The endothelial cell ecto-ADPase responsible for inhibition of platelet function is CD39. *J Clin Invest* 1997;99:1351–60

85. Marcum JA, Rosenberg RD. Anticoagulantly active heparin-like molecules from vascular tissue. *Biochemistry* 1984;23:1730–7

86. Ware JA, Heistad DD. Platelet–endothelium interactions. *N Engl J Med* 1993;328:628–35

87. Frenette PS, Wagner DD. Adhesion molecules – part 2: blood vessels and blood cells. *N Engl J Med* 1996;335:43–5

88. Cines DB, Pollak ES, Buck CA, *et al.* Endothelial cells in physiology and in the pathophysiology of vascular disorders. *Blood* 1998;91:3527–61

89. Rosenberg RD, Aird WC. Vascular-bed-specific hemostasis and hypercoagulable states. *N Engl J Med* 1999;340:1555–64

90. Ross R. Atherosclerosis – an inflammatory disease. *N Engl J Med* 1999;340:115–26.

91. Coller BS, Peerschke EI, Scudder LE, *et al.* A murine monoclonal antibody that completely blocks the binding of fibrinogen to platelets produces a thrombasthenic-like state in normal platelets and binds to glycoprotein IIb and/or IIIa. *J Clin Invest* 1983;72:325–38

92. Phillips DR, Charo IF, Scarborough RM. GPIIb-IIIa: the responsive integrin. *Cell* 1991; 65:359–62

93. Cox DA, Cohen ML. Effects of oxidized low-density lipoprotein on vascular contraction and relaxation: clinical and pharmacological implications in atherosclerosis. *Pharmacol Rev* 1996;48:3–19

94. Mendelsohn ME, Karas RH. The protective effects of estrogen on the cardiovascular system. *N Engl J Med* 1999;340:1801–11

95. Sarrel PM. The differential effects of oestrogens and progestins on vascular tone. *Hum Reprod Update* 1999;5:205–9

96. Fogelberg M, Vesterqvist O, Diczfalusy U, *et al.* Experimental atherosclerosis: effects of oestrogen and atherosclerosis on thromboxane and prostacyclin formation. *Eur J Clin Invest* 1990; 20:105–10

97. Mikkola T, Turunen P, Kristiina A, *et al.* 17β-estradiol stimulates prostacyclin, but not endothelin-1, production in human vascular endothelial cells. *J Clin Endocrinol Metab* 1995; 80:1832–6

98. Polderman KH, Stehouwer CDA, van Kamp GJ, *et al.* Influence of sex hormones on plasma endothelin levels. *Ann Intern Med* 1993;118: 429–32

99. Chen FP, Lee N, Wang CH, *et al.* Effects of hormone replacement therapy on cardiovascular risk factors in postmenopausal women. *Fertil Steril* 1998;69:267–73

100. Mitchell HC. Effect of estrogen and a progestogen on platelet adhesiveness and aggregation in rabbits. *J Lab Clin Med* 1974;83:79–89

101. Sack MN, Rader DJ, Cannon RO III. Oestrogen and inhibition of oxidation of low-density lipoproteins in postmenopausal women. *Lancet* 1994;343:269–70

102. Morales DE, McGowan KA, Grant DS, *et al.* Estrogen promotes angiogenic activity in human umbilical vein endothelial cells in vitro and in a murine model. *Circulation* 1997;95: 755–63

103. Krasinski K, Spyridipoulos I, Asahara T, *et al.* Estradiol accelerates functional endothelial recovery after arterial injury. *Circulation* 1997; 95:1768–72

104. Spyridipoulos I, Sullivan AB, Kearney M, *et al.* Estrogen receptor-mediated inhibition of human endothelial cell apoptosis: estradiol as a survival factor. *Circulation* 1997;95:1505–14

105. Caulin-Glaser T, Watson CA, Pardi R, *et al.* Effects of 17β-estradiol on cytokine-induced endothelial cell adhesion molecule expression. *J Clin Invest* 1996;98:36–42

106. Lip GY, Blann AD, Jones AF, *et al.* Effects of hormone-replacement therapy on hemostatic factors, lipid factors, and endothelial function in women undergoing surgical menopause: implications for prevention of atherosclerosis. *Am Heart J* 1997;134:764–71

15

Changes in coronary arteries with estrogen therapy

C. M. Webb, C. S. Hayward and P. Collins

INTRODUCTION

Heart disease is as common in women as in men; however, it occurs in women later in life. The menopause, and its associated estrogen deficiency, appear to be risk factors for the development of cardiovascular disease in women, and postmenopausal estrogen therapy has been shown to have beneficial effects on a number of these risk factors. The mechanisms involved include effects on metabolism, plasma lipids in particular, as well as effects on vascular physiology and pathophysiology. Estrogen decreases vascular tone by a number of mechanisms, including endothelium-derived nitric oxide and prostanoids, ion channel modulation, inhibition of constrictor factors and others. Advantageous effects on coronary blood flow by estrogen may also involve these mechanisms, and they may, at least partially, account for the beneficial effects of estrogen on atherogenesis and myocardial ischemia.

POSSIBLE MECHANISMS INVOLVED IN CORONARY ARTERY RESPONSES TO ESTROGEN

Estrogen receptor

Receptor-dependent mechanisms are involved in the response of blood vessels of the reproductive system to gonadal hormones, and estrogen receptors are found in a number of other tissues including the heart and liver[1,2]. There are conflicting data on the presence of estrogen receptors in female human coronary arteries. They have been demonstrated in normal coronary arteries; however, there is variable expression in atherosclerotic coronary arteries from premenopausal women[3]. Others have found no evidence for estrogen receptors in normal coronary arteries, using a different antibody technique[4]. Recent studies using specific monoclonal antibodies and nuclear probes have confirmed the presence of a classical estrogen receptor in a variety of vascular tissues, including cultured human umbilical, aortic and coronary artery endothelial cells[5,6]. These data would support the possibility that the cardioprotective effect of estrogen may, at least in part, be due to effects on endothelial cell function via the estrogen receptor.

A novel estrogen receptor has recently been cloned in rat prostate, called estrogen receptor-beta (ER-β)[7]. This receptor was also found in the ovary and had high affinity for 17β-estradiol. Recent work identified functional ER-α and ER-β in rat neonatal cardiac myocytes and demonstrated modulation of gene expression in these cells by 17β-estradiol[8]. At present, no such receptor has been identified in human tissue, but this finding raises the possibility of cardiac or/and vascular-specific estrogen receptors which may be involved in the modulation of vascular responses to estrogen. Recent data suggest that the acute effects of estrogen in other circulations may be independent of the classical estrogen receptor; however, receptor-dependent mechanisms may be involved in chronic vascular effects of estrogen.

Endothelium-dependent, nitric oxide-mediated effects

Long-term exposure to estrogen stimulates the nitric oxide pathway by a receptor-dependent mechanism, increasing nitric oxide synthase (NOS) activity. Nitric oxide is involved in a number of physiological processes, such as regulation of endogenous vascular tone[9], neurotransmission and immunological responses.

In vitro studies performed in the 1980s and early 1990s demonstrated a role for the endothelium in the mediation of estrogen-induced vascular relaxation[10,11]. Increased endothelium-dependent relaxation to acetylcholine and attenuation of the development of hypertension have been demonstrated in estrogen-treated spontaneously hypertensive rat aorta[12]. In cultured human umbilical vein endothelial cells, estrogen has direct, acute effects, modulating function and responses via effects on intracellular calcium concentrations[13].

Endothelium-dependent effects of estrogen were reinforced by the discovery that estrogen increased basal release of nitric oxide from the vascular endothelium of the aorta[14] and coronary arteries[15]. Wellman and colleagues[15] demonstrated that physiological levels of estradiol increased basal release of endothelium-derived nitric oxide, and caused vascular relaxation, partially through nitric oxide-mediated activation of calcium-dependent potassium channels in the smooth muscle of the coronary artery. In postmenopausal women given acute estradiol treatment, plasma nitric oxide metabolism was increased[16], demonstrating an effect of estrogen on nitric oxide production *in vivo* in humans. This has also been demonstrated in the coronary circulation of postmenopausal women with coronary atherosclerosis or risk factors for coronary artery disease[17].

Nitric oxide is synthesized in endothelial cells from L-arginine by NOS. Estrogen increases calcium-dependent NOS activity in the heart,

kidney, skeletal muscle and cerebellum in animals[18], by upregulation of endothelial NOS (eNOS) and neuronal NOS (nNOS) transcription. An increase in eNOS, associated with elevated NOS protein, has been reported in cultured human aortic endothelial cells[19]. This effect was inhibited by the estrogen receptor antagonist, tamoxifen, suggesting a receptor-dependent stimulation of NOS by estrogen. These findings have been confirmed in experiments performed using cultured human umbilical endothelial cells[20]. They demonstrated regulation of eNOS activity and basal NO release by physiological concentrations of estrogen by an estrogen receptor-dependent mechanism, independent of intracellular calcium. In fetal pulmonary artery endothelial cells, others have demonstrated estrogen receptor-dependent eNOS stimulation within 5 min of exposure to estradiol, but by a calcium-dependent pathway[21]. The classical estrogen receptor has recently been shown to be involved in non-genomic activation of NOS, most likely acting via MAP kinases[22]. This finding may explain the evidence of an acute vascular action of estrogen, both *in vitro* and *in vivo*, as discussed later in this chapter.

There is a significant association between the density of estrogen receptors and nitric oxide production by vascular endothelium in animals[23]. In human endothelial cells, physiological concentrations of estrogen stimulate eNOS activity and increase nitric oxide release via an estrogen receptor-dependent mechanism[24]. Estrogen receptors are present in cultured human coronary artery endothelial cells[24]. There is, therefore, a suggestion of a role for the estrogen receptor in the modulation of estrogen-induced stimulation of nitric oxide production, and estrogen receptor density and/or sensitivity could be a novel risk factor for coronary heart disease.

Calcium antagonistic effect

Endothelium-independent vasorelaxation by estrogen has been demonstrated *in vitro* in animal and human coronary arteries[25], suggesting an action of estrogen directly on vascular smooth muscle cells. 17β-Estradiol had similar relaxing effects on contraction induced by activation of both receptor-operated and potential-operated calcium channels in rabbit coronary arteries[26]. A calcium antagonist effect of 17β-estradiol was confirmed by experiments in isolated guinea pig myocytes, using electrophysiological and calcium indicator studies, showing a decrease in calcium current and intracellular levels of calcium in these cells[27]. These findings have been further reinforced by experiments demonstrating estrogen-induced inhibition of contraction of porcine epicardial coronary arteries, by blocking calcium influx without changing calcium sensitivity of contractile elements[28].

Most of the acute effects of estrogen in vascular smooth muscle cells occur at micromolar concentrations, which are three to four orders of magnitude greater than those achieved in the circulation of women. However, it is possible that tissues accumulate lipid-soluble steroids and local concentrations could theoretically reach these levels.

Effects on other ion channels

Ovarian steroids appear to have other regulatory roles, affecting plasma ion channels via membrane-binding sites distinct from the classical estrogen receptor and subsequent activation of intracellular second-messenger pathways(s).

Potassium channels

An *in vivo* study in dogs has demonstrated endothelium- and estrogen receptor-independent coronary dilatation and increases in blood flow induced by acute administration of 17β-estradiol[29]. Estrogen-induced dilatation, but not increases in blood flow, was attenuated by glibenclamide and by verapamil, demonstrating an effect of estrogen on ATP-sensitive potassium channels and calcium channels, respectively.

Large calcium-activated potassium (BK_{Ca}) channels are the predominant potassium channel species in coronary smooth muscle[30]. Recent studies have demonstrated an effect of estrogen on these channels. In porcine coro-

nary arteries and coronary smooth muscle cells, estrogen-induced increases in cyclic GMP phosphorylation, coupled with opening of BK_{Ca} channels, accounted for coronary relaxation[31]. Using patch-clamp techniques on rabbit aortic endothelial cells, Rusko and colleagues demonstrated a marked enhancement of activity of large BK_{Ca} channels by estrogen, and an increase in intracellular calcium concentrations[32]. Estrogen, therefore, appears to affect BK_{Ca} channels, both in vascular smooth muscle and in endothelial cells.

Endothelin-1

Endothelin is a potent vasoconstrictor released from endothelial cells. It is produced in endothelial cells by *de novo* synthesis, whereby a large messenger RNA-encoded precursor (prepro-endothelin) is converted to a smaller unit ('big' endothelin) and then into the 'mature' form, containing 21 amino acids[33]. Endothelin elicits constriction of vascular smooth muscle cells by increasing cytosolic calcium concentrations[34], in coronary arteries through slow calcium channels[35], via specific endothelin-1 binding sites[36]. Endothelin also has mitogenic properties[37] and, therefore, together with its effects on vasoconstriction and shear stress, may be involved in the process of atherosclerotic plaque formation.

Estrogen inhibits the constrictor responses to endothelin-1 in rabbit coronary arteries[38], and may regulate both eNOS and prepro-endothelin-1 at the transcriptional levels in porcine endothelial cells[39]. Physiological, but not supraphysiological, doses of 17β-estradiol inhibit release of endothelin-1 from cultured human umbilical endothelial cells[40]. In this study, the observed increases in nitric oxide synthase expression were not concomitant with inhibition of endothelin-1 release, suggesting that increased nitric oxide production is unlikely to account for the inhibition of endothelin-1 release by 17β-estradiol. Plasma endothelin-1 levels increase following acetylcholine infusion in pigs with coronary atheroma[41]. The reversal of the constrictor effect of acetylcholine in human atherosclerotic coronary arteries *in vivo* by estrogen[42–44] possibly may be partially explained by estrogen-induced inhibition of endothelin-1-induced contraction. Recent data support this hypothesis. Sudhir and colleagues demonstrated attenuation of endothelin-1-induced decreases in coronary artery cross-sectional area, average peak velocity and volume blood flow by intracoronary administration of a physiological concentration of estradiol in anesthetized female pigs[45]. This effect was possibly mediated through an effect on the endothelin-A receptor.

EFFECTS OF ESTROGEN ON CORONARY BLOOD FLOW

Estrogen induces dilatation of conductance and resistance coronary arteries in dogs, albeit at supraphysiological concentrations (> 0.1 μmol/l), when administered acutely into the coronary circulation[29] by an endothelium-independent effect. However, the majority of the data to date indicate an important role for the endothelium in the mediation of the blood flow responses to estrogen. In ovariectomized cynomolgus monkeys, long-term (2 years) estrogen replacement therapy reverses acetylcholine-induced constriction in atherosclerotic coronary arteries[46], and a similar effect is produced with a 20-min intravenous infusion of ethinylestradiol[47]. These animal data have been reproduced in a number of studies of postmenopausal women with coronary atherosclerosis. Acetylcholine-induced vasoconstriction is attenuated[42] or abolished[43,44] 15–20 min after bolus or continuous intracoronary infusion of estrogen in these women, resulting in increased coronary diameter and flow. This response of the coronary arteries to acetylcholine after exposure to 17β-estradiol appears to be gender dependent[44]. While a 20-min exposure to 17β-estradiol modulated acetylcholine-induced flow responses in postmenopausal women with coronary artery disease, there was no such effect in men with atherosclerotic coronary arteries. Current, chronic estrogen replacement has also been shown to influence endothelium-dependent and -independent coronary responsiveness to acetylcholine[48]. In this study, estrogen replacement therapy was associated with an attenuation or reversal of the coronary vasoconstrictor response to acetylcholine in postmenopausal women. This suggests a possible normalization of endothelium-dependent blood flow responses in diseased coronary vessels by estrogen.

RELEVANCE OF CORONARY VASCULAR EFFECTS OF ESTROGEN TO CARDIOVASCULAR DISEASE PREVENTION AND TREATMENT

Atherogenesis

Epidemiological studies which show that postmenopausal estrogen supplementation appears to decrease death from cardiovascular disease support the concept that it beneficially affects the atherosclerotic process[49]. Retrospective angiographic studies show a protective effect of estrogen on atheroma progression in humans. Estrogen users have less coronary artery occlusion compared to non-users[50] and less angiographically significant coronary artery disease[51]. This effect is independent of the type of menopause or other cardiovascular risk factors, except high-density lipoprotein (HDL) cholesterol. Estrogen has beneficial effects on a variety of factors involved in the atherogenic process, which may explain these clinical findings.

Effects of estrogen on atheroma development via endothelium-derived nitric oxide

Endothelial cells at sites of atherosclerosis are functionally and morphologically different from normal cells[52]. Dysfunction of the endothelium and of endothelium-derived nitric oxide release occurs at an early stage in the development of atherosclerosis[53] and may be related to alterations in endothelial G-proteins or G-protein-dependent pathways. Advanced disease may involve decreased availability of the nitric oxide precursor L-arginine, decreased sensitivity of vascular smooth muscle cells to nitric oxide, or increased breakdown of nitric oxide[52]. Endothelial damage leads to the accumulation of lipids and monocytes at the damage site[54], and may be caused by a number of factors, including blood flow disturbances, hypercholesterolemia, vasoactive amines, immunocomplexes, infection or chemical irritants, such as tobacco smoke. Attenuation by estrogen of atherosclerotic vascular disease may be explained by effects on risk factors for atherosclerosis, such as hypercholesterolemia and lipid peroxidation[55], via effects on endothelial function and the nitric oxide pathway.

Smooth muscle and endothelial cell proliferation

Nitric oxide inhibits proliferation of smooth muscle cells[56] and slows the development of atheroma, by inhibiting smooth muscle cell proliferation while stimulating proliferation of endothelial cells[57]. Estradiol has similar effects[6,58], which may be related to a nitric oxide-dependent mechanism. Recent reports demonstrate increased re-endothelialization[59,60], accelerated functional recovery of the endothelium and decreased neointimal thickening in animals subjected to carotid artery injury and given estrogen therapy[60]. These findings may explain the attenuation of restenosis after coronary angioplasty in postmenopausal women taking hormone replacement therapy[61,62]. The results of a recent study indicate that estradiol may prevent cell death of endothelial cells exposed to noxious stimuli[63]. There was a 50% decrease in apoptosis in human umbilical vein endothelial cells exposed to tumor necrosis factor-α together with estradiol, compared to cells without estrogen. This effect was reversed by the estrogen-receptor antagonist ICI 182,780, suggesting a receptor-dependent effect.

Vessel wall structure and interactions

Estrogen affects the extracellular matrix of the vessel wall by altering the proportion of collagen and elastin, enhancing the ratio of procollagen type 1 to procollagen type 3, for example[64,65]. This may contribute to plaque stability[66]. In theory, the relative rate of turnover and accumulation of collagen and elastin could affect the stiffness of the wall and, therefore, may be impli-

cated in the development of pathology of the vessel. Estrogen has the potential to enhance the development of the collateral coronary circulation in the presence of flow-limiting stenoses. *In vitro* work suggests that estrogen can enhance the migration and proliferation of endothelial cells, facilitating the organization into tubular networks, which may be critical to angiogenesis[67], a response which may limit myocardial damage should abrupt thrombotic closure of a coronary vessel occur.

Estrogen may have beneficial effects on monocyte–vessel wall interactions indirectly through preservation of the endothelium and nitric oxide production. Nitric oxide inhibits monocyte adhesion to the endothelium[68], synthesizes factors which enhance chemotaxis of monocytes[69], and reduces platelet adhesion to the endothelium[70]. Since monocyte adhesion to the blood vessel wall is one of the initiating events in the atherosclerotic process, estrogen may protect the vasculature from atheroma formation in part via this mechanism. This is further reinforced by a recent study in cultured human endothelial cells which demonstrated that 17β-estradiol can reduce surface expression and messenger RNA levels of cell adhesion molecules (involved in early atherosclerotic lesions), an effect which was mediated by the estrogen receptor[71].

Thrombogenesis

The effect of estrogen on acute vascular reactivity may be relevant to the onset of acute events, and possibly the prevention of acute events by preserving normal endothelial function and therefore decreasing the tendency to vasoconstriction and plaque rupture. Experimental and clinical studies have shown that the endothelium, in the presence of risk factors, loses the ability to produce the vasodilator NO and, therefore, may be involved in the genesis of atherosclerosis and may enhance a tendency to vasoconstriction[72–74].

Estrogen's effects on hemostatic factors, favoring a tendency towards fibrinolysis[75], do not support the widely held belief that treatment of postmenopausal women with estrogen increases arterial thrombotic tendency. In contrast, accompanied by the favorable effect of hormone therapy on platelet aggregability, these data may explain, in part, the favorable association of hormone therapy with cardiovascular disease risk.

The picture may be different for venous thrombosis. An epidemiological study suggested a slight increase in the tendency to venous thrombosis in low-risk postmenopausal women taking hormone therapy (5 per 100 000 woman-years)[76], and the recently reported Heart and Estrogen/progestin Replacement Study (HERS) showed an increase in the incidence of venous thromboembolism in the hormone-treated group versus placebo (6.3 per 1000 woman-years versus 2.2 per 1000 woman-years, respectively)[77].

Platelet function

Platelets are a vital participant in the intrinsic coagulation pathway. They adhere to subendothelial collagen fibers, where they release their intracellular contents, including thromboxane A_2 and serotonin, causing platelet aggregation and vasoconstriction, respectively. Endothelium-derived nitric oxide inhibits platelet adhesion[70], release[78] and aggregation[79] of human platelets *in vitro*. *In vivo*, stimulated release of endothelium-derived nitric oxide inhibits platelet aggregation by a cyclic GMP-mediated mechanism[80].

Estrogen-induced stimulation of basal nitric oxide synthesis and release from the endothelium may prevent initiation of thrombus generation by inhibiting platelet adhesion. 17β-Estradiol reduces platelet adherence to the endothelium *in vitro*[81]. Platelet aggregability is reduced by estrogen, which may be due to an inhibitory effect on calcium handling in human platelets[82]. Postmenopausal estrogen therapy is associated with decreased platelet aggregation and ATP release[83]. These mechanisms may contribute to protection from thrombus formation and account partially for the decreased risk of myocardial infarction and stroke in postmenopausal estrogen users.

Prostacyclin

Estrogen may indirectly affect thrombosis formation via nitric oxide-stimulated prostacyclin production, which in turn inhibits platelet aggregation, and affects aggregation by a cyclic GMP-dependent mechanism[84]. Physiological doses of estradiol increase prostacyclin production, possibly by a receptor-dependent mechanism[85].

Myocardial infarction

A tendency towards an increase in thombolysis and a decrease in platelet aggregability by estrogen could contribute to a decreased tendency to acute vascular events. Estrogen therapy reduces the risk of myocardial infarction in postmenopausal women[86–89]. The risk of myocardial infarction is also decreased in high-risk women with a previous history of cardiovascular disease or myocardial infarction[86,87,90,91]. It is plausible that the vasorelaxant effect of estrogen on the coronary arteries, coupled with a tendency toward a decrease in thrombosis, may be major contributory factors, resulting in a decrease in acute cardiovascular events such as myocardial infarction. Indeed, a report in dogs demonstrated that pretreatment with 17β-estradiol decreased infarct size and incidence of ventricular tachycardia during occlusion of the left anterior descending coronary artery. This effect was mediated by NO and opening of K_{Ca} channels[92].

The HERS study, however, using a combination of conjugated equine estrogens and medroxyprogesterone acetate, showed a null effect on the primary outcome of non-fatal myocardial infarction and coronary heart disease death in postmenopausal women with established coronary heart disease[77]. While there was a trend towards an increase in the incidence of coronary heart disease events in the 1st year of treatment in patients taking hormone replacement therapy, by years 4 and 5, this trend was reversed. This suggests that more prolonged treatment is required for conferment of cardiovascular benefit and would be in accord with atherosclerosis inhibition and plaque stabilization. Recent data suggest that the type of progestin used may be important. While medroxyprogesterone acetate in combination with conjugated estrogens has a beneficial effect on lipid profile[93], other studies suggest that medroxyprogesterone acetate may abolish the beneficial vasomotor effects of estrogen[94,95].

MYOCARDIAL ISCHEMIA

Estrogen-induced reduction in vascular resistance and increases in coronary flow may account for acute and chronic effects of estrogen on exercise-induced myocardial ischemia, where coronary stenoses become flow-limiting[96,97]. Webb and colleagues demonstrated a beneficial effect of 4 and 8 weeks' administration of transdermal 17β-estradiol versus placebo on signs of exercise-induced myocardial ischemia on the electrocardiogram (time to 1 mm ST-segment depression). This effect may be due to a direct relaxing effect on the coronary arteries[98,99], or/and peripheral vasodilatation[100], or/and a direct effect on the cardiac myocytes. Acute sublingual 17β-estradiol reduces the degree of pacing-induced myocardial ischemia in postmenopausal women with atherosclerotic coronary heart disease, as indicated by a reduction in pacing-induced coronary sinus pH shift by estradiol[101]. Using dobutamine stress-echocardiography, a recent study demonstrated a beneficial effect of acute intravenous administration of conjugated estrogens on stress-induced symptoms, summed ST-segment changes and left ventricular wall motion[102]. Further studies will be required to prove the efficacy of long-term estrogen therapy in the treatment of angina in the presence of coronary artery disease.

CONCLUSIONS

Despite the mechanistic data to support a beneficial effect of estrogen on the coronary circulation, there is still controversy over whether to prescribe estrogen to postmenopausal women for prevention of coronary heart disease. The HERS study has resulted in caution by many practitioners; however, we await the results of numerous on-going studies, using differing hormone preparations and in different patient populations, before we can make certain, evidence-based decisions.

References

1. McGill HC Jr. Sex steroid hormone receptors in the cardiovascular system. *Postgrad Med* 1989; 64–8

2. Kahn D, Zeng Q, Kajani M, Eagon PK, Lai H, Makowka L, Starzl TE, Van Theil DH. The effect of different types of hepatic injury on the estrogen and androgen receptor activity of liver. *J Invest Surg* 1989;2:125–33

3. Losordo DW, Kearney M, Kim EA, Jekanowski J, Isner JM. Variable expression of the estrogen receptor in normal and atherosclerotic coronary arteries of premenopausal women. *Circulation* 1994;89:1501–10

4. Collins P, Sheppard M, Beale CM, *et al.* The classical estrogen receptor is not found in human coronary arteries [Abstract]. *Circulation* 1995;92:1–37

5. Venkov CD, Rankin AB, Vaughan DE. Identification of authentic estrogen receptor in cultured endothelial cells. A potential mechanism for steroid hormone regulation of endothelial function. *Circulation* 1996;94:727–33

6. Kim-Schulze S, McGowan KA, Hubchak SC, Cid MC, Martin MB, Kleinman HK, Greene GL, Schnaper W. Expression of an estrogen receptor by human coronary artery and umbilical vein endothelial cells. *Circulation* 1996;94:1402–7

7. Kuiper GG, Enmark E, Pelto-Huikko M, Nilsson S, Gustafsson JA. Cloning of a novel receptor expressed in rat prostate and ovary. *Proc Natl Acad Sci USA* 1996;93:5925–30

8. Grohe C, Kahlert S, Lobbert K, Stimpel M, Karas RH, Vetter H, Neyses L. Cardiac myocytes

and fibroblasts contain functional estrogen receptors. *FEBS Lett* 1997;416:107–12

9. Moncada S, Higgs A. The L-arginine–nitric oxide pathway. *N Engl J Med* 1993;329:2002–12

10. Gisclard V, Miller VM, Vanhoutte PM. Effect of 17β-estradiol on endothelium-dependent responses in the rabbit. *J Pharmacol Exp Ther* 1988; 244:19–22

11. Bell DR, Rensberger HJ, Koritnik DR, Koshy A. Estrogen pretreatment directly potentiates endothelium-dependent vasorelaxation of porcine coronary arteries. *Am J Physiol* 1995;268: H377–83

12. Williams SP, Shackelford DP, Iams SG, Mustafa SJ. Endothelium-dependent relaxation in estrogen-treated spontaneously hypertensive rats. *Eur J Pharmacol* 1988;145:205–7

13. Gura T. Estrogen: key player in heart disease among women. *Science* 1995;269:771–3

14. Hayashi T, Fukuto JM, Ignarro LJ, Chaudhuri G. Basal release of nitric oxide from aortic rings is greater in female rabbits than in male rabbits: implications for atherosclerosis. *Proc Natl Acad Sci USA* 1992;89:11259–63

15. Wellman GC, Bonev AD, Nelson MT, Brayden JE. Gender differences in coronary artery diameter involve estrogen, nitric oxide, and Ca^{2+}-dependent K^+ channels. *Circ Res* 1996;79: 1024–30

16. Cicinelli E, Ignarro LJ, Lograno M, Matteo G, Falco N, Schonauer LM. Acute effects of transdermal estradiol administration on plasma levels of nitric oxide in postmenopausal women. *Fertil Steril* 1997;67:63–6

17. Guetta V, Quyyumi AA, Prasad A, Panza JA, Waclawiw M, Cannon RO III. The role of nitric oxide in coronary vascular effects of estrogen in postmenopausal women. *Circulation* 1997;96: 2795–801

18. Weiner CP, Lizasoain I, Baylis SA, Knowles RG, Charles IG, Moncada S. Induction of calcium-dependent nitric oxide synthases by sex hormones. *Proc Natl Acad Sci USA* 1994;91:5212–16

19. Hishikawa K, Nakaki T, Marumo T, Suzuki H, Kato R, Saruta T. Up-regulation of nitric oxide synthase by estradiol in human aortic endothelial cells. *FEBS Lett* 1995;360:291–3

20. Wilcox JG, Hatch IE, Gentzschein E, Stanczyk FZ, Lobo RA. Endothelin levels decrease after oral and nonoral estrogen in postmenopausal women with increased cardiovascular risk factors. *Fertil Steril* 1997;67:273–7

21. Asselin E, Goff AK, Bergeron H, Fortier MA. Influence of sex steroids on the production of prostaglandins F2 alpha and E2 and response to oxytocin in cultured epithelial and stromal cells of the bovine endometrium. *Biol Reprod* 1996; 54:371–9

22. Chen Z, Yuhanna IS, Galcheva-Gargova Z, Karas RH, Mendelsohn ME, Shaul PW. Estrogen receptor alpha mediates the nongenomic activation of endothelial nitric oxide synthase by estrogen. *J Clin Invest* 1999;103:401–6

23. Rubanyi GM, Freay AD, Kauser K, Sukovich D, Burton G, Lubahn DB, Couse JF, Curtis SW, Korach KS. Vascular estrogen receptors and endothelium-derived nitric oxide production in the mouse aorta. *J Clin Invest* 1997;99:2429–37

24. Hayashi T, Yamada K, Esaki T, Kuzuya M, Satake S, Ishikawa T, Hidaka H, Iguchi A. Estrogen increases endothelial nitric oxide by a receptor-mediated system. *Biochem Biophys Res Commun* 1995;214:847–55

25. Lampe JW, Martini MC, Kurzer MS, Adlercreutz H, Slavin JL. Urinary lignan and isoflavonoid excretion in premenopausal women consuming flaxseed powder. *Am J Clin Nutr* 1994;60: 122–8

26. Jiang C, Sarrel PM, Lindsay DC, Poole-Wilson PA, Collins P. Endothelium-independent relaxation of rabbit coronary artery by 17β-oestradiol *in vitro*. *Br J Pharmacol* 1991;104:1033–7

27. Jiang C, Poole-Wilson PA, Sarrel PM, Mochizuki S, Collins P, MacLeod KT. Effect of 17β-oestradiol on contraction, Ca^{2+} current and intracellular free Ca^{2+} in guinea-pig isolated cardiac myocytes. *Br J Pharmacol* 1992;106: 739–45

28. Han SZ, Karaki H, Ouchi Y, Akishita M, Orimo H. 17β-Estradiol inhibits Ca^{2+} influx and Ca^{2+} release induced by thromboxane A2 in porcine coronary artery. *Circulation* 1995;91:2619–26

29. Sudhir K, Chou TM, Mullen WL, Hausmann D, Collins P, Yock PG, Chatterjee K. Mechanisms of estrogen-induced vasodilation: *in vivo* studies in canine coronary conductance and resistance arteries. *J Am Coll Cardiol* 1995;26:807–14

30. Toro L, Scornik F, Sperelakis N, Kuriyama H, eds. *Ion Channels of Vascular Smooth Muscle Cells and Endothelial Cells*. New York: Elsevier, 1991: 111–24

31. White RE, Darkow DJ, Lang JL. Estrogen relaxes coronary arteries by opening BKCa channels through a cGMP-dependent mechanism. *Circ Res* 1995;77:936–42

32. Rusko J, Li L, van Breemen C. 17-beta-Estradiol stimulation of endothelial K+ channels. *Biochem Biophys Res Commun* 1995;214:367–72

33. Yanagisawa M, Kurihara H, Kimura S, Tomobe Y, Kobayashi M, Mitsui Y, Yazaki Y, Goto K, Masaki T. A novel potent vasoconstrictor peptide produced by vascular endothelial cells. *Nature (London)* 1988;332:411–15

34. Wallnofer A, Weir S, Ruegg U, Cauvin C. The mechanism of action of endothelin-1 as compared with other agonists in vascular smooth

muscle. *J Cardiovasc Pharmacol* 1989;13(Suppl 5):S23–31

35. Nayler WG. *The Endothelins.* Berlin: Springer-Verlag, 1990

36. Hirata Y, Yoshimi H, Emori T, Shichiri M, Marumo F, Watanabe TX, Kumagaye S, Nakajima K, Kimura T, Sakakibara S. Receptor binding activity and cytosolic free calcium response by synthetic endothelin analogs in cultured rat vascular smooth muscle cells. *Biochem Biophys Res Commun* 1989;160:228–34

37. Simon D, Preziosi P, Barrett-Connor E, Roger M, Saint-Paul M, Nahoul K, Papoz L. Interrelation between plasma testosterone and plasma insulin in healthy adult men: the Telecom Study. *Diabetologia* 1992;35:173–7

38. Jiang C, Sarrel PM, Poole-Wilson PA, Collins P. Acute effect of 17β-estradiol on rabbit coronary artery contractile responses to endothelin-1. *Am J Physiol* 1992;263:H271–5

39. Vallance P, Moncada S, Nitric oxide – from mediator to medicines. *J R Coll Phys* 1995;1994:209–19

40. Fuleihan GE. Tissue-specific estrogens – the promise for the future. *N Engl J Med* 1997;337:1686–7

41. Lerman A, Webster MWI, Chesebro JH, Edwards WD, Wei C-M, Fuster V, Burnett JC Jr. Circulating and tissue endothelin immunoreactivity in hypercholesterolemic pigs. *Circulation* 1993;88:2923–8

42. Reis SE, Gloth ST, Blumenthal RS, Resar JR, Zacur HA, Gerstenblith G, Brinker JA. Ethinyl estradiol acutely attenuates abnormal coronary vasomotor responses to acetylcholine in postmenopausal women. *Circulation* 1994;89:52–60

43. Gilligan DM, Quyyumi AA, Cannon RO III. Effects of physiological levels of estrogen on coronary vasomotor function in postmenopausal women. *Circulation* 1994;89:2545–51

44. Collins P, Rosano GMC, Sarrel PM, Ulrich L, Adamopoulos S, Beale CM, McNeill J, Poole-Wilson PA. Estradiol-17β attenuates acetylcholine-induced coronary arterial constriction in women but not men with coronary heart disease. *Circulation* 1995;92:24–30

45. Livesley B, Catley PF, Campbell RC, Oram S. Double-blind evaluation of verapamil, propranolol, and isosorbide dinitrate against a placebo in the treatment of angina pectoris. *Br Med J* 1973;17:375–8

46. Williams JK, Adams MR, Klopfenstein HS. Estrogen modulates responses of atherosclerotic coronary arteries. *Circulation* 1990;81:1680–7

47. Williams JK, Adams MR, Herrington DM, Clarkson TB. Short-term administration of estrogen and vascular responses of atherosclerotic coronary arteries. *J Am Coll Cardiol* 1992;20:452–7

48. Herrington DM, Braden GA, Williams JK, Morgan TM. Endothelial-dependent coronary vasomotor responsiveness in postmenopausal women with and without estrogen replacement therapy. *Am J Cardiol* 1994;73:951–2

49. Stampfer MJ, Colditz GA. Estrogen replacement therapy and coronary heart disease: a quantitative assessment of the epidemiologic evidence. *Prev Med* 1991;20:47–63

50. Gruchow HW, Anderson AJ, Barboriak JJ, Sobocinski KA. Postmenopausal use of estrogen and occlusion of coronary arteries. *Am Heart J* 1988;115:954–63

51. Sullivan JM, Vander Zwaag R, Lemp GF, Hughes JP, Maddock V, Kroetz FW, Ramanathan KB, Mirvis DM. Postmenopausal estrogen use and coronary atherosclerosis. *Ann Intern Med* 1988;108:358–63

52. Flavahan NA. Atherosclerosis or lipoprotein-induced dysfunction. Potential mechanisms underlying reduction in EDRF/nitric oxide activity. *Circulation* 1992;85:1927–38

53. Vita JA, Treasure CB, Nabel EG, McLenachan JM, Fish RD, Yeung AC, Vekshtein VI, Selwyn AP, Ganz P. Coronary vasomotor response to acetylcholine relates to risk factors for coronary artery disease. *Circulation* 1990;81:491–7

54. Ross R. The pathogenesis of atherosclerosis – an update. *N Engl J Med* 1986;314:488–500

55. Sack MN, Rader DJ, Cannon RO III. Oestrogen and inhibition of oxidation of low-density lipoproteins in postmenopausal women. *Lancet* 1994;343:269–70

56. Garg UC, Hassid A. Nitric oxide-generating vasodilators and 8-bromo-cyclic guanosine monophosphate inhibit mitogenesis and proliferation of cultured rat vascular smooth muscle cells. *J Clin Invest* 1989;83:1774–7

57. Dubey RK, Overbeck HW. Culture of rat mesenteric arteriolar smooth muscle cells: effects of platelet-derived growth factor, angiotensin, and nitric oxide on growth. *Cell Tissue Res* 1994;275:133–41

58. Fischer-Dzoga K, Wissler RW, Vesselinovitch D. The effect of estradiol on the proliferation of rabbit aortic medial tissue culture cells induced by hyperlipemic serum. *Exp Mol Pathol* 1983;39:355–63

59. White CR, Shelton J, Chen SJ, Darley-Usmar V, Allen L, Nabors C, Sanders PW, Chen YF, Oparil S. Estrogen restores endothelial cell function in an experimental model of vascular injury. *Circulation* 1997;96:1624–30

60. Krasinski K, Spyridopoulos I, Asahara T, van der Zee R, Isner JM, Losordo DW. Estradiol accelerates functional endothelial recovery after arterial injury. *Circulation* 1997;95:1768–72

61. O'Keefe JH Jr, Kim SC, Hall RR, Cochran VC, Lawhorn SL, McCallister BD. Estrogen

replacement therapy after coronary angioplasty in women. *J Am Coll Cardiol* 1997;29:1–5

62. O'Brien JE, Peterson ED, Keeler GP, Berdan LG, Ohman EM, Faxon DP, Jacobs AK, Topol EJ, Califf RM. Relation between estrogen replacement therapy and restenosis after percutaneous coronary interventions. *J Am Coll Cardiol* 1996;28:1111–18

63. Akhras F, Jackson G. Efficacy of nifedipine and isosorbide mononitrate in combination with atenolol in stable angina. *Lancet* 1991;338: 1036–9

64. Beldekas JC, Smith B, Gerstenfeld LC, Sonenshein GE, Franzblau C. Effects of 17 beta-estradiol on the biosynthesis of collagen in cultured bovine aortic smooth muscle cells. *Biochemistry* 1981;20:2162–7

65. Fischer GM, Swain ML. Effects of estradiol and progesterone on the increased synthesis of collagen in atherosclerotic rabbit aortas. *Atherosclerosis* 1985;54:177–85

66. Fischer GM, Cherian K, Swain ML. Increased synthesis of aortic collagen and elastin in experimental atherosclerosis. Inhibition by contraceptive steroids. *Atherosclerosis* 1981;39: 463–7

67. Morales DE, McGowan KA, Grant DS, Maheshwari S, Bhartiya D, Cid MC, Kleinman HK, Schnaper HW. Estrogen promotes angiogenic activity in human umbilical vein endothelial cells *in vitro* and in a murine model. *Circulation* 1995;91:755–63

68. Bath PM, Hassall DG, Gladwin AM, Palmer RM, Martin JF. Nitric oxide and prostacyclin. Divergence of inhibitory effects on monocyte chemotaxis and adhesion to endothelium *in vitro*. *Arterioscler Thromb* 1991;11:254–60

69. Zeiher AM, Fisslthaler B, Schray-Utz B, Busse R. Nitric oxide modulates the expression of monocyte chemoattractant protein 1 in cultured human endothelial cells. *Circ Res* 1995;76:980–6

70. Radomski MW, Palmer RMJ, Moncada S. Endogenous nitric oxide inhibits human platelet adhesion to vascular endothelium. *Lancet* 1987; 2:1057–8

71. Fukui M, Fujimoto T, Watanabe K, Endo K, Kuno K. Prostaglandin F synthase is localized to contractile interstitial cells in bovine lung. *J Histochem Cytochem* 1996;44:251–7

72. Meredith IT, Yeung AC, Weidinger FF, Anderson TJ, Uehata A, Ryan TJ, Selwyn AP, Ganz P. Role of impaired endothelium-dependent vasodilation in ischemic manifestations of coronary artery disease. *Circulation* 1993;87(Suppl V):56–66

73. Ludmer PL, Selwyn AP, Shook TL, Wayne RR, Mudge GH, Alexander RW, Ganz P. Paradoxical vasoconstriction induced by acetylcholine in atherosclerotic coronary arteries. *N Engl J Med* 1986;315:1046–51

74. Gimbrone MA Jr, Cybulsky MI, Kume N, Collins T, Resnick N. Vascular endothelium. An integrator of pathophysiological stimuli in atherogenesis. *Ann NY Acad Sci* 1995;748: 122–31

75. Gebara OCE, Mittleman MA, Sutherland P, Lipinska I, Matheney T, Xu P, Welty FK, Wilson PWF, Levy D, Muller JE, *et al.* Association between increased estrogen status and increased fibrinolytic potential in the Framingham Offspring Study. *Circulation* 1995;91:1952–8

76. Grodstein F, Stampfer MJ, Goldhaber SZ, Manson JE, Colditz GA, Speizer FE, Willett WC, Hennekens CH. Prospective study of exogenous hormones and risk of pulmonary embolism in women. *Lancet* 1996;348:983–7

77. Hulley S, Grady D, Bush T, Furberg C, Herrington D, Riggs B, Vittinghoff E. Randomized trial of estrogen plus progestin for secondary prevention of coronary heart disease in postmenopausal women. *J Am Med Assoc* 1998;280: 605–12

78. Lieberman EH, O'Neill S, Mendelsohn ME. *S*-nitrosocysteine inhibition of human platelet secretion is correlated with increases in platelet cGMP levels. *Circ Res* 1991;68:1722–8

79. Alheid U, Frolich JC, Forstermann U. Endothelium-derived relaxing factor from cultured human endothelial cells inhibits aggregation of human platelets. *Thromb Res* 1987;47: 561–71

80. Hogan JC, Lewis MJ, Henderson AH. *In vivo* EDRF activity influences platelet function. *Br J Pharmacol* 1988;94:1020–2

81. Miller ME, Dores GM, Thorpe SL, Akerley WL. Paradoxical influence of estrogenic hormones on platelet–endothelial cell interactions. *Thromb Res* 1994;74:577–94

82. Raman BB, Standley PR, Rajkumar V, Ram JL, Sowers JR. Effects of estradiol and progesterone on platelet calcium responses. *Am J Hypertens* 1995;8:197–200

83. Bar J, Tepper R, Fuchs J, Pardo Y, Goldberger S, Ovadia J. The effect of estrogen replacement therapy on platelet aggregation and adenosine triphosphate release in postmenopausal women. *Obstet Gynecol* 1993;81:261–4

84. Radomski MW, Palmer RM, Moncada S. The role of nitric oxide and cGMP in platelet adhesion to vascular endothelium. *Biochem Biophys Res Commun* 1987;148:1482–9

85. Mikkola T, Ranta V, Orpana A, Ylikorkala O, Viinikka L. Effect of physiological concentrations of estradiol on PGI_2 and NO in endothelial cells. *Maturitas* 1996;25:141–7

86. Henderson BE, Paginini-Hill A, Ross RK. Decreased mortality in users of estrogen replacement therapy. *Arch Intern Med* 1991;151:75–8

87. Henderson BE, Paganini-Hill A, Ross RK. Estrogen replacement therapy and protection from

acute myocardial infarction. *Am J Obstet Gynecol* 1988;159:312–17

88. Jick H, Dinan B, Rothman KJ. Noncontraceptive estrogens and nonfatal myocardial infarction. *J Am Med Assoc* 1978;239:1407–9

89. Falkeborn M, Persson I, Adami HO, Bergstrom R, Eaker E, Lithell H, Mohsen R, Naessen T. The risk of acute myocardial infarction after oestrogen and oestrogen–progestogen replacement. *Br J Obstet Gynaecol* 1992;99:821–8

90. Bush TL, Barrett-Connor E, Cowan LD, Criqui MH, Wallace RB, Suchindran CM, Tyroler HA, Rifkind BM. Cardiovascular mortality and noncontraceptive use of estrogen in women: results from the Lipid Research Clinics Program Follow-up Study. *Circulation* 1987;75:1102–9

91. Ross RK, Paganini-Hill A, Mack TM, Arthur M, Henderson BE. Menopausal oestrogen therapy and protection from death from ischaemic heart disease. *Lancet* 1981;1:858–60

92. Johnston SD, Lu B, Dowsett M, Liang X, Kaufmann M, Scott GK, Osborne CK, Benz CC. Comparison of estrogen receptor DNA binding in untreated and acquired antiestrogen-resistant human breast tumors. *Cancer Res* 1997;57:3723–7

93. The Postmenopausal Estrogen/Progestin Interventions Trial Writing Group. Effects of estrogen or estrogen/progestin regimens on heart disease risk factors in postmenopausal women. *J Am Med Assoc* 1995;273:199–208

94. Miyagawa K, Rosch J, Stanczyk F, Hermsmeyer K. Medroxyprogesterone interferes with ovarian steroid protection against coronary vasospasm. *Nature Med* 1997;3:324–7

95. Rosano GMC, Sarrel PM, Chierchia SL, *et al.* Medroxyprogesterone (MPA) but not natural progesterone reverses the beneficial effect of estradiol-17β upon exercise induced myocardial ischemia. A double-blind cross-over study [Abstract]. *Circulation* 1996;94:1–18

96. Rosano GMC, Sarrel PM, Poole-Wilson PA, Collins P. Beneficial effect of oestrogen on exercise-induced myocardial ischaemia in women with coronary artery disease. *Lancet* 1993;342:133–6

97. Webb CM, Rosano GMC, Collins P. Oestrogen improves exercise-induced myocardial ischaemia in women. *Lancet* 1998;351:1556–7

98. Mugge A, Riedel M, Barton M, Kuhn M, Lichtlen PR. Endothelium independent relaxation of human coronary arteries by 17 beta-oestradiol *in vitro*. *Cardiovasc Res* 1993;27:1939–42

99. Chester AH, Jiang C, Borland JA, Yacoub MH, Collins P. Estrogen relaxes human epicardial coronary arteries through non-endothelium-dependent mechanisms. *Cor Art Dis* 1995;6:417–22

100. Volterrani M, Rosano GMC, Coats A, Beale C, Collins P. Estrogen acutely increases peripheral blood flow in postmenopausal women. *Am J Med* 1995;99:119–22

101. Rosano GMC, Caixeta AM, Chierchia SL, Arie S, Lopez-Hidalgo M, Pereira WI, Leonardo F, Webb CM, Pileggi F, Collins P. Acute anti-ischemic effect of estradiol-17β in postmenopausal women with coronary artery disease. *Circulation* 1997;96:2837–41

102. Alpaslan M, Shimokawa H, Kuroiwa-Matsumoto M, Harasawa Y, Takeshita A. Short-term estrogen administration ameliorates dobutamine-induced myocardial ischemia in postmenopausal women with coronary artery disease. *J Am Coll Cardiol* 1997;30:1466–71

16

Stroke, postmenopausal women and estrogen

M. Perez Barreto and A. Paganini-Hill

INTRODUCTION

Stroke attacks an American every 53 seconds and annually claims the lives of 160 000[1]. Despite declines in the death rate due to stroke over the past several decades, stroke remains the third leading killer (after heart disease and cancer) of women in the USA and most developed countries. Each year the absolute number of strokes and deaths from stroke in women increases, owing to the growing size of the elderly population.

Because incidence increases with age, there is a need for greater awareness of the importance of stroke and other cardiovascular diseases as a major public health issue for older women. Stroke represents a significant healthcare burden, with an estimated cost of more than $45 billion per year in the USA (Table 1)[1]. It accounts for more than half of all patients hospitalized for acute neurological diseases and, together with ischemic heart disease, ranks

first among all disease categories in hospital discharges. Leaving many survivors with mental and physical impairment, stroke is the leading cause of serious, long-term disability. Stroke is also the second leading cause of dementia (after Alzheimer's disease). However, in the very old it remains second in men but ranks first in women[2]. Depression also occurs in more than 30% of stroke patients, with an increased risk in women[3,4]. Thus, the magnitude of the epidemic in women and its consequences necessitate a strong emphasis on primary prevention to reduce the burden of stroke and other cardiovascular diseases in our society.

Unfortunately, misconceptions still exist that cardiovascular disease is not a real problem for women. Many women are far more fearful of breast or ovarian cancer than of stroke or heart disease. Yet one in three women will die of heart disease and one in six from stroke, while one in

Table 1 Estimated public health impact of stroke in the USA. Adapted from reference 1

Incidence	Prevalence	Mortality	Cost ($ billion)

600 000 strokes per year
   500 000 new strokes
   100 000 recurrent
     strokes
1 stroke every 53 s
	4 400 000 survivors
	2 150 000 men
	2 250 000 women
		160 000 stroke deaths
		   per year
		62 500 men
		97 500 women
		1 death from stroke
		   every 3.3 min
		1 of every 14.5 deaths
		proportion dying
		   within 1 year 29%
			direct
			   hospital/nursing: $24.2
			   physicians/other professionals: $2.2
			   drugs: $0.3
			   home health/other medical: $2.8
			   total direct: $29.5
			indirect
			   lost productivity/morbidity: $5.4
			   lost productivity/mortality: $10.4
			   total indirect: $15.8
			total: $45.3

nine will develop breast carcinoma and one in 25 will eventually die of it[5].

Here we review the recent advances in knowledge of stroke in postmenopausal women, with principal emphasis on hormone replacement therapy and its effects on the vascular system and potential neuroprotective action. Other aspects of stroke, including its clinical presentation, diagnosis and general management, are basically the same for men and women. For a review of these, see Barnnet and colleagues[6].

PREVALENCE, INCIDENCE AND MORTALITY

Both the prevalence and the incidence of stroke are higher in men than in women, increase with age and are greater in blacks than whites or Hispanics[1]. In both men and women, the incidence rate approximately doubles every 10 years after the age of 55 years (Figure 1)[7]. However, the gender difference disappears among older (> 80 years) adults[7,8]. Today, approximately 4 400 000 stroke victims in the USA are alive, and over half of them are female (Table 1)[1].

Although the lifetime risk of stroke is 20% higher in men, women are more likely to die of stroke (16% vs. 8%)[9]. Black women are roughly twice as likely to die of stroke as white women[10,11]. In fact, stroke is the single largest contributor to the black–white mortality difference[12]. However, nearly 40% of the race-related risk for stroke may be due to environmental or other stroke risk factors[12]. Among Hispanics, stroke mortality is similar to that for non-Hispanic whites at young ages and is marginally lower at older ages.

STROKE SUBTYPES

Stroke consists of a group of etiologically and clinically heterogeneous diseases that can be classified by their pathology as ischemic or hemorrhagic. About 70% of strokes are ischemic, 27% hemorrhagic and 3% of other etiologies, with similar frequencies in men and women[13]. The mechanism of ischemia (hemodynamic or thromboembolic) and the site of the vascular lesion can classify ischemic infarction as large vessel atherothrombotic (10% of all strokes), lacunar (19%), cardioembolic (14%) and of undetermined cause (28%). Intracranial hemorrhage can be further divided about equally into subarachnoid hemorrhage (SAH) or intracerebral hemorrhage, depending on the site and origin of the blood.

STROKE RISK FACTORS

Although most stroke risk factors are the same for men and women (Table 2)[14–17], a few exhibit gender differences. Below we discuss those risk factors that differ between men and women, may be modified by estrogen use, or are particularly relevant to postmenopausal women.

Hypertension

Hypertension is the leading stroke risk factor in both sexes and is one of the few risk factors common to all stroke subtypes[15–18]. Hypertension affects approximately 43 million men and women in the USA[19]. However, while a greater percentage of men younger than 60 years than women have high blood pressure, after age 60 more women than men are affected[20].

The benefit of lowering blood pressure for primary stroke prevention is overwhelming. In prospective observational studies, a difference of 5–6 mmHg in usual diastolic blood pressure (DBP) is associated with 35–40% less stroke, even among 'normotensive' individuals[21]. Similarly, prospective randomized trials indicate that a 5–6 mmHg decrease in DBP reduces

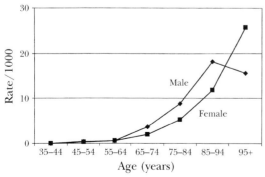

Figure 1 Annual incidence of stroke in men and women. Cardiovascular Health Study[8]

Table 2 Risk factors for ischemic stroke

Non-modifiable risk factors
Increasing age
Male gender
Black race
Family history of stroke

Disease history
Hypertension
Diabetes and impaired glucose tolerance
Hypercholesterolemia
Cardiac disease
    atrial fibrillation
    coronary heart disease
    left ventricular hypertrophy
    cardiac failure
Transient ischemic attack
Previous stroke
Asymptomatic carotid bruit

Lifestyle factors
Cigarette smoking
Alcohol consumption
Physical inactivity
Obesity
Diet
Stress
Street drugs

stroke risk by 33–55%[22], suggesting that just a few years of blood pressure lowering reduces stroke risk. However, results of some randomized clinical trials have suggested that treatment in women may not offer the same protection against stroke that it does in men[20,23].

There is little evidence to suggest that hormone replacement therapy (HRT) increases blood pressure in postmenopausal women. The 3-year Postmenopausal Estrogen and Progestin Interventions (PEPI) Trial found no effect of hormone therapy (unopposed estrogen or estrogen plus progestin) on blood pressure levels[24]. Hypertension should not be a relative contraindication to hormone therapy.

Diabetes and glucose metabolism

Diabetes mellitus affects six million Americans and nearly as many may be undiagnosed[25]. Epidemiological studies confirm diabetes as an independent risk factor for ischemic stroke, increasing the risk roughly 2–4 times[15,25–28]. However, diabetes is both more prevalent and a stronger risk factor in women than in men[26,27].

In addition, the risk of thromboembolic stroke increases with worsening glucose intolerance category (mildly elevated blood sugar, asymptomatic hyperglycemia, diabetes)[29]. Both hyperinsulinemia and increased insulin resistance are also risk factors for atherothrombotic infarction among subjects with normal glucose status[30].

The PEPI trial found that postmenopausal women taking oral estrogen or combined estrogen plus progestin had increased 2-h glucose levels compared with the placebo group[24]. Fasting insulin and glucose levels were lower in women assigned active treatment in this and other trials[31], as were fasting insulin levels in women treated with transdermal estrogen[32].

Serum cholesterol levels

About 40% of women aged 55 years and older have serum cholesterol levels that are considered high (≥ 240 mg/dl)[33]. However, the relationship between serum cholesterol and stroke is not clear and data on women are scant. A meta-analysis of 45 prospective epidemiological studies found no significant association between total serum cholesterol level and total stroke incidence[34]. Nonetheless, some studies in men have found that total cholesterol level measured years previously was directly related to incidence of and death from ischemic stroke[35,36]. Intervention trials have also given mixed results. A pooled analysis of 11 cholesterol-lowering trials (diet, drugs, or ileal bypass surgery) found no significant effect on all stroke (RR = 1.0) or fatal stroke (RR = 1.1)[37]. However, two of the trials with stroke subtype information suggested a possible lower risk of ischemic stroke (RR = 0.6; 95% CI 0.3–1.1). In addition, several clinical trials in patients with cardiovascular disease (myocardial infarction, coronary heart disease (CHD) or coronary artery disease) found stroke frequency significantly reduced by 30–60% in those treated with various statins vs. placebo[38–41].

After the menopause, low-density lipoprotein (LDL) cholesterol levels rise (commonly exceeding those of age-matched men) with a shift to smaller, denser and potentially more atherogenic particle sizes, while high-density lipoprotein (HDL) cholesterol levels decline[42,43]. Several randomized clinical trials have shown that oral administration of estrogen reduces LDL and total cholesterol levels and increases HDL, principally HDL_2, cholesterol levels in postmenopausal women[24,31,44,45]. The PEPI trial found that 3 years of daily use of 0.625 mg of unopposed oral conjugated equine estrogen (CEE) raised HDL cholesterol by 5.6 mg/dl[24]. With cyclic or sequential medroxyprogesterone acetate the increase was 1.2–1.6 mg/dl; and with micronized progesterone, 4.1 mg/dl. All active treatments decreased total cholesterol by 7.6–14.1 mg/dl, decreased LDL cholesterol by 14.5–17.7 mg/dl and increased triglycerides by 11.4–13.7 mg/dl. Thus, the beneficial action of CEE on lipids, and subsequently on atherosclerosis, should reduce the lipoprotein-associated risk of ischemic stroke. However, transdermal estrogen has little effect on lipoprotein levels, suggesting that the hepatic effects of estrogen absorbed through the gut are important for changes in lipoprotein levels[44].

Cardiac disease

Several cardiac diseases are associated with increased stroke risk. CHD, left ventricular hypertrophy and cardiac failure increase stroke risk about two-, three- and four-fold, respectively[8,28,46]. Atrial fibrillation increases stroke risk nearly five-fold and becomes increasingly important in the elderly[46]. In women, stroke risk associated with atrial fibrillation is almost twice that in men[46,47].

Cigarette smoking

Although the prevalence of smoking has decreased, progress in smoking control continues to be slower among women. Currently, about one-fourth of women in the USA smoke[48], and in the next millennium women smokers will exceed male smokers[49]. Cigarette smoking nearly doubles the risk of all forms of stroke, with a higher risk among women than men[50]. The number of cigarettes smoked increases the

risk in a clear dose–response relationship, and smoking cessation leads to a reduction in stroke risk. Women who smoke have an earlier age at natural menopause[51,52] and lower estrone and estradiol levels after receiving estrogen replacement therapy (ERT) than non-smokers[52].

HORMONE REPLACEMENT THERAPY AND STROKE

Millions of postmenopausal women use HRT – either unopposed ERT or combined estrogen plus progestin therapy. In 1992, over 39 million prescriptions were written for menopausal estrogens in the USA[53]. Although ERT has been available for 50 years, the indications for use have gradually widened from relief of current menopausal symptoms to prevention of future osteoporotic fractures or CHD. ERT has been associated with a 35% reduction in risk of CHD in observational studies[54,55]. Since stroke shares many risk factors with CHD, ERT may reduce stroke risk through modification of intervening risk factors in the same way as it lowers the risk of CHD. However, studies of HRT and stroke are limited.

The epidemiological evidence

In the past 25 years, 26 observational studies (in 37 articles) have evaluated the effect of HRT on stroke risk in postmenopausal women. Three designs have been used:

(1) Case–control studies comparing estrogen use among women with stroke to those without stroke[56–63];

(2) Uncontrolled cohort studies comparing the stroke rate in estrogen users to that in the general population[64–70];

(3) Internally controlled cohort studies comparing the stroke rate among estrogen users to that of non-users in the same sample[47,71–91].

All five case–control studies examining the association of HRT and risk of all stroke or ischemic stroke reported essentially null effects, with relative risks ranging from 0.97 to 1.20[57,58,60,62,63].

The four uncontrolled cohort studies[65,66,68,70] found a 20–50% reduced risk of stroke among estrogen users, which was statistically significant in two[68,70]. Twelve[71,73,75–77,79,81,84,85,89–91] of the 15 internally controlled cohort studies found a reduction of 30% or more in stroke risk among estrogen users, which was significant in four[71,77,81,84]. Two found a statistically significantly increased risk[47,74], and another no overall effect of estrogen[86].

Clearly, the association of estrogen and stroke is not as consistent as that of estrogen and CHD. The relative risks for total stroke (principally ischemic stroke) from all studies ranged from 0 to 3.2 (Figure 2). In 1993, Psaty and colleagues summarized the literature on estrogen and stroke and concluded that there was little, if any, association[92]. Grady and co-workers[55] derived a summary RR of stroke in ERT users of 0.96 (95% CI 0.82–1.13), but pointed out evidence of statistical heterogeneity among the studies. However, at the time of these summaries, few studies on estrogen and stroke had been published.

Evaluating the epidemiological evidence

Unfortunately, the studies of HRT and stroke are fraught with difficulties and potential biases:

(1) Data are derived from observational studies, not randomized trials;

(2) Crude and varying definitions of stroke end-points were used; few studies considered specific stroke subtypes;

(3) Often the only comparison made was between ever and never users of estrogen;

(4) The populations studied had different estrogen-use patterns including different estrogens, progestogens and combinations as well as different doses, durations and recency of HRT;

(5) Confounding factors were often not considered;

(6) The number of cases was often small, resulting in low statistical power.

Although stroke consists of a group of etiologically and clinically heterogeneous diseases, most epidemiological studies have grouped together all stroke subtypes. If HRT affects the risks of subtypes differently, combining them would mask the effect. Six studies looked specifically at ischemic or thromboembolic stroke[47,58,62,63,70,88], finding relative risks of 1.0–3.2. However, even ischemic stroke is a heterogeneous condition, both clinically and

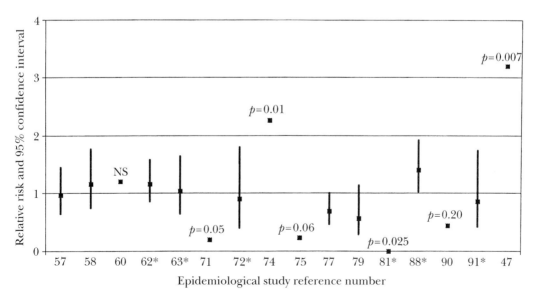

Figure 2 Epidemiological studies: hormone replacement therapy (HRT) and risk of total or ischemic stroke. Asterisks indicate current users of HRT

169

pathologically, originating not only from thromboembolic disease in the heart or carotid artery, but also from *in situ* arteriolar disease and lacunar infarction. The six studies that looked separately at SAH are also inconsistent[59,61,62,70,72,88]. Although three case–control studies[59,61,62] found a 35–50% reduced risk among estrogen users (significant in one[61]), three prospective studies[70,72,88] found no significant effect of estrogen, with relative risks ranging from 0.9 to 1.6. In all SAH studies, the number of cases was small (11–160). The low incidence makes the study of SAH difficult, especially in cohort studies.

Some of the conflicting results on estrogen use and stroke may be due to the grouping of all estrogen users together, regardless of dose, duration, recency of use, or type of estrogen. High doses may increase the stroke risk by a procoagulant effect; lower doses may decrease the risk by retarding atherosclerosis, and continuous and long-term therapy may be necessary. Unfortunately, detailed information on estrogen and stroke risk is limited. Paganini-Hill[84] found that the risk of fatal stroke was reduced in both long-term (≥ 15 years) and short-term (≤ 3 years) users. Petitti and associates[63] found no clear trend of increasing or decreasing risk of ischemic stroke in relation to duration of current hormone use. However, Longstreth and colleagues[61] found a decreasing risk of SAH with increasing duration (for trend $p < 0.002$). MacMahon[66] stated that the highest stroke risk was among women taking the larger doses, whereas Paganini-Hill[84] found that a dose of 1.25 mg or more of CEE offered about the same protection (RR = 0.37) against fatal stroke as did 0.625 mg or less (RR = 0.41). Both findings were based on small numbers. Schairer and co-workers[70] classified estrogens by potency and found that, for acute stroke, both potent estrogens (estradiol and conjugated estrogens) and weak estrogens (primarily estriol) were associated with a 20% reduction in risk. Although weak estrogens were not associated with intracerebral hemorrhage (RR = 0.9), a marked and significant reduction in risk was seen with potent estrogens (RR = 0.4).

If current estrogen users enjoy greater protection against stroke than past users, combining current and past into 'ever' use will produce a misleading risk estimate, since the proportion of current users (which will differ among studies) will affect the results. Eleven studies looked at current users separately from past users[58,61–63,72,81,84–86,88,89,91]. Six[58,62,63,72,86,91] found essentially no effect of current use on stroke risk (RR 0.86–1.17), and one[81] found a significantly reduced risk (RR = 0). For fatal stroke, all but one[86] of five studies[84–86,89,91] found at least a 30% reduced risk in current users (Figure 3). For SAH, one study[61] found a significantly reduced risk (RR = 0.38), another[88] essentially no effect (RR = 0.90) and a third[72] a non-significantly increased risk (RR = 1.6). A fourth[62] found that current users of ERT had a non-significantly reduced risk of SAH (RR = 0.52), while current users of combined HRT had a non-significantly increased risk (RR = 1.22). As the addition of progestin to the hormone regimen has been relatively recent, few studies[62,88] have been able to examine the risk of stroke in combined HRT users and ERT users separately.

As all these epidemiological studies associating estrogen use and stroke are non-experimental investigations without random assignment of subjects to estrogen or placebo, recall bias, selection bias and confounding are possible. A major concern of studies of the effects of HRT on disease is the possible self-selection of HRT by women with other health-promoting habits and the differential interaction with the medical care system between users and non-users. Although many investigators have adjusted their analyses for potential confounders, the possibility exists that women who use HRT are different from non-users in some unquantified but confounding way. Estrogen use may be a marker, rather than a cause, of good health.

A clinical trial with random assignment of women to estrogen and placebo groups would ensure that the estrogen and not some characteristic of estrogen users accounts for the beneficial effects observed among estrogen users. The only randomized clinical trial of

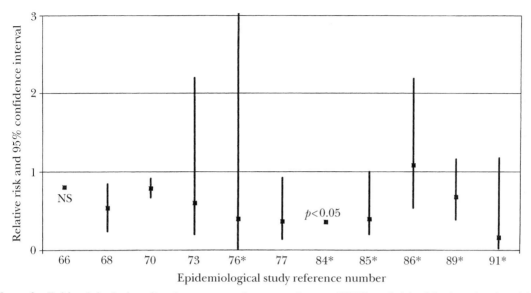

Figure 3 Epidemiological studies: hormone replacement therapy (HRT) and risk of fatal stroke. Asterisks indicate current users of HRT

HRT that looked at stroke end-points is the HERS trial[45]. A total of 2763 postmenopausal women with CHD were randomized to receive 0.625 mg CEE plus 2.5 mg medroxyprogesterone acetate or placebo daily. With an average follow-up of 4.1 years, treated women exhibited no difference in incidence of stroke or transient ischemic attack compared with controls (RR = 1.13, 95% CI 0.85–1.48). The study, however, did not examine unopposed estrogen or other estrogen and progestin regimens. It also did not study the use of HRT in postmenopausal women without CHD.

Although not completely consistent, the preponderance of evidence suggests that HRT does not increase stroke risk, and some evidence suggests that estrogen may decrease the risk. Overall, estrogen users appear to have a moderately lower risk of fatal stroke (Figure 3).

Hormone replacement therapy in women with stroke

Few studies have evaluated the risk of recurrent stroke in women using HRT. A secondary analysis of one clinical trial of aspirin in patients with transient ischemic attacks found that women who used estrogens had a significantly reduced risk of stroke, retinal infarction and death

(RR = 0.20; $p = 0.06$)[75]. In contrast, a reanalysis of another clinical trial of aspirin found that ERT was associated with a higher rate of ischemic stroke (RR = 3.2; $p = 0.007$)[47].

EFFECTS OF ESTROGEN ON THE VASCULAR SYSTEM

The vascular system is an important target for the action of estrogen. In addition to systemic effects (on serum lipid concentrations, coagulation, fibrinolysis and antioxidant activity), data suggest that estrogen acts directly on the vessel wall (promoting vasodilatation and inhibiting the development and progression of atherosclerosis) and protects the brain (increasing cerebral blood flow and reducing ischemia) (Table 3). Here, we review recent information about the mechanisms by which estrogen may reduce the incidence of vascular disease and ischemic stroke.

Systemic effects

Lipoprotein effects

In addition to effects on LDL and HDL cholesterol levels, estrogen reduces lipoprotein(a) levels in postmenopausal women[93,94]. Elevated

Table 3 Estrogen actions: effects against ischemic stroke

Systemic effects
Lipoprotein concentrations
    decreases LDL
    increases HDL, especially HDL_2
    decreases lipoprotein(a)
Coagulation and fibrinolytic systems
    decreases fibrinogen
    decreases plasminogen-activator inhibitor-1
    decreases tissue plasminogen activator antigen
Antioxidant systems
    inhibits LDL oxidation

Direct effects on the arterial wall
Vasodilatory effects
    promotes flow of potassium, sodium and
        calcium ions in vascular smooth-muscle cells
    enhances activity of the endothelium-derived
        relaxing factor nitric oxide
    increases prostacyclin production
Anti-inflammatory effects against vascular injury
    and atherosclerosis
    inhibits expression of cellular adhesion
        molecules
    inhibits proliferation of vascular smooth-muscle
        cells
    accelerates growth of endothelial cells

Neuroprotective effects
Increases cerebral blood flow
Reduces experimental ischemia

lipoprotein(a) is an independent risk factor for atherosclerosis and may promote thrombosis[95]. However, its importance as an independent risk factor for stroke is controversial[96].

Effects on the coagulation and fibrinolytic systems

In normal circumstances the coagulation system is a balance between maintaining flow in the vessels and stemming vessel leaks. Activation of blood coagulation with thrombosis is an obligatory event in almost all ischemic strokes. Several proteins are responsible for changes in blood coagulation and fibrinolysis, and many of these are affected by estrogen. Postmenopausal women have increased serum levels of fibrinogen, plasminogen-activator inhibitor-1 (PAI-1) and tissue plasminogen activator (tPA) antigen[97]. As the activity of the fibrinolytic system is dependent principally on the balance between

tPA and PAI-1, this finding may indicate an attenuation of fibrinolytic activity during the menopause. Oral estrogen therapy, alone or with progestin, has been associated with reduced plasma levels of PAI-1 and tPA antigen and with enhanced systemic fibrinolysis[97–100]. The PEPI and other studies found significantly lower fibrinogen levels in women taking estrogen than in untreated women[24,93,101,102]. However, estrogen also decreases the anticoagulant proteins antithrombin III and protein S[93,102], which may predispose to venous thrombosis. Transdermal administration of estrogen has not been associated with similar coagulation and fibrinolytic changes[98].

Antioxidant effects

Oxidation of lipoproteins plays a key role in atherogenesis. In cell culture[103–105] and in postmenopausal women[106,107], estradiol inhibits LDL oxidation, which may prevent the conversion of macrophages to foam cells and reduce lipid accumulation and plaque formation within the vessel wall. Likewise, all three conjugated equine estrogens (estrone sulfate, equilin sulfate and 17α-dihydroequilin sulfate) administered orally for 30 days prolonged the oxidative lag time[108].

Direct effects on the arterial wall

The ability of the arteries to vasodilate begins to decline after 50 years of age in women compared with age 40 in men[109,110], suggesting a beneficial effect of naturally occurring estrogens. Estrogens, administered orally, intravenously and intra-arterially to postmenopausal women, improve vasodilatation[111–115]. As blood vessels are complex structures, with walls containing smooth-muscle cells and an endothelial cell lining, estrogens can cause vasodilatation by various means.

Nitric oxide, ion channels and other derived factors

Two mechanisms for the rapid vasodilatory effects of estrogens are effects on ion-channel function and effects on nitric oxide[116]. First, ion channels direct the flow of potassium, sodium and calcium ions in and out of vascular smooth-muscle cells, determining the electrical potential of the membrane at rest and the contractile state of smooth muscle. Estrogen stimulates the opening of calcium-activated potassium channels, causing smooth muscle to relax and blood vessels to dilate. Second, normal endothelium in response to various stimuli releases nitric oxide, which both relaxes vascular smooth muscle and inhibits platelet activation. In cultured endothelial cells, estrogen causes a rapid release of nitric oxide. This release is blocked by estrogen receptor-α antagonists, suggesting that these effects may be mediated by estrogen receptor-α.

Estrogens also have long-term effects by increasing the expression of the genes for important vasodilatory enzymes such as prostacylin synthase and for the inducible form of nitric oxide synthase[117,118].

Vascular injury and atherosclerosis: anti-inflammatory effects

Atherosclerosis is increasingly recognized as a chronic inflammatory process associated with endothelial damage and dysfunction[119]. The changes preceding the formation of atherosclerotic lesions include increased endothelial permeability to lipoproteins and other plasma constituents (mediated in part by nitric oxide, prostacyclin and endothelin), up-regulation of leukocytes and endothelial adhesion molecules, migration of leukocytes into the artery wall (mediated in part by oxidized LDL-cholesterol) and proliferation of vascular smooth-muscle cells.

Estrogen may have a favorable effect on vascular inflammation and its atherogenic consequences, by inhibiting the proliferation of vascular smooth-muscle cells and accelerating the growth of endothelial cells. In postmenopausal women with coronary artery disease or hypercholesterolemia, those taking ERT have significantly lower levels of cellular adhesion molecules than do those not receiving ERT, and men[100,120]. Estrogens also accelerate endothelial cell growth *in vitro* and *in vivo*[121,122] and reduce the size of vascular lesions in carotid arteries and the aorta[122]. After vascular injury, the rapid re-endothelialization induced by estrogen may be partly due to increased local expression of vascular endothelial growth factor[122]. Early restoration of endothelial integrity by estrogen may contribute to the attenuation of the response to injury by increasing the availability of nitric oxide and thereby inhibiting the proliferation of smooth-muscle cells[123].

Estrogen appears to reduce subclincical atherosclerosis as measured by intimal–medial and plaque characteristics. In the Cardiovascular Health Study, current use of estrogen and estrogen plus progestin was associated with reduced carotid intimal–medial thickness[124]. In a 3-year lovastatin trial, investigators found that, in the placebo group, intimal–medial thickness tended to regress in ERT users but to progress among non-users[125].

Neuroprotective effects

Cerebral blood flow

Because estrogens have well-known vasoactive properties and their levels decrease after the menopause, changes in cerebral blood flow and vasomotor reactivity may occur after the menopause. Increasing evidence demonstrates that estrogen improves blood flow. Studies using transcranial Doppler ultrasonography have found estrogen-related differences in blood flow velocity, pulsatility index (PI) and vasomotor reactivity (VMR). VMR is lower in postmenopausal women compared to premenopausal women[126] and flow resistance of the internal carotid and middle cerebral arteries is increased[127]. In addition, time since menopause correlates with the PI in the cerebral circulation[127,128]. Both transdermal and oral estradiol given to postmenopausal women improves the PI in the internal carotid and middle cerebral arteries[128–131]. Some investigators have shown that estradiol replacement therapy increases the blood velocity and decreases resistance in the cerebral microcirculation (central retinal artery)[132]. Cyclic progestational supplementation does not modify the positive effect on reactivity of the blood vessels[129,131]. Likewise, single photon emission computed tomography (SPECT) scans of 15 postmenopausal women with Alzheimer's disease showed that the mean cerebral blood flow increased after 3–5 weeks of treatment with 0.625 mg of CEE[133].

Experimental ischemia

Estrogens seem to exert neuroprotective effects, improving stroke outcome. After experimental carotid occlusion, female rats showed smaller cerebral infarcts and less tissue damage than age-matched males[134]. In addition, pretreatment of ovariectomized rats with estradiol significantly reduced infarct volume following middle cerebral artery occlusion, although acute treatment did not[135]. These findings provide evidence for gender-specific responses to cerebrovascular occlusion and suggest a dual neuroprotective and flow-preserving effect of estrogen in the setting of cerebral ischemia and stroke.

CONCLUSION

An enduring half-truth about stroke and other cardiovascular diseases is that they are 'a man's disease'. However, as women approach the menopause, their risk of stroke begins to rise and increases steadily with age. Stroke is the third leading killer of women (and men). In fact, each year stroke claims the lives of more females than males. If women underestimate their risk of cardiovascular disease, they may not take the steps necessary to reduce their risk of these deadly – but to some extent preventable – diseases.

Because stroke is often fatal and the impact of treatment on prognosis is limited, control of the disease must be through primary prevention. The risk factors for stroke are similar for men and women. However, some (diabetes, atrial fibrillation) are more potent contributing factors for women in general, while others (hypertension, smoking, high cholesterol levels) are more frequent problems for older women. Today, women need to recognize the seriousness of stroke and other cardiovascular diseases and modify their risk factors to reduce the likelihood of stroke.

There is no strong evidence that HRT increases stroke risk and some evidence that it may moderately reduce the risk of fatal stroke. However, the epidemiological studies of estrogen and stroke are virtually all observational studies with all their inherent limitations. Clinical trials are needed to demonstrate more clearly the benefits of estrogen on the cardiovascular system. Nonetheless, potential biological mechanisms for a protective role of estrogen against stroke are plentiful. Further characterization of the cellular and molecular mechanisms by which estrogen inhibits cardiovascular disease will lead to the development of drugs free of unwanted side-effects.

References

1. American Heart Association. *1999 Heart and Stroke Statistical Update*. Dallas, TX: American Heart Association, 1998
2. Skoog I, Nilsson L, Palmertz B, *et al.* A population-based study of dementia in 85-year-olds. *N Engl J Med* 1993;328:153–8
3. Vestergaard AG, Ingemann-Nielsen M, Lauritzen L. Risk factors for post-stroke depression. *Acta Psychiatr Scand* 1995;92:193–8
4. Kotila M, Numminen H, Waltimo O, Kaste M. Depression after stroke. Results of the FINNSTROKE Study. *Stroke* 1998;29:368–72
5. American Heart Association. *1997 Heart and Stroke Statistical Update*. Dallas, TX: American Heart Association, 1996
6. Barnnet H, Mohr JP, Stein BM, Yatsu F, eds. *Stroke: Pathophysiology, Diagnosis, and*

Management, 3rd edn. Philadelphia, PA: Churchill Livingstone, 1998

7. Brown RD Jr, Whisnant JP, Sicks JRD, *et al.* Stroke incidence, prevalence, and survival. Secular trends in Rochester, Minnesota, through 1989. *Stroke* 1996;27:373–80

8. Manolio TA, Kronmal RA, Burke GL, *et al.* Short-term predictors of incident stroke in older adults. The Cardiovascular Health Study. *Stroke* 1996;27:1479–86

9. Bonita R. Epidemiology of stroke. *Lancet* 1992; 339:342–4

10. Howard G, Anderson R, Sorlie P, *et al.* Ethnic differences in stroke mortality between non-Hispanic whites, Hispanic whites, and blacks. The National Longitudinal Mortality Study. *Stroke* 1994;25:2120–5

11. Gillum RF. Stroke in blacks. *Stroke* 1988;19:1–9

12. Otten MW Jr, Teutsch SM, Williamson DF, Marks JS. The effect of known risk factors on the excess mortality of black adults in the United States. *J Am Med Assoc* 1990;263:845–50

13. Sacco R, Toni D, Mohr JP. Classification of ischemic stroke. In Barnnet H, Mohr JP, Stein BM, Yatsu F, eds. *Stroke: Pathophysiology, Diagnosis, and Management*, 3rd edn. Philadelphia, PA: Churchill Livingstone, 1998:341–54

14. Ostfeld AM, Wilk E. Epidemiology of stroke, 1980–1990: a progress report. *Epidemiol Rev* 1990;12:253–6

15. Bronner LL, Kanter DS, Manson JE. Primary prevention of stroke. *N Engl J Med* 1995;333: 1392–400

16. Thrift AG, Donnan GA, McNeil JJ. Epidemiology of intracerebral hemorrhage. *Epidemiol Rev* 1995;17:361–81

17. Teunissen LL, Rinkel GJE, Algra A, van Gijn J. Risk factors for subarachnoid hemorrhage. A systematic review. *Stroke* 1996;27:544–9

18. Marmot MG, Poulter NR. Primary prevention of stroke. *Lancet* 1992;339:344–7

19. Burt VL, Whelton P, Roccella EJ, *et al.* Prevalence of hypertension in the US adult population. Results from the Third National Health and Nutrition Examination Survey, 1988–1991. *Hypertension* 1995;25:305–13

20. Hayes SN, Taler SJ. Hypertension in women: current understanding of gender differences. *Mayo Clin Proc* 1998;73:157–65

21. MacMahon S, Peto R, Cutler J, *et al.* Blood pressure, stroke, and coronary heart disease. Part 1. Prolonged differences in blood pressure: prospective observational studies corrected for the regression dilution bias. *Lancet* 1990;335: 765–74

22. Collins R, Peto R, MacMahon S, *et al.* Blood pressure, stroke, and coronary heart disease. Part 2. Short-term reductions in blood pressure: overview of randomised drug trials in their epidemiological context. *Lancet* 1990;335:827–38

23. Reynolds E, Baron RB. Hypertension in women and the elderly. Some puzzling and some expected findings of treatment studies. *Postgrad Med* 1996;100:58–70

24. The Writing Group for the PEPI Trial. Effects of estrogen or estrogen/progestin regimens on heart disease risk factors in postmenopausal women. The Postmenopausal Estrogen/Progestin Interventions (PEPI) Trial. *J Am Med Assoc* 1995;273:199–208

25. Biller J, Love BB. Diabetes and stroke. *Med Clin North Am* 1993;77:95–110

26. Wolf PA, D'Agostino RB, Belanger AJ, Kannel WB. Probability of stroke: a risk profile from the Framingham study. *Stroke* 1991;22:312–18

27. Tuomilehto J, Rastenyte D, Jousilahti P, *et al.* Diabetes mellitus as a risk factor for death from stroke. Prospective study of the middle-aged Finnish population. *Stroke* 1996;27:210–15

28. Whisnant JP, Wiebers DO, O'Fallon WM, *et al.* A population-based model of risk factors for ischemic stroke: Rochester, Minnesota. *Neurology* 1996;47:1420–8

29. Burchfiel CM, Curb JD, Rodriguez BL, *et al.* Glucose intolerance and 22-year stroke incidence. The Honolulu Heart Program. *Stroke* 1994;25:951–7

30. Shinozaki K, Naritomi H, Shimizu T, *et al.* Role of insulin resistance associated with compensatory hyperinsulinemia in ischemic stroke. *Stroke* 1996;27:37–43

31. Lobo RA, Pickar JH, Wild RA, *et al.* Metabolic impact of adding medroxyprogesterone acetate to conjugated estrogen therapy in postmenopausal women. *Obstet Gynecol* 1994;84: 987–95

32. Cagnacci A, Soldani R, Carriero PL, *et al.* Effects of low doses of transdermal 17β-estradiol on carbohydrate metabolism in postmenopausal women. *J Clin Endocrinol Metab* 1992;74: 1396–400

33. Sempos CT, Cleeman JI, Carroll MD, *et al.* Prevalence of high blood cholesterol among US adults. An update based on guidelines from the Second Report of the National Cholesterol Education Program Adult Treatment Panel. *J Am Med Assoc* 1993;269:3009–14

34. Prospective Studies Collaboration. Cholesterol, diastolic blood pressure, and stroke: 13 000 strokes in 450 000 people in 45 prospective cohorts. *Lancet* 1995;346:1647–53

35. Benfante R, Yano K, Hwang L-J, *et al.* Elevated serum cholesterol is a risk factor for both coronary heart disease and thromboembolic stroke in Hawaiian Japanese men. Implications of shared risk. *Stroke* 1994;25:814–20

36. Iso H, Jacobs DR Jr, Wentworth D, *et al.* Serum cholesterol levels and six-year mortality from stroke in 350,977 men screened for the Multiple Risk Factor Intervention Trial. *N Engl J Med* 1989;320:904–10

37. Herbert PR, Gaziano JM, Hennekens CH. An overview of trials of cholesterol lowering and risk of stroke. *Arch Intern Med* 1995;155:50–5

38. Scandinavian Simvastatin Survival Study Group. Randomised trial of cholesterol lowering in 4444 patients with coronary heart disease: the Scandinavian Simvastatin Survival Study (4S). *Lancet* 1994;344:1383–9

39. Byington RP, Jukema JW, Salonen JT, *et al.* Reduction in cardiovascular events during pravastatin therapy. Pooled analysis of clinical events of the Pravastatin Atherosclerosis Intervention Program. *Circulation* 1995;92:2419–25

40. Sacks FM, Pfeffer MA, Moye LA, *et al.* The effect of pravastatin on coronary events after myocardial infarction in patients with average cholesterol levels. *N Engl J Med* 1996;335:1001–9

41. Plehn JF, Davis BR, Sacks FM, *et al.* Reduction of stroke incidence after myocardial infarction with pravastatin: the Cholesterol and Recurrent Events (CARE) Study. *Circulation* 1999;99: 216–23

42. Stevenson JC, Crook D, Godsland IF. Influence of age and menopause on serum lipids and lipoproteins in healthy women. *Atherosclerosis* 1993;98:83–90

43. Brown SA, Hutchinson R, Morrisett J, *et al.* Plasma lipid, lipoprotein cholesterol, and apoprotein distributions in selected US communities. The Atherosclerosis Risk in Communities (ARIC) Study. *Arterioscler Thromb* 1993;13: 1139–58

44. Walsh BW, Schiff I, Rosner B, *et al.* Effects of postmenopausal estrogen replacement therapy on the concentration and metabolism of plasma lipoproteins. *N Engl J Med* 1991;325: 1196–204

45. Hulley S, Grady D, Bush T, *et al.* Randomized trial of estrogen plus progestin for secondary prevention of coronary heart disease in postmenopausal women. *J Am Med Assoc* 1998;280: 605–13

46. Wolf PA, Abbott RD, Kannel WB. Atrial fibrillation as an independent risk factor for stroke: the Framingham Study. *Stroke* 1991;22:983–8

47. Hart RG, Pearce LA, McBride R, *et al.* Factors associated with ischemic stroke during aspirin therapy in atrial fibrillation. Analysis of 2012 participants in the SPAF I–III clinical trials. *Stroke* 1999;30:1223–9

48. Department of Health and Human Services. *Healthy People 2010 Objectives: Draft for Public Comments.* Item No. 0445; Sub Docs No. HE 20.2:P39 Tobacco use. Overview. DHHS publication.

Washington, DC: Government Printing Office, 1999

49. Pierce JP, Fiore MC, Novotny TE, *et al.* Trends in cigarette smoking in the United States. Projections to the year 2000. *J Am Med Assoc* 1989;261: 61–5

50. Shinton R, Beevers G. Meta-analysis of relation between cigarette smoking and stroke. *Br Med J* 1989;298:789–94

51. Midgette AS, Baron JA. Cigarette smoking and the risk of natural menopause. *Epidemiology* 1990;1:474–80

52. Gindoff PR, Stillman RJ. Influence of cigarette smoking on age at menopause, estrogen-related disease, and hormone replacement therapy. In Lobo RA, ed. *Treatment of the Postmenopausal Woman. Basic and Clinical Aspects.* New York, NY: Raven Press, 1994:295–300

53. Wysowski DK, Golden L, Burke L. Use of menopausal estrogens and medroxyprogesterone in the United States, 1982–1992. *Obstet Gynecol* 1995;85:6–10

54. Grodstein F, Stampfer M. The epidemiology of coronary heart disease and estrogen replacement in postmenopausal women. *Prog Cardiovasc Dis* 1995;38:199–210

55. Grady D, Rubin SM, Petitti DB, *et al.* Hormone therapy to prevent disease and prolong life in postmenopausal women. *Ann Intern Med* 1992;117: 1016–37

56. Pfeffer RI, Van den Noort S. Estrogen use and stroke risk in postmenopausal women. *Am J Epidemiol* 1976;103:445–56

57. Pfeffer RI. Estrogen use, hypertension and stroke in postmenopausal women. *J Chron Dis* 1978;31:389–98

58. Rosenberg SH, Fausone V, Clark R. The role of estrogens as a risk factor for stroke in postmenopausal women. *West J Med* 1980;133: 292–6

59. Adam S, Williams V, Vessey MP. Cardiovascular disease and hormone replacement treatment: a pilot case–control study. *Br Med J* 1981;282: 1277–8

60. Thompson SG, Meade TW, Greenberg G. The use of hormonal replacement therapy and the risk of stroke and myocardial infarction in women. *J Epidemiol Community Health* 1989;43: 173–8

61. Longstreth WT Jr, Nelson LM, Koepsell TD, van Belle G. Subarachnoid hemorrhage and hormonal factors in women. A population-based case–control study. *Ann Intern Med* 1994;121: 168–73

62. Pedersen AT, Lidegaard Ø, Kreiner S, Ottesen B. Hormone replacement therapy and risk of non-fatal stroke. *Lancet* 1997;350:1277–83

63. Petitti DB, Sidney S, Quesenberry CP Jr, Bernstein A. Ischemic stroke and use of

estrogen and estrogen/progestogen as hormone replacement therapy. *Stroke* 1998;29:23–8

64. Burch JC, Byrd BF Jr, Vaughn WK. The effects of long-term estrogen on hysterectomized women. *Am J Obstet Gynecol* 1974;118:778–82

65. Byrd BF Jr, Burch JC, Vaughn WK. The impact of long term estrogen support after hysterectomy. A report of 1016 cases. *Ann Surg* 1977;185: 574–80

66. MacMahon B. Cardiovascular disease and noncontraceptive oestrogen therapy. In Oliver MF, ed. *Coronary Heart Disease in Young Women.* New York, NY: Churchill Livingstone, 1978:197–207

67. Hunt K, Vessey M, McPherson K, Coleman M. Long-term surveillance of mortality and cancer incidence in women receiving hormone replacement therapy. *Br J Obstet Gynaecol* 1987; 94:620–35

68. Hunt K, Vessey M, McPherson K. Mortality in a cohort of long-term users of hormone replacement therapy: an updated analysis. *Br J Obstet Gynaecol* 1990;97:1080–6

69. Falkeborn M, Persson I, Terént A, *et al.* Hormone replacement therapy and the risk of stroke. Follow-up of a population-based cohort in Sweden. *Arch Intern Med* 1993;153:1201–9

70. Schairer C, Adami H-O, Hoover R, Persson I. Cause-specific mortality in women receiving hormone replacement therapy. *Epidemiology* 1997;8:59–65

71. Hammond CB, Jelovsek FR, Lee KL, *et al.* Effects of long-term estrogen replacement therapy. I. Metabolic effects. *Am J Obstet Gynecol* 1979;133:525–36

72. Petitti DB, Wingerd J, Pellegrin F, Ramcharan S. Risk of vascular disease in women. Smoking, oral contraceptives, noncontraceptive estrogens, and other factors. *J Am Med Assoc* 1979; 242:1150–4

73. Petitti DB, Perlman JA, Sidney S. Noncontraceptive estrogens and mortality: long-term follow-up of women in the Walnut Creek Study. *Obstet Gynecol* 1987;70:289–93

74. Wilson PWF, Garrison RJ, Castelli WP. Postmenopausal estrogen use, cigarette smoking, and cardiovascular morbidity in women over 50. The Framingham Study. *N Engl J Med* 1985; 313:1038–43

75. The American–Canadian Co-operative Study Group. Persantine aspirin trial in cerebral ischemia – Part III: risk factors for stroke. *Stroke* 1986;17:12–18

76. Bush TL, Barrett-Connor E, Cowan LD, *et al.* Cardiovascular mortality and noncontraceptive use of estrogen in women: results from the Lipid Research Clinics Program Follow-up Study. *Circulation* 1987;75:1102–9

77. Finucane FF, Madans JH, Bush TL, *et al.* Decreased risk of stroke among postmenopausal

hormone users. Results from a national cohort. *Arch Intern Med* 1993;153:73–9

78. Boysen G, Nyboe J, Appleyard M, *et al.* Stroke incidence and risk factors for stroke in Copenhagen, Denmark. *Stroke* 1988;19:1345–53

79. Lindenstrøm E, Boysen G, Nyboe J. Lifestyle factors and risk of cerebrovascular disease in women. The Copenhagen City Heart Study. *Stroke* 1993;24:1468–72

80. Lafferty FW, Helmuth DO. Post-menopausal estrogen replacement: the prevention of osteoporosis and systemic effects. *Maturitas* 1985;7: 147–59

81. Lafferty FW, Fiske ME. Postmenopausal estrogen replacement therapy: a long-term cohort study. *Am J Med* 1994;97:66–77

82. Paganini-Hill A, Ross RK, Henderson BE. Postmenopausal oestrogen treatment and stroke: a prospective study. *Br Med J* 1988;297:519–22

83. Henderson BE, Paganini-Hill A, Ross RK. Decreased mortality in users of estrogen replacement therapy. *Arch Intern Med* 1991;151: 75–8

84. Paganini-Hill A. Morbidity and mortality changes with estrogen replacement therapy. In Lobo RA, ed. *Treatment of the Postmenopausal Woman: Basic and Clinical Aspects.* New York, NY: Raven Press, 1994:399–404

85. Sturgeon SR, Schairer C, Brinton LA, *et al.* Evidence of a healthy estrogen user survivor effect. *Epidemiology* 1995;6:227–31

86. Folsom AR, Mink PJ, Sellers TA, *et al.* Hormonal replacement therapy and morbidity and mortality in a prospective study of postmenopausal women. *Am J Public Health* 1995;85:1128–32

87. Stampfer MJ, Colditz GA, Willett WC, *et al.* Postmenopausal estrogen therapy and cardiovascular disease. Ten-year follow-up from the Nurses' Health Study. *N Engl J Med* 1991;325: 756–62

88. Grodstein F, Stampfer MJ, Manson JE, *et al.* Postmenopausal estrogen and progestin use and the risk of cardiovascular disease. *N Engl J Med* 1996;335:453–61

89. Grodstein F, Stampfer MJ, Colditz GA, *et al.* Postmenopausal hormone therapy and mortality. *N Engl J Med* 1997;336:1769–75

90. O'Keefe JH, Kim SC, Hall RR, *et al.* Estrogen replacement therapy after coronary angioplasty in women. *J Am Coll Cardiol* 1997;29:1–5

91. Sourander L, Rajala T, Räihä I, *et al.* Cardiovascular and cancer morbidity and mortality and sudden cardiac death in postmenopausal women on oestrogen replacement therapy (ERT). *Lancet* 1998;352:1965–9

92. Psaty BM, Heckbert SR, Atkins D, *et al.* A review of the association of estrogens and progestins with cardiovascular disease in postmenopausal women. *Arch Intern Med* 1993;153:1421–7

93. Nabulsi AA, Folsom AR, White A, *et al.* Association of hormone replacement therapy with various cardiovascular risk factors in postmenopausal women. *N Engl J Med* 1993;328: 1069–75

94. Sacks FM, McPherson R, Walsh BW. Effect of postmenopausal estrogen replacement on plasma Lp(a) lipoprotein concentrations. *Arch Intern Med* 1994;154:1106–10

95. MBewu AD, Durrington PN. Lipoprotein (a): structure, properties and possible involvement in thrombogenesis and atherogenesis. *Atherosclerosis* 1990;85:1–14

96. Hachinski V, Graffagnino C, Beaudry M, *et al.* Lipids and stroke. A paradox resolved. *Arch Neurol* 1996;53:303–8

97. Gebara OCE, Mittleman MA, Sutherland P, *et al.* Association between increased estrogen status and increased fibrinolytic potential in the Framingham Offspring Study. *Circulation* 1995; 91:1952–8

98. Scarabin PY, Alhenc-Gelas M, Plu-Bureau G. Effects of oral and transdermal estrogen/ progesterone regimens on blood coagulation and fibrinolysis in postmenopausal women. A randomized controlled trial. *Arterioscl Thromb Vasc Biol* 1997;17:3071–8

99. Koh KK, Mincemoyer R, Bui MN, *et al.* Effects of hormone-replacement therapy on fibrinolysis in postmenopausal women. *N Engl J Med* 1997; 336:683–90

100. Koh KK, Cardillo C, Bui MN, *et al.* Vascular effects of estrogen and cholesterol-lowering therapies in hypercholesterolemic postmenopausal women. *Circulation* 1999;99:354–60

101. Meilahn EN, Kuller LH, Matthews KA, Kiss JE. Hemostatic factors according to menopausal status and use of hormone replacement therapy. *Ann Epidemiol* 1992;2:445–55

102. The Writing Group for the Estradiol Clotting Factors Study. Effects on haemostasis of hormone replacement therapy with transdermal estradiol and oral sequential medroxyprogesterone acetate: a 1-year, double-blind, placebo-controlled study. *Thromb Haemost* 1996;75: 476–80

103. Mazière C, Auclair M, Ronveaux M-F, *et al.* Estrogens inhibit copper and cell-mediated modification of low density lipoprotein. *Atherosclerosis* 1991;89:175–82

104. Subbiah MTR, Kessel B, Agrawal M, *et al.* Antioxidant potential of specific estrogens on lipid peroxidation. *J Clin Endocrinol Metab* 1993;77: 1095–7

105. Nègre-Salvayre A, Pieraggi M-T, Mabile L, Salvayre R. Protective effect of 17β-estradiol against the cytotoxicity of minimally oxidized LDL to cultured bovine aortic endothelial cells. *Atherosclerosis* 1993;99:207–17

106. Sack MN, Rader DJ, Cannon RO III. Oestrogen and inhibition of oxidation of low-denisty lipoproteins in postmenopausal women. *Lancet* 1994;343:269–70

107. Guetta V, Panza JA, Waclawiw MA, Cannon RO III. Effect of combined 17β-estradiol and vitamin E on low-density lipoprotein oxidation in postmenopausal women. *Am J Cardiol* 1995; 75:1274–6

108. Wilcox JG, Sevanian A, Hwang J, *et al.* Cardioprotective effects of individual conjugated equine estrogens through their possible modulation of insulin resistance and oxidation of low-density lipoprotein. *Fertil Steril* 1997;67: 57–62

109. Celermajer DS, Sorensen KE, Spiegelhalter DJ, *et al.* Aging is associated with endothelial dysfunction in healthy men years before the age-related decline in women. *J Am Coll Cardiol* 1994;24:471–6

110. Taddei S, Virdis A, Ghiadoni L, *et al.* Menopause is associated with endothelial dysfunction in women. *Hypertension* 1996;28:576–82

111. Gilligan DM, Badar DM, Panza JA, *et al.* Acute vascular effects of estrogen in postmenopausal women. *Circulation* 1994;90:786–91

112. Reis SE, Gloth ST, Blumenthal RS, *et al.* Ethinyl estradiol acutely attenuates abnormal coronary vasomotor responses to acetylcholine in postmenopausal women. *Circulation* 1994;89:52–60

113. Herrington DM, Braden GA, Williams JK, Morgan TM. Endothelial-dependent coronary vasomotor responsiveness in postmenopausal women with and without estrogen replacement therapy. *Am J Cardiol* 1994;73:951–2

114. Lieberman EH, Gerhard MD, Uehata A, *et al.* Estrogen improves endothelium-dependent, flow-mediated vasodilation in postmenopausal women. *Ann Intern Med* 1994;121:936–41

115. Collins P, Rosano GMC, Sarrel PM, *et al.* 17β-estradiol attenuates acetylcholine-induced coronary arterial constriction in women but not men with coronary heart disease. *Circulation* 1995;92:24–30

116. Mendelsohn ME, Karas RH. The protective effects of estrogen on the cardiovascular system. *N Engl J Med* 1999;340:1801–11

117. Binko J, Majewski H. 17β-estradiol reduces vasoconstriction in endothelium-denuded rat aortas through inducible NOS. *Am J Physiol* 1998;274:H853–9

118. Weiner CP, Lizasoain I, Baylis SA, *et al.* Induction of calcium-dependent nitric oxide synthases by sex hormones. *Proc Natl Acad Sci USA* 1994;91:5212–16

119. Ross R. Atherosclerosis – an inflammatory disease. *N Engl J Med* 1999;340:115–26

120. Caulin-Glazer T, Farrell WJ, Pfau SE, *et al.* Modulation of circulating cellular adhesion

molecules in postmenopausal women with coronary artery disease. *J Am Coll Cardiol* 1998; 31:1555–60

121. Morales DE, McGowan KA, Grant DS, *et al.* Estrogen promotes angiogenic activity in human umbilical vein endothelial cells *in vitro* and in a murine model. *Circulation* 1995;91:755–63

122. Krasinski K, Spyridopoulos I, Asahara T, *et al.* Estradiol accelerates functional endothelial recovery after arterial injury. *Circulation* 1997; 95:1768–72

123. Cornwell TL, Arnold E, Boerth NJ, Lincoln TM. Inhibition of smooth muscle cell growth by nitric oxide and activation of cAMP-dependent protein kinase by cGMP. *Am J Physiol* 1994;267: C1405–13

124. Jonas HA, Kronmal RA, Psaty BM. Current estrogen–progestin and estrogen replacement therapy in elderly women: association with carotid atherosclerosis. *Am J Epidemiol* 1996;6: 314–23

125. Espeland MA, Applegate W, Furberg CD, *et al.* Estrogen replacement therapy and progression of intimal–medial thickness in the carotid arteries of postmenopausal women. *Am J Epidemiol* 1995;142:1011–19

126. Matteis M, Troisi E, Monaldo BC, *et al.* Age and sex differences in cerebral hemodynamics. A transcranial doppler study. *Stroke* 1998;29: 963–7

127. Penotti M, Farina M, Sironi L, *et al.* Cerebral artery blood flow in relation to age and menopausal status. *Obstet Gynecol* 1996;88:106–9

128. Gangar KF, Vyas S, Whitehead M, *et al.* Pulsatility index in internal carotid artery in relation to transdermal oestradiol and time since menopause. *Lancet* 1991;338:839–42

129. Penotti M, Nencioni T, Gabrielli L, *et al.* Blood flow variations in internal carotid and middle cerebral arteries induced by postmenopausal hormone replacement therapy. *Am J Obstet Gynecol* 1993;169:1226–32

130. Penotti M, Sironi L, Miglierina L, *et al.* The effect of tamoxifen and transdermal 17β-estradiol on cerebral arterial vessels: a randomized controlled study. *Am J Obstet Gynecol* 1998;178:801–5

131. Cacciatore B, Paakkari I, Toivonen J, *et al.* Randomized comparison of oral and transdermal hormone replacement on carotid and uterine artery resistance to blood flow. *Obstet Gynecol* 1998;92:563–8

132. Belfort MA, Saade GR, Snabes M, *et al.* Hormonal status affects the reactivity of the cerebral vasculature. *Am J Obstet Gynecol* 1995; 172:1273–8

133. Ohkura T, Isse K, Akazawa K, *et al.* Evaluation of estrogen treatment in female patients with dementia of the Alzheimer's type. *Endocr J* 1994;41:361–71

134. Li K, Futrell N, Tovar JS, *et al.* Gender influences the magnitude of the inflammatory response within embolic cerebral infarcts in young rats. *Stroke* 1996;27:498–503

135. Dubal DB, Kashon ML, Pettigrew LC, *et al.* Estradiol protects against ischemic injury. *J Cerebral Blood Flow Metab* 1998;18:1253–8

17

The lower urinary tract in menopause: the contributions of aging and estrogen deficiency

L. Hoyte and E. Versi

INTRODUCTION: ESTROGEN AND THE LOWER URINARY TRACT

Anatomy

The primary functions of the lower urinary tract are the storage and emptying of urine. It consists of the bladder, the urethra and the fascial tissues which normally support them. The bladder wall consists of the detrusor smooth muscle, lined by transitional bladder epithelium. The urethra comprises four tissue layers, as shown in Figure 1. Starting from the mucosal side, these are non-keratinized squamous epithelium, blood vessels and connective tissue, smooth muscle and striated muscle. The external urethral sphincter comprises a ring of striated muscle, possibly deficient posteriorly, which encircles the mid-urethra. Continence is thought to be maintained primarily by the external urethral sphincter, aided by the pelvic floor muscles, bladder neck and the seal provided by the urethral vascularity, collagen and mucosa[1,2].

Embryology

The bladder, urethra and trigone originate from the cloaca, cloacal membrane and the ureteric bed of the mesonephric duct. The urogenital sinus is divided into rostral and caudal portions by the entrance of the mesonephric ducts. The rostral portion gives rise to the

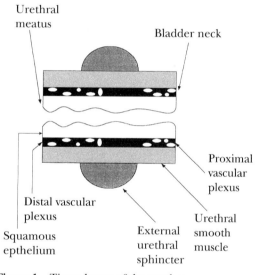

Figure 1 Tissue layers of the urethra

bladder and proximal urethra, and the caudal portion to the distal urethra and vestibule of the vagina. Accordingly, the embryonic relationship between the lower genital and lower urinary tracts is evident[3]. Furthermore, anomalies in one system often occur in association with congenital malformations in the other, emphasizing the common developmental pathway[4]. This makes it reasonable to assume that sex hormones may influence the lower urinary tract in addition to their well-known influence on the genital tract.

Histology

Mucosa/submucosa

In adult women, the bladder mucosa consists of transitional epithelium, and in the neonate, the proximal urethra is also lined with transitional epithelium[5]. The distal urethra is lined with non-keratinized squamous epithelium, which extends proximally during the reproductive period[5] and may cover the entire urethra and trigone[6]. The distal urethra is sensitive to estrogen in some species, including humans[7-9], and correlation between atrophic urethritis and vaginitis has been shown by Smith[10]. It has also been shown that distal urethral and vaginal smears undergo similar changes during the menstrual cycle, pregnancy and menopause[11-13]. Before the menopause, the softness and multiple folds in the urethral mucosa permit it to provide a hermetic seal to aid continence[14,15]. This softness is probably under estrogenic influence[16], because the mucosal folds are lost after menopause and a decrease in mucus is also observed[5]. The pliability and rugation of the urethral mucosa probably account for part of the total continence mechanism.

Vascular structures

There are two submucosal vascular plexuses which underlie the urethral mucosa[5]. One is the distal plexus and is situated directly above the external urethral meatus and is unaltered by aging. The other plexus is proximal, and is located beneath the bladder neck. It becomes wider and loses its tortuosity after the menopause. In women, vascular pulsations, synchronous with the heart beat, can be recorded during urethral pressure studies. These pulsations have been noted to decrease in amplitude after the menopause, a finding which is reversible with estrogen replacement therapy[17,18]. Furthermore, it has been shown that estrogen treatment increases blood flow in the rabbit urethra[19], arguing for the contribution of estrogen in the submucosal vascular bed. In fact, it has been shown in dogs[20] and humans[21] that the vascular component accounts for approximately one-third of the maximal urethral

closure pressure. Based on these findings, it is fair to conclude that estrogen could influence continence by acting on this proximal urethral closure mechanism.

Connective tissue

Underneath the urethral vascular plexus is found a layer of smooth muscle and connective tissue. This area stains strongly for collagen, and these fibrils predominate over the smooth muscle in mice[22] and dogs[23], with elastin fibers prominent near the bladder neck[24]. For some time it has been known that skin collagen decreases after the menopause and that this is reversed by estrogen replacement[25]. Proximal urethral pressures correlate with skin collagen, suggesting a link with urethral collagen[26]. However, Falconer and colleagues have recently shown that periurethral collagen concentration and cross-linking increase after menopause. To them, this suggested a decrease in collagen elasticity[27]. They further showed that estrogen reversed the rise in collagen concentration and decreased cross-linking to premenopausal levels, suggesting that estrogen replacement can restore collagen elasticity. They also showed evidence of increased synthesis of types I and III collagen with estrogen therapy in postmenopausal women, as has been shown for skin[28]. Falconer and co-workers concluded that, in menopause, the periurethral collagen is less elastic compared to premenopause, and that estrogen replacement partially restores the elasticity to premenopausal levels, and increases collagen synthesis and turnover. These findings are summarized in Table 1. Notwithstanding their conclusions, it is clear that collagen function in the lower urinary tract is complex and as yet unresolved.

Collagen occurs in many structural forms, and at the time of writing 14 different types have been identified. The major types in skin are types I and III, and it has been shown that hormone replacement with percutaneous estrogen and testosterone implants results in an increase in the proportion of type III collagen[28]. Abnormal collagen ratios have been found in many conditions involving structural weakness, including recurrent inguinal hernia, vascular aneurysms and the Ehlers–Danlos syndrome[29]. These abnormal ratios may result in weaker structures, and may explain why certain individuals develop genital prolapse.

Falconer and co-workers compared collagen biochemistry between normal controls and women with stress urinary incontinence in the pre- and postmenopause, looking for effects of estrogen on collagen. The results, summarized in Table 2, suggest that premenopausal women with stress urinary incontinence have a different underlying periurethral collagen biochemistry compared to those with postmenopausal stress urinary incontinence[30,31]. Premenopausal stress incontinence seems to be associated with collagen stiffening and increased synthesis when

compared to age-matched controls, whereas postmenopausally it seems to occur in the absence of relative structural changes to periurethral collagen. These findings raise the possibility that premenopausal-onset stress urinary incontinence may have a different etiology than stress urinary incontinence of postmenopausal onset.

In contrast, however, Falconer and colleagues found that, in postmenopausal women with stress urinary incontinence, estrogen replacement decreased periurethral collagen cross-linking by a greater percentage, when compared to women without incontinence[31]. This, and other findings, are summarized in Table 3 and suggest that estrogen restores collagen elasticity to a greater degree in postmenopausal women with stress urinary incontinence, compared to age-matched controls without incontinence. The significance of these findings remains to be elucidated, but it may suggest a biochemical collagen abnormality specific to women who develop stress urinary incontinence.

Table 1 Periurethral collagen: postmenopausal changes among continent women

Collagen parameter	Postmenopausal changes	Effect of postmenopausal estrogen
Cross-linking	↑	↓
Concentration	↑	↓
mRNA for collagens types I, III	unchanged	↑
Proteoglycan (PG)	unchanged	unchanged
PG : collagen ratio	↓	↑

Effect of menopause and estrogen replacement on periurethral collagen biochemistry in continent women without pelvic organ prolapse (after Falconer et al.[27]). Proteoglycans are modified proteins which interact with collagen fibrils and are thought to affect the mechanical properties of collagen. The PG : collagen ratio is thought to be related to collagen stiffness and elasticity. Increased mRNA levels suggest increased synthesis

Smooth muscle

The detrusor smooth muscle appears to be sexually differentiated[32]. The relationship between actinomycin content of the uterine smooth muscle and estrogen status has been demonstrated[33], and the profound effect of estrogen on smooth muscle has been shown[34]. It is reasonable to infer that the detrusor may also be sensitive to estrogen. Gap junctions, which play an important role in synchronizing smooth

Table 2 Periurethral collagen and stress urinary incontinence (SUI) in pre- and postmenopausal women

Collagen parameter	Premenopausal, SUI vs. normals (after Falconer et al.[30])	Postmenopausal, SUI vs. normals (after Falconer et al.[31])
Cross-linking	↑	unchanged
Concentration	↑ (30%)	unchanged
Fibril diameter	↑ (30%)	↑ (trend only, not significant)
mRNA for collagens I, III	↑ (I & III)	↓ (I), ↑ (III)
Proteoglycan concentration	unchanged	↑
PG : collagen ratio	↓	↑

Effect of menopause and estrogen replacement on periurethral collagen biochemistry in stress urinary incontinence versus continent women in pre- and postmenopause

Table 3 Periurethral collagen, stress urinary incontinence (SUI) and estrogen replacement therapy (ERT) among postmenopausal women

Collagen parameter	Postmenopausal SUI, on ERT compared to no ERT	Postmenopausal continent, on ERT compared to no ERT
Cross-linking	↓↓	↓
Concentration	↓	↓
Fibril diameter	unchanged	unchanged
mRNA for collagen I, III	↓(I), ↑(III)	unchanged
Proteoglycan (PG) concentration	↓	unchanged
PG : collagen ratio	unchanged	↑

Effect of menopause and estrogen replacement on periurethral collagen biochemistry in stress urinary incontinence versus continent women (after Falconer *et al.*)[31]

muscle contractions, are composed of proteins called connexins, and it is thought that expression of these proteins is controlled by sex hormones[35]. Because smooth muscle contributes to the resting tone of the urethra, we may infer that urethral resting tone is in part influenced by estrogen.

Striated muscle

We have noted the influence of estrogen on collagen, but there is no evidence that estrogen strengthens striated muscle[36,37]. Bernstein has shown that the thickness of the pelvic floor muscles decreases with age, probably unrelated to estrogen status, because they were unable to identify estrogen receptors by immunohisto-analysis of pelvic floor biopsy specimens[38]. Furthermore, the same group found that this atrophy could be reversed by pelvic floor exercises, but that the increase in muscle bulk could not be correlated with subjective or objective improvement in urinary incontinence.

Physiology

Urinary function is controlled via autonomic and somatic branches of the central nervous system. The storage function is achieved when the urethra closes and the detrusor smooth muscle relaxes to accommodate urine during filling. The emptying function is facilitated via relaxation of the urethra and contraction of the detrusor. Detrusor contraction is achieved via activation of cholinergic (S2–S4) and inhibition of adrenergic (T10–L1$_{[LH1]}$) fibers[39,40].

Urethral closure is achieved via activation of the somatic (S2–S4) fibers from Onuf's [LH2] nucleus to the external urethral sphincter; somatic (S2–S4) activation of the levator ani muscles; and activation of α-adrenergic fibers to the urethral smooth muscle. Storage is maintained by a greater sympathetic drive, in concert with somatic activation of the striated muscles. Voiding is achieved by a greater parasympathetic drive, together with somatic inhibition of the striated muscles of the external urethral sphincter and levator ani[41]. In addition to the above modes of control, many other transmitter receptors have been identified in the lower urinary tract, including those for nitric oxide and substance P[42]. High-affinity estrogen receptors have been demonstrated in the lower urinary tract of female animals[43] and humans[44], with receptor concentrations highest in the urethra, followed by the trigone, and negligible levels in the remainder of the bladder. These data offer evidence of direct estrogen action in the urethra and the trigone.

Biomechanics and control of urinary tract function

As noted previously, normal control of lower urinary tract function is obtained via the interaction of the smooth detrusor muscle with the urethra, striated external sphincter and perhaps the levator ani muscles, in concert with the intra-abdominal pressures generated by valsalva maneuvers. Continence is maintained when urethral closure pressure exceeds bladder pressure, and emptying occurs when urethral pressure is less than bladder pressure. Bladder pressure is the sum of detrusor and intra-abdominal pressure, and urethral pressure is a composite of pressures generated by the urethra, external sphincter and abdominal pressure transmitted to a portion of the urethra.

Stress continence mechanisms

In normal continent women under stress, abdominal pressure is transmitted to the urethra and bladder simultaneously. The 'pressure transmission ratio' is the ratio of pressures transmitted to the bladder and urethra under stress events. It has been known for some time that the pressure transmission ratio is significantly lower in women with genuine stress incontinence, when compared to those without genuine stress incontinence[45–47]. The exact mechanism of continence has not been clearly defined, but many hypotheses have been proposed[2]. During stress (e.g. coughing, sneezing), urethral reinforcement action is thought to have a passive component caused by transmission of the abdominal pressure created by the cough impulse, and an active component mediated by the striated muscles of the external urethral sphincter and/or levator ani[48]. Constantinou and Govan showed that this active component can precede the actual stress impulse by up to 0.25 seconds[48], ample time for the striated muscle to tighten and prevent leakage. Three factors combine to maintain continence under stress. These are simultaneous transmission of intra-abdominal pressure to urethra and bladder, contraction of the external urethral sphincter/levator ani, and tone of the urethral smooth muscle. Transmission of intra-abdominal pressure to the urethra can be affected by hypermobility of the bladder neck, leading to stress incontinence. Bladder neck hypermobility is thought to be due to torn or lax collagen bladder neck supports, and is not thought to be responsive to estrogen therapy. Contraction of the external urethral sphincter can be absent or inadequate due to nerve or sphincteric damage, e.g. due to vaginal delivery or pelvic surgery. In either case, estrogen therapy would not be expected to restore function to the external urethral sphincter. Finally, urethral smooth muscle tone can be diminished, either due to damage from prior surgery or radiation (intrinsic sphincteric deficiency), or as a side-effect of α-adrenergic blocker therapy[49]. Combination estrogen/α-agonist therapy has been shown objectively to improve genuine stress incontinence due to intrinsic sphincteric deficiency[50,51]. The impact of estrogen on stress continence mechanisms are shown in Table 4.

Resting continence mechanisms

As noted previously, resting continence is achieved via several factors:

(1) Urethral mucosa;

(2) Submucosal vascular plexuses;

(3) Periurethral collagen;

(4) Striated muscle of the external urethral sphincter and perhaps levator ani;

(5) Urethral smooth muscle (internal sphincter);

(6) Relaxation of the detrusor muscle.

The impact of estrogen on each of these structures is summarized in Table 5.

Estrogen can aid the rugation and pliability of the mucosa, and contribute to the submucosal vascular fullness, as discussed previously. Estrogen can therefore have influence on the resting continence mechanism, as

Table 4 Estrogen effects on stress incontinence

Parameter	Effect of estrogen	Effect on continence
Pressure transmission ratio	possibly increases proximally	probably minimal
Contraction of external urethral sphincter/levator ani	no evidence of direct effect	none
Urethral tone	possibly increases baseline tone	unclear

Table 5 Impact of estrogen on resting continence

Tissue	Effect of estrogen	Effect on continence
Urethral mucosa	softens, increases pliability	aids hermetic seal, aids continence
Submucosal vascular plexuses	increases fullness and tortuosity of proximal plexus / no effect on distal plexus	increased closing pressure, aids resting continence
Periurethral collagen	increases elasticity, collagen synthesis	effect on continence unclear
Striated muscle	no effect	no direct effect
Urethral smooth muscle	may increase tone synergistically with α-agonist	effect unclear when used alone
Detrusor smooth muscle	probably decreased irritability	possible decrease in urge incontinence

suggested by the results of Versi[52] and Sartori and colleagues[53].

Local factors which influence continence

Irritation of the detrusor muscle can cause isolated detrusor contractions which could lead to urge incontinence. Cystitis can be one such cause of bladder irritation. It is known that recurrent cystitis occurs in low estrogen states, and the prospective randomized controlled study by Raz and Stamm showed that estrogen replacement reduces the incidence of urinary tract infections in postmenopausal women[54].

LOWER URINARY TRACT MALFUNCTION: THE RELATIVE ROLES OF AGING AND ESTROGENS

Epidemiology

Incontinence: symptoms and prevalence

Women are more commonly subject to urinary incontinence than men[55], with the prevalence increasing with age[56]. We present data from several studies, which suggest an overall rate of incontinence of 14–24% in the general female population, and 45–47% among peri- and postmenopausal women. These data show that the prevalence of incontinence symptoms is inversely proportional to their severity, with 20–50% of responders calling their incontinence 'frequent', or claiming it as a social or hygiene problem. These findings are summarized in Table 6.

Incontinence: age at peak prevalence

Urological symptoms appear most commonly around the time of the climacteric, as is summarized in Table 7. Symptoms of incontinence have also been to noted to rise following surgically induced menopause[64]. Together, these data point to declining or absent ovarian function in the etiology of the onset of stress urinary incontinence.

These studies show an agreement in timing between clinical diagnosis and patient symptoms of urinary incontinence, and this implicates the climacteric as the time of peak incontinence in women. However, the lack of a continuing increase in prevalence with age (see Figure 2) suggests a multifactorial etiology. It is possible that decreasing activity levels in the elderly produce fewer 'stress' events which could trigger incontinence.

Complaints of urge-related incontinence continue to rise in the years beyond the menopause. As shown in Figure 3, the data show an increasing prevalence with age[57].

Irritative symptoms

Women may experience a number of irritative urinary symptoms. These include frequency (more than seven times per day), nocturia (more than once per night), urgency and painful urination. These are the classic symptoms of infection, but they often occur in the presence of a negative urine culture. This symptomatology was recognized long ago in patients with senile atrophic urethritis[9] and is complicated by

Table 6 Prevalence of incontinence symptoms

Study group	Ref.	Urinary incontinence	Stress symptoms	Urge symptoms	Notes
1636 Japanese women	57		29%	11%	
833 British women from a general practice	58	41%			rates higher among parous and premenopausal subjects
4206 women aged 70–90 years	59	16% at time of study 22% current or previous	24% of urinary incontinence sufferers	49% of urinary incontinence sufferers	50% of current urinary incontinence sufferers had daily incontinence
1500 Chinese women, telephone survey	60	14%	10%	4%	
1250 Turkish outpatient general gynecology patients	61	24%			85% of symptomatic women never sought help
285 women attending menopause clinic	62		45% occasional 9% frequent	21% occasional 5% frequent	
489 subjects, aged 50–74, population-based study	63	47% occasional 37% regular			objective incontinence demonstrated in only 19% 19% claimed symptoms as social/hygiene problem

Table 7 Urinary incontinence symptoms: age at peak prevalence

Ref.	Age at peak prevalence (years)	Prevalence	Study group
65	40–60	40%	750 patients referred to urodynamic clinic
61	40–44 (This was the oldest group surveyed)	36%	1250 patients attending general gynecology outpatient clinic
66	45–49 (2nd peak of 30% in 55–59 age group)	35%	600 British women surveyed in a store
58	45–55	60%	833 British women from a general practice
63	55–64	20–25%	489 women, population-based study. ICS definition

the fact that pH increases associated with atrophic changes may increase susceptibility to urinary tract infections.

Molander and associates, in a survey of 4206 women aged 70–90 years, found that urinary tract infections appear to increase in frequency with advancing age, as shown in Figure 4[59]. The continued rise so long after the menopause suggests that age may have a significant influence. The incidence of bacteriuria was only 3.2% in a group aged 45–64 years, compared to 3.5% in a group aged 20–64 years[67]. However, a 19% bacteriuria rate was found in a group of 511 patients over the age of 65 years[68].

The 'urethral syndrome' is defined as recurrent episodes of frequency, urgency and dysuria without bacteriuria. The onset of such symptoms with menopause has been noted by Smith[69]. It is known, however, that the condition occurs most commonly during the reproductive years[70], and the association with sexual activity is recognized[71]. Versi and colleagues found that only 2% of climacteric women had the urethral syndrome[62]. Smith was able to correlate symptoms of dysuria with changes in urethral cytology in postmenopausal women and showed that both responded to estrogen therapy[69]. He suggested that senile atrophic urethritis may progress to produce partial obstruction, resulting in ascending infection. Because of this hypothesis, estrogen therapy

and urethral dilatation have been advocated as standard management for this condition, with little in the way of scientific evaluation.

Frequency and urgency symptoms can appear at any age[72]. The symptoms show a pattern similar to stress incontinence, in that they rise and peak at 45–50 years of age, and decline thereafter. This relationship is shown in Figure 5.

In the study by Versi and colleagues, half of the women admitted to urgency, with 20% calling it a frequent problem[62]. Their incidence of urgency also peaked in the perimenopause, paralleling vasomotor symptoms, but showed no definitive pattern therafter. These results are summarized in Figure 6.

Voiding frequency shows a different pattern. Thirty per cent of Versi's study patients had urinary frequency and voided more than seven times per day at perimenopause. The frequency was slightly increased 3 years postmenopausally, as shown in Figure 7[62].

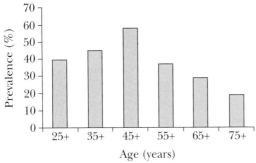

Figure 2 Prevalence of stress incontinence and age; after Jolleys[58]

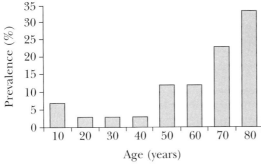

Figure 3 Prevalence of urge incontinence with age; after Kondo[57]

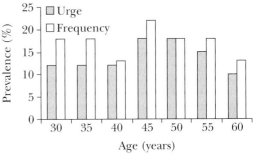

Figure 5 Frequency/urgency with age; after Bungay and colleagues[72]

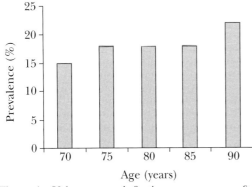

Figure 4 Urinary tract infections versus age; after Molander[59]

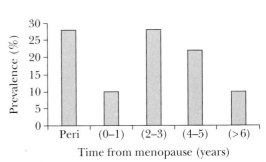

Figure 6 Urgency symptoms versus menopausal age; after Versi[62]

Nocturia increased steadily with age in the group studied by Glenning[73] (Figure 8); however, Osborne[66], and subsequently Versi[62], found that nocturia appeared to increase following the menopause, suggesting that estrogen deprivation leads to a lower sensory threshold in the bladder. However, many times a climacteric woman will be awoken with night sweats, at which time she may decide to urinate. Care should be taken not to count these events when evaluating nocturia.

Voiding difficulty

The problems of voiding relate to outlet obstruction, inadequate detrusor contractions, detrusor/sphincter dyssynergia, or a combination of the three. The symptoms include poor stream, straining to void, incomplete emptying, post-micturation dribble and painful voiding. It has been suggested in the past that estrogen deficiency may contribute to distal urethral stenosis[74], and so estrogen therapy was advocated for its management. Voiding difficulties were present in 33% of 600 women presenting to a London urogynecology clinic for urological complaints[75], whereas data from our study point to a rate of 10–15% in women presenting for climacteric symptoms[62]. We were unable in our study to correlate voiding difficulty with the time of the menopause. In a study of women who underwent surgery for pelvic organ prolapse, Theofrastous and co-workers showed that women on preoperative estrogen replacement therapy required significantly fewer days of postoperative catheterization when compared to those who were not on estrogen replacement therapy[76]. This result suggests that detrusor contractility may be amenable to estrogen therapy.

EVALUATION OF THE URINARY TRACT IN CLIMACTERIC WOMEN

Investigation of lower urinary tract dysfunction in climacteric women is the same as for women at other stages of their reproductive life. Available techniques include uroflowmetry[77] and video-urodynamics[78]. If fluoroscopy is not available, then flow studies combined with three-channel cystometry[79] will suffice. Urethral pressure profilometry data may be useful to diagnose a low-pressure urethra[80].

Urodynamic findings during the climacteric

Incontinence: clinical diagnoses

Major urodynamics findings in the climacteric women visiting our menopause clinic are presented in Table 8[62]. Interestingly, only two-thirds of climacteric women could be considered to be urodynamically 'normal'. Genuine stress incontinence and idiopathic detrusor instability were the the two leading diagnoses.

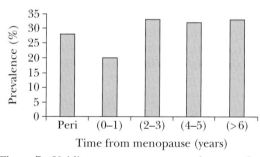

Figure 7 Voiding versus menopausal age; after Versi[62]

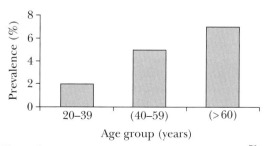

Figure 8 Prevalence of nocturia; after Glenning[73]

Table 8 Urodynamic findings among climacteric women

Urodynamic diagnosis	Prevalence
Normal	59%
Genuine stress incontinence	22%
Detrusor instability	10%
Voiding difficulties	7%
Sensory urgency	4%

Prevalence of urodynamic diagnoses among 285 women attending a menopause clinic; after Versi[62]

Versi and associates observed that the prevalence of genuine stress incontinence falls off with increasing time from menopause, whereas the prevalence of detrusor instability rises with patients' age. The ratio of genuine stress incontinence to detrusor instability inverts at 6 years after the menopause, suggesting that detrusor instability is an age-related phenomenon. This relationship is shown in Figure 9.

Urethral sphincter: clinical diagnoses

The conventional thinking is that continence is maintained at the level of the internal spincter (bladder neck) with the external urethral sphincter as a back-up. We noted in our series, however, that, of the climacteric women who were continent on pad testing and videourodynamics, 50% had an incompetent bladder neck[81]. These findings appear to demote the role of the bladder neck in maintaining continence[82]. Furthermore, we note that there is no significant difference in the prevalence of bladder neck incompetence in pre- and postmenopausal women[83], suggesting that this failure may not be estrogen-related. In normal women, the maximum urethral closure pressure and functional urethral length increase from birth to age 20–25 years, and fall thereafter[84]. Data suggest that estrogen replacement may increase urethral closure pressure in postmenopausal women. Resting urethral closure may be estrogen dependent, but this is not yet supported by conclusive data[52].

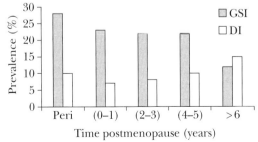

Figure 9 Age distribution of genuine stress incontinence and detrusor instability; after Versi and co-workers[62]

The effects of estrogens on urinary function in the climacteric and menopause

Stress incontinence: uncontrolled clinical trials

The use of estrogens in the treatment of lower urinary tract symptoms has been reported for over 50 years, with varying levels (30–80%) of symptomatic improvement[85–87]. More recent studies were performed, with urodynamic variables as the outcome parameters. In their meta-analysis, Fantl and co-workers found 17 such studies in the literature[88]. According to them, the studies collectively point to subjective improvement in urinary incontinence symptoms, but they fail conclusively to demonstrate estrogen-induced improvement in the urethral pressure profile variables. These studies all suffered from the lack of appropriate placebo-controlled groups, which probably inflated the subjective findings, especially given the up to 56% placebo effect noted among the placebo-controlled trials which they also analyzed. A selected subset of these studies is summarized in Table 9.

Stress incontinence: controlled clinical trials

Estrogen only Since the first randomized placebo-controlled trial was published in 1969 by Judge[90], five double-blind, randomized placebo-controlled studies have reported on the effect of estrogens in stress incontinence. These results are summarized in Table 10. The largest and most significant of these is the double-blind, randomized placebo-controlled trial of 83 postmenopausal women by Fantl and colleagues, which demonstrates the absence of objective improvement after 3 months of oral estrogen therapy. This result is significant because they demonstrated that the estrogen was sufficient to re-estrogenize adequately the vaginal and urethral tissues, but that this did not change the objective measure of genuine stress incontinence, as had been suggested by the results of uncontrolled trials. Fantl's study confirmed that estrogen produces a significant improvement in subjective symptoms of

Table 9 Estrogen therapy in stress incontinence: uncontrolled trials

Ref.	Subjects	Type	Outcome variable	Intervention	Result	Notes
45	11 PM, GSI	cohort	MUCP PTR	2 g vaginal conjugated E_2 daily × 4 weeks	significant improvement in MUCP and PTR, non-significant improvement in symptoms	
89	11 PM, GSI	cohort	UPP	2 g vaginal conjugated E_2 daily × 6 weeks	6/11 cured or improved. Improved UPP in cured patients	no UPP changes in patients who were not cured
8	10 PM, GSI	cohort	UPP	vaginal conjugated E_2 × 6 weeks	5/10 improved. Improved urethral cytology only among improved GSI	proposes 'urethral mucosal factor' to explain results
53	30 PM, GSI	cohort	leakage at maximum capacity	Premarin 0.625/ Provera 2.5 oral qd × 3 months	70% had no leaking at maximum bladder capacity	no discussion of their GSI criteria. Significant subjective improvement

PM, postmenopausal; GSI, genuine stress incontinence; UPP, urethral pressure profile; MUCP, maximum urethral closure pressure; PTR, pressure transmission ratio

Table 10 Estrogen and stress incontinence; randomized placebo-controlled trials

Ref.	Subjects	Study type	Outcome variable	Intervention	Result
90	20 PM hospital-based geriatric patients	R	incontinence	quinestrol po qd × 5 weeks	significant reduction in frequency of incontinence at 5th week placebo had no effect
91	29 PM with UI	R	SI, UPP	cyclic po E_2/E_3 × 20 days	no improvement in SI or UPP
92	34 PM with UI	R	SI	po estriol × 3 months	no significant change in SI
93	36 PM with SI	R	SI, F, pad change frequency	po estrone × 3 months	no significant change in no. of pad changes, UPP, or frequency
51	12 PM with GSI	R	urine leakage	po estriol 4 mg qd plus α-agonist	significant objective decrease in amount of urine loss
94	83 PM, GSI, hypoestrogenism	R	GSI, hypoestrogenism, subjective	po estrogen × 3 months	no improvement in GSI vs. placebo significant improvement in vaginal and urethral estrogenization significant improvement in subjective symptoms

PM, postmenopausal; SI, stress incontinence; UI, urinary incontinence; F, frequency; GSI, genuine stress incontinence; UPP, urethral pressure profile; R, randomized, double-blind, placebo-controlled incontinence, as had been found by previous studies.

Fantl and associates, in their meta-analysis of estrogen and incontinence, also analyzed six randomized controlled trials[88]. They found that estrogen replacement subjectively improved urinary incontinence in postmenopausal women by an average of 64% over placebo, but that the improvement was reduced when only women with genuine stress urinary incontinence were considered. Improved urethral pressure profile variables were also noted, but this effect was influenced by a single study with a large effect. The objective quantity of fluid loss was not significantly different, according to their analysis.

Accepting that meta-analytic studies are subject to a publication bias of positive results, convincing evidence is lacking to support estrogen replacement alone as a treatment for urodynamically proven genuine stress urinary incontinence.

Estrogen plus α-agonist Estrogens are thought to potentiate the effects of α-adrenergic drugs in the proximal urethra. Data from multiple studies show improvement in stress incontinence and other objective variables when estrogen is used in combination with α-agonist therapy. These studies are summarized in Table 11.

Urge incontinence

Study data on estrogen and urge incontinence are summarized in Table 12. Results suggest that estrogen therapy may ameliorate urge incontinence when given in adequate quantities. More data are needed to confirm these results.

Voiding difficulties

Hilton and Stanton noted a significant decrease in symptoms of voiding difficulty following the

Table 11 Estrogen plus α-agonist therapy in treating urinary incontinence

Ref.	Subjects	Type	Outcome variable	Intervention	Result
95	13 PM UI, USI	R	symptoms, UPP	oral E_2 versus oral E_2 & PPA	8/13 became continent with combination therapy vs E_2 alone. Significantly improved UPP with combination therapy
96	20 PM UI, USI	R, X	UPP	PPA 50 mg po bid vaginal estriol 1 mg qd	8 cured, 9 improved with combination therapy
97	36 PM, GSI	R	UPP, leakage	oral E_2 vs oral E_2 & PPA	significant objective improvement with combination therapy vs E_2 alone
98	60 PM, GSI	R	GSI, frequency, nocturia, subjective	oral E_2 vs oral E_2 & PPA	significant objective improvement with combination therapy vs E_2 alone frequency, nocturia improved more with combined vs single therapy
51	12 PM with GSI	R	urine leakage	po estriol 4 mg qd plus α-agonist	significant objective decrease in amount of urine loss
50	29 PM, GSI	R	UPP, symptoms	oral E_3 placebo vs oral E_3 & PPA	significant subjective improvement in E_3 + PPA vs E_3 + placebo significant objective improvement in UPP variables in E_3 + PPA group vs E_3 + placebo significant decrease in leakage episodes, decrease in urine loss on standard stress test

PM, postmenopausal; UI, urinary incontinence; GSI, genuine stress incontinence; R, randomized, double-blind, placebo-controlled; X, cross-over; UPP, urethral pressure profile; USI, urethral sphincter insufficiency (low urethral closure pressure); PPA, phenylpropanolamine (α-adrenergic agonist); E_2, estradiol; E_3, estriol

Table 12 Estrogen therapy for urinary frequency and urge incontinence

Ref.	Subjects	Type	Outcome variable	Intervention	Result
91	21 PM, F, UI	R	UI, F	estrogen vs placebo × 6 weeks	7/11 study subjects improved 1/10 controls improved ($p < 0.05$)
92	34 PM with UI	R	urge, mixed	po estriol × 3 months	significant improvement in urge symptoms and mixed incontinence symptoms
99	64 PM	R	UI, F	oral estriol	no significant difference between estriol and placebo both groups showed significant improvement over pre-intervention
100	154 PM	R	UI, F, SI, dysuria	vaginal estradiol tablets	significant improvement in study group over placebo

PM, postmenopausal; R, randomized, double-blind, placebo-controlled; UI, urge incontinence; SI, stress incontinence; F, frequency

use of vaginal Premarin cream[45]. Sartori and co-workers reported significant improvement in average flow rate and maximum bladder capacity when they treated 30 postmenopausal women with conjugated estrogens and cyclic progestin for 3 months[53]. Together with the results of Theofrastous and colleagues, noted previously[76], these data suggest that estrogen may reduce the prevalence of voiding difficulties.

Urethral syndrome

Salmon and colleagues, in 1940, reported improvement in urgency, dysuria and stress incontinence in 12 out of 16 postmenopausal women treated with 2 weeks of estradiol[101]. They noted that the symptomatic improvements correlated with changes in the vaginal mucosa. Smith correlated symptoms with changes in urethral cytology and showed that both responded to estrogen therapy in postmenopausal women[10,69]. Schleyer-Saunders, in a retrospective study, claimed a 30% improvement in urgency and dysuria with estrogen implant therapy[87]. Hilton and Stanton also reported improvement in frequency and urgency in ten patients with detrusor stable incontinence who were treated with vaginal Premarin cream[45]. The limited available data seem to indicate that

estrogen improves the symptoms of frequency and urgency.

Recurrent urinary tract infections

When estrogen levels fall after ovarian failure, atrophic changes in the vagina result in a reduced production of glycogen. This reduces the colonization of lactobacilli, reducing the vaginal acidity due to decreased lactic acid production. The increasing vaginal pH permits the overgrowth by fecal flora, and it is possible that estrogen replacement therapy would reverse this overgrowth by reversing vaginal atrophy. In 41 elderly women with recurrent urinary tract infections, Brandberg showed that oral estriol restored vaginal flora to the premenopausal state, and these patients required fewer antibiotics[102]. Privette and colleagues retrospectively examined the outcome of 12 women on estrone (0.625 mg), over a period of 2–8 years[103]. Before therapy, the women had an average of four urinary tract infections per year, but the entire group had only four urinary tract infections whilst receiving therapy. There are few randomized controlled trials of the effect of estrogen in the treatment of recurrent urinary tract infections. The results of four published trials are summarized in Table 13. Two of the studies showed a significant reduction in the incidence of urinary tract infection in the

Table 13 Controlled trials of estrogen therapy for recurrent urinary tract infections

Ref.	Subjects	Type	Outcome variable	Intervention	Result
105	23 PM, R-UTI	R	frequency of UTI	vaginal estriol × 5 months	no significant improvement in study vs placebo significant improvement in vaginal cytology
106	40 PM R-UTI	R	frequency of UTI	oral estriol × 12 weeks	significant reduction in UTI vs placebo
107	93 PM R-UTI	R	frequency of UTI	vaginal estriol vs placebo × 8 months	reduction in UTI in study group vs placebo improvement in vaginal cytology in study group
104	72 PM R-UTI	R	frequency of UTI	oral estriol vs placebo × 3 months	improvement in study and placebo groups; no significant difference between 2 groups. Insufficient power to detect difference

PM; postmenopausal; R-UTI; recurrent urinary tract infection; R; randomized, double-blind placebo-controlled trial

estrogen group, and the smallest study found no difference in study and control groups. The fourth study (Cardozo and associates) also failed to show a reduction relative to placebo, but acknowledged insufficient power to detect relevant differences between study and control groups[104]. Overall, however, the data appear to support the use of estrogen therapy to decrease the incidence of recurrent urinary tract infections in the menopause.

Urethral pressure profile changes

The effects of estrogen on the urethral pressure profile have been studied, with inconsistent findings. They are summarized in Table 14. Perhaps these inconsistent results are due to small sample sizes in the setting of a wide range of normal urethral pressure profile values in the general population.

CONCLUSION

There are anatomical, embryological and physiological reasons to expect that estrogen status should affect the female urinary system. The prevalence of symptoms and urodynamic abnormalities is high in the climacteric, and so it

Table 14 Trials of estrogen effects on urethral pressure variables

Reference	Study size	Effect of estrogen
86	41	improved resting UPP
45	10	improved PTR
96	20	improved resting UPP
108	64	no changes in UPP
109	6	enhanced PTR to proximal mid-urethra
110	12	no changes in UPP
111	12	no change in UPP after GnRH-induced menopause
112	80	improved pressure to proximal urethra. No change in other UPP variables

UPP, urethral pressure profile; GnRH, gonadotropin releasing hormone

is easy to suspect low estrogen status as the responsible factor. Despite this relationship, epidemiological data suggest that urinary symptoms are at least multifactorial in origin, and that age plays a major role, with important contributions from obstetric history, obesity and prior gynecological surgery.

Notwithstanding this, the sensory symptoms appear to increase after menopause, and there appears to be an improvement with estrogen replacement. Estrogen replacement may decrease the recurrence of urinary tract infections in the menopause. Estrogen therapy may also help symptoms of urge incontinence, but there is no evidence that it cures stress incontinence. However, in combination with α-adrenergic drugs, estrogen therapy may be useful in the medical management of genuine stress incontinence. The effects of estrogen in the lower urinary tract are summarized in Table 15.

As a preoperative treatment before bladder neck surgery, estrogen probably improves the periurethral tissues, possibly aiding the success of the procedure. The possibility remains that the observed improvements of estrogen in the lower urinary tract are an 'add on' effect of the improvement in vasomotor and psychological symptoms. Data are needed from large placebo-controlled trials to evaluate this. It would appear that recurrent urinary tract infections may be treated, or even prevented, by the use of estrogen therapy.

Table 15 Summary of estrogen effects in the postmenopausal lower urinary tract

Parameter	Effect of estrogen
Symptoms of urinary incontinence	improved
Genuine stress incontinence (objective diagnosis)	not improved with estrogen alone objective improvement with combination estrogen and α-agonist therapy
Urge incontinence	probably improved
Recurrent urinary tract infections	improved
Urethral pressure profile	inconclusive
Nocturia	improved
Frequency	probably improved
Voiding difficulty	probably improved

References

1. DeLancey JO. Anatomy and physiology of urinary continence. *Clin Obstet Gynecol* 1990; 33:298–307
2. Delancey JOL. Three dimensional analysis of urethral support: 'the hammock hypothesis'. *Neurourol Urodyn* 1992;11:306–8
3. Gosling JA. Anatomy. In Stanton SI, ed. *Clinical Gynecologic Urology*. St Louis: CV Mosby, 3–12
4. Metts JC 3rd, *et al.* Genital malformations and coexistent urinary tract or spinal anomalies in patients with imperforate anus. *J Urol* 1997;158:1298–300
5. Huisman AB. Aspects on the anatomy of the female urethra with special relation to urinary incontinence. *Obstet Gynecol* 1983;10:1–31
6. Packham DA. The epithelial lining of the female trigone and urethra. *Br J Urol* 1971;43:201–5
7. Zuckerman S. Histogenesis of tissue sensitive to oestrogens. *Biol Rev Cambridge Philos Soc* 1940;15:231–71
8. Bergman A, Karram MM, Bhatia N. Changes in urethral cytology following estrogen administration in 10 postmenopausal women with genuine stress urinary incontinence. *Gynecol Obstet Invest* 1990;29:211–13
9. Everett HS. Urology in the female. *Am J Surg* 1941;52:521–30
10. Smith P. Age changes in the female urethra. *Br J Urol* 1972;44:667–76
11. Soloman S, Panagotopolous P, Oppenheim A. Urinary cytology studies as an aid to diagnosis. *Am J Obstet Gynecol* 1958;76:57–62
12. McCallin PE, Stewart-Tatlor E, Whitehead RW. A study of the changes in the cytology of urinary sediment during the menstrual cycle and pregnancy. *Am J Obstet Gynecol* 1950;60:64–74
13. del Castillo EB, Argonz J, Galli Mainini CG. Cytological cycle of the urinary sediment and its parallelism with the vaginal cycle. *J Clin Endocrinol Metab* 1948;8:76–87
14. Zinner NN, Sterling AM, Ritter RC. The role of urethral softness in urinary incontinence. *Urology* 1980;16:115–17
15. Zinner NN, Sterling AM, Ritter RC. Evaluation of inner urethral softness. *Urology* 1983;22:446–8

16. Versi E. Incontinence in the climacteric. *Clin Obstet Gynecol* 1990;33:392–8

17. Asmussen M, Miller A. *Clinical Gynaecological Urology*. Oxford: Blackwell Scientific Publications, 1983:21

18. Versi E, Cardozo LD. Urethral vascular pulsations. *Proc Int Cont Soc* 1985;15:503–4

19. Batra S, Bjellin L, Iosif S, *et al.* Effects of oestrogen and progesterone on the blood flow in the lower urinary tract of the rabbit. *Acta Physiol Scand* 1985;123:191–4

20. Raz S, Caine M, Zeigler M. The vascular component in the production of intraurethral pressure. *J Urol* 1972;108:93–8

21. Rud T, Andersson M, *et al.* Factors maintaining the urethral pressure in women. *Invest Urol* 1980;17:343–7

22. Phillips JI, Davies I. A comparative morphometric analysis of the component tissues of the urethra in young and old female C57BL/ICRFA mice. *Invest Urol* 1981;18:422–5

23. Cullen WC, Fletcher TF, Bradley WE. Histology of the canine urethra. I. Morphometry of the female urethra. *Anat Rec* 1981;199:177–86

24. Lapides J. Structure and function of the internal vesical sphincter. *J Urol* 1958;50:341–53

25. Brincat M, *et al.* Skin collagen changes in postmenopausal women receiving oestradiol gel. *Maturitas* 1987;9:1–5

26. Versi E, *et al.* Correlation of urethral physiology and skin collagen in postmenopausal women. *Br J Obstet Gynaecol* 1988;95:505–6

27. Falconer C, *et al.* Changes in paraurethral connective tissue at menopause are counteracted by estrogen. *Maturitas* 1996;24:197–204

28. Savvas M, *et al.* Type III collagen content in the skin of postmenopausal women receiving oestradiol and testosterone implants. *Br J Obstet Gynaecol* 1993;100:154–6

29. Norton P, *et al.* Reduced type I : type III collagen ratios in men with recurrent inguinal hernias. *Surg Forum* 1991;42:369

30. Falconer C, *et al.* Different organization of collagen fibrils in stress incontinent women of fertile age. *Acta Obstet Gynecol Scand* 1998;77:87–94

31. Falconer C, *et al.* Paraurethral connective tissue in stress-incontinent women after menopause. *Acta Obstet Gynecol Scand* 1998;77:95–100

32. Gosling JA. The structure of the bladder and urethra in relation to function. *Urol Clin North Am* 1979;6:31–8

33. Csapo A. Actinomycin content of the uterus. *Nature (London)* 1948;162:218–19

34. Batra S. Oestrogen and smooth muscle function. *Trends Pharmacol Soc* 1980;1:388–96

35. Andersen J, *et al.* Expression of connexin-43 in human myometrium and leioma. *Am J Obstet Gynecol* 1993;169:1266–76

36. Armstrong AL, *et al.* Effects of hormone replacement therapy on muscle performance and balance in post-menopausal women. *Clin Sci (Colch)* 1996;91:685–90

37. Seeley DG, *et al.* Is postmenopausal estrogen therapy associated with neuromuscular function or falling in elderly women? Study of Osteoporotic Fractures Research Group. *Arch Intern Med* 1995;155:293–9

38. Bernstein IT. The pelvic floor muscles: muscle thickness in healthy and urinary-incontinent women measured by perineal ultrasonography with reference to the effect of pelvic floor training. Estrogen receptor studies. *Neurourol Urodyn* 1997;16:237–75

39. Rushton DN. Sexual and sphincter dysfunction. In Bradley DR, *et al.*, eds. *Neurology in Clinical Practice: Principles of Diagnosis and Management.* Boston: Butterworth-Heinemann, 1996:407–20

40. de Groat WC. A neurologic basis for the overactive bladder. *Urology* 1997;50(Suppl 6A):36–52

41. Blaivas JG. The neurophysiology of micturition: a clinical study of 550 patients. *J Urol* 1982;127:958–63

42. de Groat W. Anatomy and physiology of the lower urinary tract. *Urol Clin North Am* 1993;20:383–401

43. Batra S, Iosif CS. Female urethra: a target for estrogen action. *J Urol* 1983;129:418–20

44. Iosif CS, *et al.* Estrogen receptors in the human lower urinary tract. *Am J Obstet Gynecol* 1981;141:817–20

45. Hilton P, Stanton SL. The use of intravaginal oestrogen cream in genuine stress incontinence. *Br J Obstet Gynaecol* 1983;90:940–4

46. Versi E, Cardozo L, Cooper DJ. Urethral pressures; analysis of pressure transmission ratios. *Br J Urol* 1991;68:266–70

47. Wijma J, Tinga DJ, Visser GH. Compensatory mechanisms which prevent urinary incontinence in aging women. *Gynecol Obstet Invest* 1992;51:102–4

48. Constantinou CE, Govan DE. Spatial distribution and timing of transmitted reflexly generated urethral pressures in healthy women. *J Urol* 1982;127:964

49. Dwyer PL, Teele JS. Prazosin: a neglected cause of genuine stress incontinence. *Obstet Gynecol* 1979;79:117–21

50. Ahlstrom K, *et al.* Effect of combined treatment with phenylpropanolamine and estriol compared with estriol treatment alone, in postmenopausal women with stress urinary incontinence. *Gynecol Obstet Invest* 1990;30:37–43

51. Walter S, *et al.* Stress urinary incontinence in postmenopausal women treated with oral estrogen (estriol) and alpha adrenoceptor stimulating agent (phenylpropanolamine): a

randomized double blind placebo controlled study. *Int Urol J* 1990;12:74–9

52. Versi E. The bladder in menopause: lower urinary tract dysfunction during the climacteric. *Curr Probl Obstet Gynecol* 1994;17:193–232

53. Sartori MG, *et al*. Menopausal genuine stress urinary incontinence treated with conjugated estrogens plus progestogens. *Int J Gynaecol Obstet* 1995;49:165–9

54. Raz R, Stamm W. A controlled trial of intravaginal estriol in postmenopausal women with recurrent urinary tract infection. *N Engl J Med* 1993;329:153–6

55. Thomas TM, *et al*. Prevalence of urinary incontinence. *Br Med J* 1980;281:1243–5

56. Brocklehurst JC. Urinary incontinence in the community – analysis of a MORI poll. *Br Med J* 1993;306:832–4

57. Kondo A, *et al*. Prevalence of handwashing and urinary incontinence in healthy subjects in relation to stress and urge incontinence. *Neurourol Urodyn* 1992;11:519–23

58. Jolleys JV. Reported prevalence of urinary incontinence in women in general practice. *Br Med J* 1988;296:1300–2

59. Molander UM, Ekelund P, *et al*. An epidemiological study of urinary incontinence and related urogenital symptoms in elderly women. *Maturitas* 1990;12:51–60

60. Brieger GM, HL, Mongelli M, Chung TK. The epidemiology of urinary dysfunction in Chinese women. *Int Urogynecol J Pelvic Floor Dysfunct* 1997; 8:191–5

61. Turan C, *et al*. Urinary incontinence in women of reproductive age. *Gynecol Obstet Invest* 1996; 41:132–4

62. Versi E, *et al*. Urinary disorders and the menopause. *Menopause* 1995;2:89–95

63. Holtedahl K, Hunsaker S. Prevalence, 1 year incidence and factors associated with urinary incontinence; a population based study of women 50–74 years of age in primary care. *Maturitas* 1998;28:205–11

64. Rekers H, *et al*. The menopause, urinary incontinence and other symptoms of the genito urinary tract. *Maturitas* 1992;15:101–11

65. Hilton P, Varmna R. The menopause. In Stanton SL, ed. *Clinical Gynecologic Urology*. St. Louis: CV Mosby, 1984:

66. Osborne JL, Postmenopausal changes in micturition habits and in urine flow and urethral pressure studies. In Campbell S, ed. *The Management of the Menopause and Postmenopausal Years*. Lancaster: MTP Publications, 1976: 285–9

67. Sussman M, *et al*. Asymptomatic significant bacteriuria in the non pregnant woman. *Br Med J* 1969;1:799–803

68. Brocklehurst JC, *et al*. The prevalence and symptomatology of urinary infection in an aged population. *Gerontol Clin* 1968;10:242–53

69. Smith PJB. The effect of oestrogens on bladder function in the female. In Campbell S, ed. *The Management of the Menopause and Postmenopausal Years*. Lancaster: MTP Press, 1976:291–8

70. Jolleys JV. Factors associated with regular episodes of dysuria among women in one rural general practice. *Br J Gen Pract* 1991;41:241–3

71. Cardozo LD. Sex and the bladder. *Br Med J* 1988;296:587–8

72. Bungay GT, Vessey MP, McPherson CK. A study of symptoms in middle life with special reference to the menopause. *Br Med J* 1980;281: 181–3

73. Glenning PP. Urinary voiding patterns of apparently normal women. *Aust NZ J Obstet Gynaecol* 1985;25:62–5

74. Roberts M, Smith PJB. Non-malignant obstruction of the female urethra. *Br J Urol* 1968;40: 694–702

75. Stanton SL, Oszoy C, Hilton P. Voiding difficulties in the female: prevalence, clinical and urodynamic review. *Obstet Gynecol* 1983;61:144–7

76. Theofrastous JP, Addison WA, Timmons MC. Voiding function following prolapse surgery. Impact of estrogen replacement. *J Reprod Med* 1996;41:881–4

77. Haylen BT, *et al*. Maximum and average flow rates in normal male and female populations – the Liverpool nomograms. *Br J Urol* 1989;64: 30–8

78. Bates CP, Whiteside CG, Tumer-Warwick R. Synchronous cine/pressure/flow cystourethrography with special reference to stress and urge incontinence. *Br J Urol* 1970;42:714–23

79. Sand PK. Evaluation of the incontinent female. *Curr Probl Obstet Gynecol Fertil* 1992;15:105–52

80. Versi E, Cardozo LD. The predictive value of symptoms and urethral pressure profilometry for the diagnosis of genuine stress incontinence. *J Obstet Gynaecol* 1988;9:168–9

81. Versi E, Cardozo LD. Perineal pad weighing versus videographic analysis in genuine stress incontinence. *Br J Obstet Gynaecol* 1986;93:364–6

82. Versi E, *et al*. The urinary sphincter in the maintenance of female continence. *Br Med J* 1986; 292:166–7

83. Versi E, Cardozo LD, Studd J. Distal urethral compensatory mechanisms in women with an incompetent bladder neck who remain continent. *Neurourol Urodyn* 1990;9:679–90

84. Rud T. Urethral pressure profile in continent women from childhood to old age. *Acta Obstet Gynecol Scand* 1980;59:331–5

85. Rud T. The effect of oestrogens and gestagens on the urethral pressure profile in urinary

continent and stress incontinent women. *Acta Obstet Gynecol Scand* 1980;59:265–70

86. Faber P, Heidenreich J. Treatment of stress incontinence with estrogen in postmenopausal women. *Urol Int* 1977;32:221–3

87. Schleyer-Saunders E. Results of hormone implants in the treatment of the climacteric. *J Am Geriatr Soc* 1971;19:114–21

88. Fantl JA, *et al.* Estrogen therapy in the management of urinary incontinence in postmenopausal women: a meta-analysis. First report of the Hormones and Urogenital Therapy Committee. *Obstet Gynecol* 1994;83:12–18

89. Bhatia NN, Bergman A, Karrarn MM. Effects of estrogen on urethral function in women with stress incontinence. *Obstet Gynecol* 1989;160:176–81

90. Judge TG. The use of quinestrol in elderly incontinent women: a preliminary report. *Gerontol Clin* 1969;11:159–64

91. Walter S, *et al.* Urinary incontinence in postmenopausal women treated with estrogens: a double blind clinical trial. *Urol Int* 1978;33:135–43

92. Samsioe G, *et al.* Occurrence, nature and treatment of urinary incontinence in a 70 year old female population. *Maturitas* 1985;7:335–42

93. Wilson PD, *et al.* Treatment with oral piperazine oestrone sulphate for genuine stress incontinence in post-menopausal women. *Br J Obstet Gynaecol* 1987;94:568–74

94. Fantl JA, *et al.* Efficacy of estrogen supplementation in the treatment of urinary incontinence. The Continence Program for Women Research Group. *Obstet Gynecol* 1996;88:745–9

95. Beisland HO, *et al.* On incompetent urethral closure mechanism: treatment with estriol and phenylpropanolamine. *Scand J Urol Nephrol* 1981;60(Suppl):67–9

96. Beisland HO, *et al.* Urethral sphincteric insufficiency in postmenopausal females; treatment with phenylpropanolamine and oestriol separately and in combination. *Urol Int* 1984;39:211–16

97. Kinn AC, Liskog M. Estrogens and phenylpropanolamine in combination for stress urinary incontinence in postmenopausal women. *Urology* 1988;32:273–80

98. Hilton P, Tweddel AL, Mayne C. Oral and intravaginal estrogens alone and in combination with alphaadrenergic stimulation in genuine stress incontinence. *Int J Urol* 1990;12:80–6

99. Cardozo LD, *et al.* Oestriol in the treatment of postmenopausal urgency: a multicentre study. *Maturitas* 1993;18:47–53

100. Eriksen PS, Rasmussen H. Low-dose 17 beta estradiol vaginal tablets in the treatment of atrophic vaginitis: a double-blind placebo controlled study. *Eur J Obstet Gynaecol Reprod Biol* 1992;44:137–44

101. Salmon UJ, Walter RI, Geist SH. The use of estrogens in the treatment of dysuria and incontinence in postmenopausal women. *Am J Obstet Gynecol* 1941;42:845–51

102. Brandberg A, Mellstrom D, Samsioe G. Per oral estriol treatment of older women with urogenital infections. *Lakartidningen* 1985;82:3399–401

103. Privette M, *et al.* Prevention of recurrent urinary tract infections in postmenopausal women. *Nephron* 1988;50:24–7

104. Cardozo L, Benness C, Abbott D. Low dose oestrogen prophylaxis for recurrent urinary tract infections in elderly women. *Br J Obstet Gynaecol* 1998;105:403–7

105. Kjaergaard B, *et al.* Treatment with low dose vaginal estradiol in postmenopausal women: a double-blind controlled trial. *Ugeskr Laeger* 1990;152:658–9

106. Kirkengen AL, *et al.* Oestriol in the prophylactic treatment of recurrent urinary tract infections in post menopausal women. *Scand J Prim Health Care* 1992;10:139–42

107. Raz R, Stamm WE. A controlled trial of intravaginal estriol in postmenopausal women with recurrent urinary tract infections. *N Engl J Med* 1993;329:753–6

108. Fantl JA, *et al.* Postmenopausal urinary incontinence: comparison between non-estrogen supplemented and estrogen supplemented women. *Obstet Gynecol* 1988;71:823–6

109. Karram MM, *et al.* Urodynamic changes following hormonal replacement therapy in women with premature ovarian failure. *Obstet Gynecol* 1989;74:208–11

110. Versi E, Cardozo L, Studd JWW. Long-term effect of estradiol implants on the female urinary tract during the climacteric. *Int Urogynaecol J* 1990;1:87–90

111. Langer R, *et al.* The absence and effect of induced menopause by gonadotrophin releasing hormone analogs on lower urinary tract symptoms and urodynamic parameters. *Fertil Steril* 1991;55:751–3

112. Iosif CS. Effects of protracted administration of estriol on the lower genitourinary tract in postmenopausal women. *Arch Gynecol Obstet* 1992;251:115–20

18

Intravaginal estriol and the bladder

R. Raz

Urinary tract infection (UTI) remains one of the most common bacterial infections seen in women, with 6–10% of girls and young women having bacteriuria. Furthermore, the incidence rises dramatically in the elderly population; in elderly, non-institutionalized women, for example, the presence of bacteriuria reaches at least 20%[1] and of women aged 80 years or more, 25–50% have bacteriuria[2]. Despite the high prevalence of bacteriuria in the elderly, the factors predisposing such women to UTI have been little explored or compared to those identified in premenopausal women.

We conducted a case–control study comparing healthy non-institutionalized postmenopausal women with recurrent UTI with a control group of women without UTI (Raz and associates; submitted for publication). In this study, we showed that several urological factors, particularly cystocele, the presence of a post-void residual volume and incontinence, were all strongly associated with recurrent UTI. Additionally, urogenital surgery often preceded the onset of UTI and was a risk factor for recurrent UTI. Finally, the same genetic factor associated with recurrent UTI in some groups of premenopausal women, namely non-secretor status, was also strongly associated with recurrent UTI in these women.

Another important factor in postmenopausal women is the potential role that estrogen deficiency plays in the development of bacteriuria.

Postmenopausal women frequently present with genitourinary symptoms. Among women aged 61 years or more, half of them had genitourinary disorders and 29% had urinary incontinence[3].

Postmenopause is characterized by a significant reduction of ovarian estrogen secretion, which is often associated with vaginal atrophy. Clinically it manifests as a syndrome consisting of vaginal dryness, itching, irritation and dyspareunia. UTI and urinary incontinence are also frequent postmenopausal conditions (Table 1)[4,5].

Estrogen stimulates the proliferation of lactobacillus in the vaginal epithelium, reduces pH and avoids the vaginal colonization of Enterobacteraceae, which are the main pathogens of the urinary tract (Figure 1). In addition, the absence of estrogen decreases the volume of the vaginal muscles, resulting in slackness of the ligaments holding the uterus, the pelvic floor and the bladder, resulting in the development of prolapse of the internal genitalia[6].

Kicovic and colleagues[7] showed that vaginal estriol cream is safe and improved urogenital complaints associated with atrophic vaginitis. Atrophy of the meatal epithelium and the trigonum area in the bladder disappeared after treatment with oral or vaginal estrogen.

Table 1 Clinical consequences of estrogen deficiency

Atrophy of:	Predisposes to:
Vaginal mucosa	Atrophic vaginitis
Urethral mucosa	Urinary tract infection
	Urinary incontinence
Bladder mucosa	Urinary incontinence

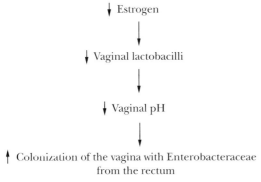

Figure 1 Pathophysiology of urinary tract infections in elderly women

Several studies described changes of the vaginal flora in women receiving small doses of oral estriol. The use of estriol orally or vaginally was also related to a reduction of recurrent UTI and urge incontinence in postmenopausal women[3,8,9].

We demonstrated in a randomized, double-blind, placebo controlled study that vaginal estrogen treatment dramatically reduced the incidence of UTI in elderly women. In addition, after 1 month of therapy, significant changes were observed in the vagina of the women who received estriol; lactobacilli appeared in 60% of these women, but not in the placebo group. In addition, the vaginal pH decreased from 5.5 ± 0.7 before treatment to 3.6 ± 1.0 later[9]. Our study corroborates the impression that estriol replacement is not only effective in the treatment of urogenital complaints related to menopause, but also in the prevention of recurrent UTI.

Intravaginal estriol is well absorbed, and peak levels of unconjugated estriol after insertion of 0.5 mg of cream are comparable with those obtained after 8–12 mg administered orally. In women without liver disease, estriol is rapidly metabolized[10]. Estriol administered locally has the advantage over an oral preparation in that lower doses are required, because the entero-hepatic recirculation is less important, the first liver passage is avoided, and we can obtain similar clinical effects[10].

The optimal dosage of estriol and the induced effect varied according to different studies[7–12]. The actual recommended dosage is

Table 2 Indications and contraindications of estrogen therapy

Indications	
Oral therapy	*Vaginal therapy*
Young postmenopausal women	Elderly women (≥ 60 years old)
Contraindications	*Contraindications*
endometrial carcinoma	high blood pressure
breast carcinoma	diabetes mellitus
thromboembolic disorders	gallstones
liver disease	

Difficulties in vaginal therapy
Physical limitations
Tremor
Obesity
S/P cerebrovascular accident
Dementia
Psychological problems
Educational/cultural behavior

0.5 mg of vaginal estriol twice weekly after a loading dose of 14 days' application. The optimal duration of treatment must also be evaluated in prospective studies in the future. Semmens and co-workers[13] established that correction of vaginal blood flow and pH requires 18–24 months of estrogen therapy. However, we obtained significant changes in the vaginal pH and flora after 1 month of therapy[9].

Two of the questions regarding the prolonged use of estriol are its possible side-effects and its carcinogenicity.

While estradiol is the naturally occurring estrogenic hormone during the premenopausal period, estrone is the predominant hormone in postmenopausal women. Both have receptors in the vagina and endometrium, therefore, they produce proliferation of the mucosa of the endometrium and their use is related to bleeding and they are potentially carcinogenic hormones. Several potential risks of estrogen therapy are endometrial carcinoma, breast cancer, thromboembolic disease, increased blood pressure, gallstones and hyperglycemia[14]. In order to avoid some of these undesirable events, progesterone is added to the estrogen therapy[15]. This continued therapy produces periodic endometrial bleedings.

Estriol is one of the metabolic end products of estradiol. It has specially a specific urogenital activity. Since there are only estriol receptors in the vagina estriol treatment does not cause endometrial proliferation. Therefore, women treated with estriol do not need progesterone replacement.

Moreover, estriol has been used for more than four decades and there is no evidence of carcinogenic effects[16]. Its local use had minimal side-effects such as burning or pruritus, that generally disappeared after several days of treatment.

The use of intravaginal estriol therapy has several difficulties, especially in elderly women with physical limitations, such as tremor, obesity, dementia, neurological deficits, and sometimes educational and cultural behavior. In these cases, a low dose of oral estriol can be given (Table 2).

ACKNOWLEDGEMENT

We would like to thank Mrs Frances Nachmani for her secretarial assistance in typing this manuscript.

References

1. Abruptyn E, Biscia JA, Kaye D. The treatment of asymptomatic bacteriuria in the elderly. *J Am Geriatr Soc* 1988;36:473–5
2. Sourander LB. Urinary tract infection in the aged – an epidemiological study. *Am Med Intern Fenn* 1966;55:7–55
3. Iosif CS, Bekassy Z. Prevalence of genito-urinary symptoms in the late menopause. *Acta Obstet Gynecol Scand* 1984;63:257–60
4. Haspels AA, Luisi M, Kicovic PM. Endocrinological and clinical investigations in post-menopausal women following administration of vaginal cream containing oestriol. *Maturitas* 1981;3:321–7
5. Thomas TM, Plymat KR, Blannin J, *et al.* Prevalence of urinary incontinence *Br Med J* 1980;281:1243–5
6. Raz R. Role of estriol therapy for women with recurrent urinary tract infections: advantages and disadvantages. *Inf Dis Clin Pract* 1999;8:64–6
7. Kicovic PM, Cortes-Prieto J, Milojevic S, *et al.* The treatment of postmenopausal vaginal atrophy with Ovestin vaginal cream or suppositories: clinical, endocrinological and safety aspects. *Maturitas* 1980;2:275–82
8. Brocklehurst JC, Dillane JB, Griffiths L, *et al.* The prevalence and symptomatology of urinary infection in an aged population. *Gerontology* 1968;10:242–53
9. Raz R, Stamm WE. A controlled trial of intra-vaginal estriol in postmenopausal women with recurrent urinary tract infections. *N Engl J Med* 1993;329:753–6
10. Mattson LA, Cullberg G. Vaginal absorption of two estriol preparations: a comparative study in postmenopausal women. *Acta Obstet Gynecol Scand* 1983;62:393–6
11. Heimer GM. Estriol in the postmenopause. *Acta Obstet Gynecol Scand (Suppl)* 1987;139:1–23
12. Haskins AL, Moszkowski EF, Whitelock VP. The estrogenic potential of estriol. *Am J Obstet Gynecol* 1968;1:665–7
13. Semmens JP, Tsai CC, Curtis Semmens E, *et al.* Effects of estrogen therapy on vaginal physiology during menopause. *Obstet Gynecol* 1985;66:15–18
14. Lauritzen C. Erfahrungen mit einer östriol-vaginal creme (experiences with an estriol cream). *Ther Ggw* 1979;118:567–7
15. Gambrell RD Jr. The prevention of endometrial cancer in postmenopausal women with progestogens. *Maturitas* 1978;1:107–12
16. Puck AV. Wirkung von Östriol bei dysmenorrhoe, entzündungen im weiblichen genitale, pruritus und beschwerden der climax. *Munch Med Wochenschr* 1957;99:1505–7

19

Menopause and sexual functioning

L. Dennerstein, P. Lehert, H. Burger, C. Garamszegi and E. Dudley

INTRODUCTION

Women attending menopause clinics often complain of sexual problems[1]. Clinicians have been concerned to sort out whether any aspect of female sexual functioning is linked to hormonal change as this may indicate that hormone therapy would have a role in the treatment of such disorders. While double-blind randomized trials of hormone therapy provide results of the pharmacological properties of various compounds, often used in supraphysiological doses, they indicate little about the physiological etiology of any changes in sexual behavior experienced by women in midlife. Clinicians are also concerned about the relative role of hormonal factors to those of aging, health and psychosocial factors on human sexuality. Population-based surveys can help address the question of a link between aging, menopause and sexuality. Yet relatively few of the population-based studies of the menopausal transition in mid-aged women have assessed sexual functioning. Even fewer have used a validated questionnaire to assess the different aspects of sexuality. Differing measures of sexual functioning have been used with studies often failing to offer any data on the validity or reliability of these measures in their local population. Some of the assessments have been very vague constructs indeed. For example, Osborn and colleagues[2] asked a general practice population if they suffered from 'sexual dysfunction' while Koster and Garde[3] asked women whether sexual desire was decreased or infrequent compared with 11 years previously. Even fewer

studies have undertaken any hormonal determinations and these have either been of small sample size[4] or are still in progress. Studies of the role of menopausal status often use a comparison of the health outcome measure before and after women have reached menopause (12 months of amenorrhea). Yet endocrine change occurs for some years prior to cessation of menopause so it would seem important to examine for changes in health outcomes also some years before menses cease. Exogenous hormones may mask the effects of changing ovarian function so that women taking the oral contraceptive pill or any sort of hormone therapy must be documented when the objective is to examine the role of the natural menopausal transition. Population-based studies often suffer from being cross-sectional in design. Cross-sectional studies can only indicate whether associations exist and are unable to determine the direction of causality. Cross-sectional studies are also unable to establish a difference between cohort membership (effects of social change on different age groups) and aging. Aging and length of the relationship are known to affect sexual functioning of both men and women. For example, James[5] used cross-sectional and longitudinal data to show that coital rate halved over the first year of marriage and then took another 20 years to halve again. The role of aging *per se* has to be disentangled from that of menopause, with which it is confounded. Longitudinal studies of samples derived from the general population are in the best position to sort out whether there is a change in sexual functioning, and if so whether this reflects aging, health status, or hormonal or psychosocial factors.

Other methodological issues include the need for an appropriate age band which covers the menopausal transition (45–55 years); use of standardized objective definitions of menopausal status; distinctions between women in the natural menopausal transition and those with an induced menopause; limitations imposed on women by questionnaire design; and need for appropriate data analysis techniques[6]. Most studies have only utilized univariate analysis and thus have been unable to take into account the role of confounding or interacting factors.

With these limitations in mind, this chapter utilizes the results of a population-based study of mid-aged Australian-born women to explore the impact of the menopause on women's sexual functioning.

THE MELBOURNE WOMEN'S MIDLIFE HEALTH PROJECT

The Melbourne Women's Midlife Health Project is one of the few longitudinal population-based studies to have measured the relationship between sexuality, mood, menopausal status and a range of other variables, including hormone levels and psychosocial factors.

Study design and sampling

The Melbourne Women's Midlife Health Project involves a community-based cohort of mid-aged women. The study began in 1991 with population sampling by random telephone digital dialling to find 2001 Australian-born women aged between 45 and 55 years and resident in Melbourne. There was a 71% response rate to participation in a telephone interview used to acquire baseline data[7,8]. The study was approved by the Human Research Ethics Committee of the University of Melbourne. All subjects provided written informed consent for their participation in the study. All those women who had experienced menses in the prior 3 months, and who were not taking the oral contraceptive pill

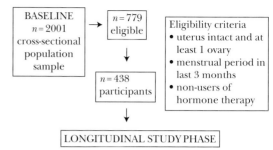

Figure 1 Study design for the Melbourne Women's Midlife Health Project

or hormone therapy were invited to participate in a longitudinal study. Of those eligible to enter the longitudinal study, only 56% chose to do so ($n = 438$) (see Figure 1).

Volunteers for the longitudinal study were more likely than non-participants to report: better self-rated health, paid employment, more than 12 years of education, having ever had a Papanicolaou smear, exercising at least once a week, and having undergone dilatation and curettage[9].

The retention rate of the 438 women who volunteered for the longitudinal study was 97% for year 2, 94% for year 3, 91% for years 4 and 5 and 90% for year 6.

Measures and procedures

The Melbourne research team was allowed access to questionnaires carefully constructed by the groups of Kaufert and McKinlay and used in cross-sectional and longitudinal studies in North America[10,11]. The core questionnaire was modified for use in Australia after advice from co-investigators and a community advisory committee. Additional references are given below for specific variables and for those questions or instruments which supplemented the core questionnaire.

The cross-sectional questionnaire utilized in the initial telephone interview included socio-demographic data, health status, history of premenstrual complaints, lifestyle behaviors, and attitudes to aging and to menopause. Questions pertaining to bothersome symptoms were included in a list of other health-related symptoms[7]. Menstrual status and use of any hormone therapy was determined. Premenopausal status was assigned to women who reported no change in menstrual frequency. Perimenopausal status was used when women reported change in menstrual frequency. Women were deemed to be postmenopausal when there had been amenorrhea for at least 12 months. Separate categories were assigned to women who were taking hormone therapy or had an induced menopause. Well-being was assessed by a validated scale[12,13]. Three questions related to sexual functioning[8]. Women were asked whether, with regard to the last 12 months: sexual intercourse had occurred at all; whether sexual intercourse had been associated with unusual pain or discomfort; or whether there had been any change in sexual interest (increased, no change, or decreased).

The longitudinal study involves annual face-to-face assessments in the women's own homes, with interviews and physical measures. Interview information is collected annually on the following variables: menstrual status; sociodemographic factors (age, marital status, paid work status); health status; symptoms (total score used)[7]; daily hassles[14,15]; stress[13]; well-being[12,13]; and use of hormone replacement therapy (HRT). The longitudinal study provided the opportunity to include a detailed assessment of sexual functioning. The Personal Experiences Questionnaire (PEQ)[16], derived from the McCoy Female Sexual Questionnaire[17], was handed to women to self-complete and return to field workers in a closed envelope. The PEQ focuses on current sexual experience and uses a 5-point Likert scale. Women were also asked to indicate their sexual preference and whether or not they had a sexual partner. Using cross-sectional data from the third year of study, the psychometric properties of the PEQ were assessed[16]. Six factors were extracted by principal components factor analysis and these explained 70% of the variance. Two of these factors related to possible determinants of sexual functioning: Feelings for Partner; and Partner Problems. The other four factors were considered to be indicators of different aspects of sexual functioning. These were named: Sexual Responsivity, Sexual Frequency, Libido and Vaginal Dryness/Dyspareunia. Internal consistency was considered adequate with a Cronbach's alpha of 0.71. Items included in each factor are shown in Table 1.

Blood samples for hormone assays and measurement of cholesterol were taken between days 4 and 8 for those still cycling or after 3 months of amenorrhea. Estradiol, follicle stimulating hormone (FSH) and immunoreactive inhibin were determined by radioimmunoassay[9].

Table 1 The Personal Experiences Questionnaire (PEQ)

PEQ factor	Item
Factor 1. Feelings for Partner	Companionable love for partner
	Satisfied with partner as friend
	Passionate love for partner
	Satisfied with partner as lover
	Resentment towards partner
	Hostility towards partner
Factor 2. Sexual Responsivity	Arousal during sexual activities
	Orgasm during sexual activities
	Enjoyment of sexual activities
Factor 3. Frequency of Sexual Activities	Sexual intercourse in last month (frequency)
	Sexual activities in the last two weeks (frequency)
	Satisfied with frequency of sexual activity
Factor 4. Libido	Sexual thoughts/fantasies in last month (frequency)
	Masturbation (frequency)
Factor 5. Partner Problems	Partner difficulties in sexual performance
Factor 6. Vaginal Dryness/Dyspareunia	Lack vaginal wetness during sexual activity
	Pain during intercourse

RESULTS

Cross-sectional baseline study[8]

The majority of women for whom data were available ($n = 1879$) reported no change in sexual interest over the 12 months in question (62.3%), although 31.1% reported a decline in sexual interest and a smaller group reported an increase (6.6%). Most women engaged in sexual intercourse in the previous year (84.2%) and, of these, only 11.9% reported experiencing unusual pain on intercourse. The natural menopausal transition was significantly associated with a decline in sexual interest, decreased likelihood of sexual intercourse and increased dyspareunia. Of the reasons offered for a decline in sexual interest, most were vague (e.g. no desire, bored, no interest) whereas increase in sexual interest was most commonly associated with a new partner[8]. Logistic regression was used to identify explanatory variables for change in sexual interest. Decline in sexual interest was significantly associated with natural menopause, decreased well-being, decreasing employment and presence of bothersome symptoms. Eleven to 12 years of education was associated with a lower risk of decreased sexual functioning.

Longitudinal study[18]

Longitudinal data from the first 6 years of annual assessments were included in the following analysis. Women were excluded from the analysis for the following reasons: drop-outs ($n = 49$), surgical menopause during the study ($n = 29$), oral contraceptive use during any year ($n = 6$). This left a sample size of 354 women.

Measures were selected for inclusion in this analysis based on significant relationships with sexual interest in the baseline cross-sectional study[8] and review of the literature. Structural equation modelling (SEM)[19,20] was chosen as a particularly suitable technique for assessing the whole model by means of a unique global goodness-of-fit test. This enables the relative role of hormonal, physical and psychosocial factors to be assessed. The results are summarized below from Dennerstein and colleagues[18].

Changes in sexuality factors with aging

The following factors significantly diminished ($p < 0.001$) with time (years in study): Feelings for Partner; Sexual Responsivity; Frequency of Sexual Activities; Libido. The following factors significantly increased ($p < 0.001$) with time (years in study): Vaginal Dryness/Dyspareunia; Partner Problems.

Structural modelling

Using the set of 354 women, we tested a global model using *a priori* hypotheses which included the sexual outcome factors measured by the PEQ, and possible determinants: aging, menopausal status, HRT use, symptoms, hormone levels, social factors (education, paid work, stress, daily hassles), well-being, Feelings about Partner and Partner Problems.

The best-fit model is shown in Figure 2, reprinted with permission from Dennerstein and co-workers[18]. The Normal-Fit Index was 0.92, which means that the fit was not too far from the perfect fit, taking the independence model as the zero fit. Rectangles represent the measured variables. The circle denotes the latent variable (ovarian functioning) and arrows designate a causal path and its direction. Two directional arrows indicate covariance between two variables. Age was confounded with menopausal status and has thus not been included in Figure 2. Menopausal status does directly affect two aspects of sexual functioning (Vaginal Dryness/Dyspareunia and Sexual Responsivity). The effect on Sexual Responsivity appears to be indirect, with significant effects of menopausal status on bothersome symptoms, which then affect well-being, which in turn influences Sexual Responsivity. No direct effects of hormonal variables or HRT on sexual outcome measures were evident.

Social factors, such as stress, daily hassles, educational level and paid work, have only indirect effects on sexual functioning, through effects on well-being and experience of problematic symptoms, both of which affect parameters of sexual functioning. Women's increasing positive Feelings for Partner have significant and powerful positive effects on their Libido,

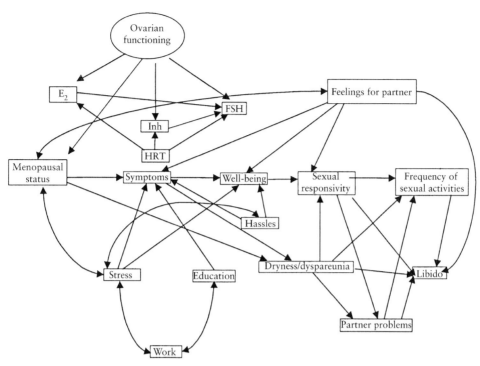

Figure 2 Global model of factors affecting sexual functioning. Reprinted with permission from reference 18. FSH, follicle stimulating hormone; E_2, estradiol; Inh, inhibin; HRT, hormone replacement therapy

Sexual Responsivity and well-being, and protect against experience of symptoms. The covariance between Feelings for Partner and menopausal status may indicate a vulnerability during the menopausal transition. This close relationship during the menopausal transition is also evident for experience of stress. Similarly, covariance is evident between stress and daily hassles, stress and paid work, and paid work and educational status. Decreasing Sexual Responsivity and increasing Vaginal Dryness/Dyspareunia increase partner problems. The presence of Partner Problems leads to lower Frequency of Sexual Activities but increased Libido (a measure of autoeroticism). Increasing Vaginal Dryness/Dyspareunia has a significant negative effect on Sexual Responsivity and Libido. The reader is referred to Dennerstein and colleagues[18] for details of the regression weights which indicate the strength of each set of equations.

DISCUSSION

This study set out to determine whether women's sexual functioning declined in midlife, and if so the relative roles of biological and psychosocial factors. The initial cross-sectional analysis suggested that a substantial minority of women were aware of a decline in their sexual interest and that sexual interest, intercourse occurrence and dyspareunia were affected by the natural menopausal transition. Psychosocial and health status variables, including well-being and experience of bothersome symptoms, were also found to be significantly associated with a decline in sexual interest. The baseline study used only three questions about sexual functioning and a long recall period. The prospective study was able to include a detailed questionnaire (PEQ), a shorter recall period and annual hormone measures. The statistical analysis (SEM) chosen allowed an overall appraisal of the relative roles of various factors as well as pathways of interrelationships to be demonstrated. The SEM model provides an adequate way of controlling confounding, concomitant factors which may affect separate linear regressions. When this is done and most of the important determinants included in the model, the effects of hormone levels are relatively weak. Some effects of hormone levels are still present (indicated through a significant effect of menopausal status on Vaginal Dryness/Dyspareunia and direct effects of menopausal status on the number of bothersome symptoms. The number of symptoms then affects well-being, which influences Sexual Responsivity, which in turn influences Frequency of Sexual Activities and Libido. This highlights the need for analytic models to include most of the variables rather than just a few. A powerful effect of Feelings for Partner on Libido was found, confirming our preliminary analysis which found that the effect of Feelings about Partner on Libido was much more significant ($p = 0.003$) than that of hormones ($p = 0.02$)[21]. Other social factors, such as educational level, experience of interpersonal stress and daily hassles, affect sexual functioning indirectly, by influencing symptoms and/or well-being.

Previous longitudinal analysis using repeated measures for multivariate analysis of covariance also found no direct effect of menopausal status, FSH, estradiol, or inhibin on the negative mood subscale of the well-being score[15]. However, negative mood was significantly adversely affected by bothersome symptoms, negative feelings for the partner, daily hassles and high interpersonal stress. The menopausal transition had an indirect effect in amplifying the effect of stressors and poor health[15].

The findings of the preliminary analysis[21] taken together with the current findings indicate that any effects of the hormones estradiol, FSH and inhibin on female sexual functioning are relatively weak compared to the effects of other variables, such as feelings for partner, symptoms, well-being and partner problems. Only a single blood sample for each woman was collected on an annual basis. Given the variability of menstrual cycles at this time and the

associated variability of hormonal levels during the perimenopause[9], a great deal of variance in hormone levels would be expected. This, and the level of sensitivity of the estradiol assay, may limit the ability of annual single plasma hormone assays to detect relationships with parameters of sexual functioning. Furthermore, the current statistical modelling involves pooling data and this involves a loss of power. Future longitudinal modelling using change measures in structural equation modelling will provide a more sensitive confirmatory analysis. Techniques such as cluster analysis may identify particular groups of women who may be vulnerable to change in sexual functioning during the transition.

No relationship was evident between HRT use and any of the parameters of sexual functioning, even Vaginal Dryness/Dyspareunia. This may suggest that the type of HRT used may not be well adapted towards providing optimal sexual outcomes. The same seems to be true for effects of HRT on well-being and symptoms. However, we did not have measures of these health status variables just prior to use of HRT. Measures taken immediately prior to use of HRT and then some months into the use of HRT would be needed to adequately determine the effects of HRT. Clearly, double-blind controlled trials remain the best way to assess the effects of HRT.

Qualitative data

How do these findings relate to what women themselves say? The PEQ does have a place for further comments. All the comments provided by the women relating to changes in their sexual behavior during the longitudinal phase of the study were downloaded and subjected to a preliminary content analysis. There were a variety of responses listed but these fell predominantly into four groups. Some comments which are typical of women in each of these groups are described below.

No partner

'No current partner.'

'I have been widowed for 2 years.'

'Have been divorced for some time – no partner for the last 5 years.'

Husband's problems

'My partner is impotent so I don't have sex with him.'

'Some things have changed since my husband's operation for bowel cancer 1 year ago.'

'Husband currently working overseas with infrequent visits home.'

Her decreased interest

'The last 5 years have been quieter in the sex department than were the previous years.'

'We seldom have sex. Our relationship is good but not sexual these days.'

'Sexual intercourse is less exciting now than earlier years and I seem to find other things take time that my partner and I spend together e.g. children, friends, work. Put less effort into making it fun.'

'At 47 I don't feel like instigating sex.'

Increased interest

'I was separated 3 years ago. I have a new partner (9 months' duration). My new partner has transformed my life and love life.'

'I don't think I have changed. The difference between now and 5 years ago is that I have a different partner.'

'My sex life with the same partner has improved greatly from being satisfactory before in the past 5 years because we have deliberately made time for each other, such as going away for weekends once or twice a year.'

IMPLICATIONS FOR CLINICIANS

Population-based studies such as the Melbourne Women's Midlife Health Project suggest a deterioration in several aspects of female sexual functioning associated with the midlife years. This study provides further evidence about the direct and indirect roles of the hormonal changes of the menopausal transition. The analysis also demonstrates that hormonal change is only one aspect of the many factors that impact on sexual functioning. These include the woman's own premorbid level of sexual functioning, presence of bothersome symptoms, well-being, stress and the presence and quality of the sexual relationship with a partner.

When mid-aged women report sexual problems, the clinician must engage in detailed history taking involving the woman and her partner, alone and together. Given the range of factors affecting sexual functioning and the significantly more powerful effect of partner factors over that of hormonal factors, a broadly based biopsychosocial approach is needed. Bothersome symptoms which are known to be responsive to hormone therapy should be treated, as these impact on aspects of sexual functioning as well as causing distress in their own right. But hormonal prescription alone is rarely enough! Attention is needed to the relationship with the partner, and other stressors in the woman's life. Inspection of women's own comments reveals that the midlife transition allows the opportunity for positive change in relationships, if couples increase their intimacy at this time.

ACKNOWLEDGEMENTS

This study was supported by grants from the Public Health & Research Development Committee of the National Health & Medical Research Council and the Victorian Health Promotion Foundation. Prince Henry's Institute of Medical Research, Monash Medical Centre, received grants from Organon Pty Ltd, for hormone assays, and Pharmacia & Upjohn, grant-in-aid.

References

1. Sarrel P, Whitehead M. Sex and menopause: defining the issues. *Maturitas* 1985;7:217–24

2. Osborn M, Hawton K, Gath D. Sexual dysfunction among middle aged women in the community. *Br Med J* 1988;296:959–62

3. Koster A, Garde K. Sexual desire and menopausal development. A prospective study of Danish women born in 1936. *Maturitas* 1993;16:49–60

4. McCoy N, Davidson J. A longitudinal study of the effects of menopause on sexuality. *Maturitas* 1985;7:203–10

5. James W. Decline in coital rates with spouses' ages in duration of marriage. *J Biosoc Sci* 1983;15:83–7

6. Dennerstein L. Well-being, symptoms and the menopausal transition. *Maturitas* 1966;23:147–57

7. Dennerstein L, Smith A, Morse C, *et al*. Menopausal symptoms in Australian women. *Med J Aust* 1993;159:232–6

8. Dennerstein L, Smith A, Morse C, *et al*. Sexuality and the menopause. *J Psychosom Obstet Gynaecol* 1994;15:59–66

9. Burger H, Dudley M, Hopper J, *et al*. The endocrinology of the menopausal transition: a cross-sectional study of a population-base sample. *J Clin Endocrinol Metab* 1995;80:3537–45

10. Kaufert P, Syrotuik J. Symptom reporting at the menopause. *Soc Sci Med* 1981;15:173–84

11. McKinlay J, McKinlay S, Brambilla D. Health status and utilization behavior associated with menopause. *Am J Epidemiol* 1987;125:110–21

12. Kammann R, Flett R. Affectometer 2: a scale to measure current level of general happiness. *Aust J Psychol* 1983;35:259–65

13. Dennerstein L, Dudley E, Burger H. Wellbeing and the menopausal transition. *J Psychosom Obstet Gynaecol* 1994;18:95–101

14. Kanner A, Coyne J, Schaefer C, *et al*. Comparison of two modes of stress measurement: daily hassles and uplifts versus major life events. *J Behav Med* 1981;4:1–39

15. Dennerstein L, Lehert P, Burger H, *et al*. Mood and the menopausal transition. *J Nerv Mental Dis* 1999;187:in press

16. Dennerstein L, Dudley E, Hopper J, *et al*. Sexuality, hormones and the menopausal transition. *Maturitas* 1997;26:83–93

17. McCoy N, Matyas J. Oral contraceptives and sexuality in university women. *Arch Sex Behav* 1996;25:73–9

18. Dennerstein L, Lehert P, Burger H, *et al*. Factors affecting sexual functioning of women in the mid-life years. *Climacteric* 1999;2:in press

19. Bentler PM, Stein JA. Structural equation models in medical research. *Stat Methods Med Res* 1992;1:159–81

20. Hoyle R. Introduction to special section: structural equation modelling in clinical research. *J Consult Clin Psychol* 1994;62:427–8

21. Dennerstein L, Lehert P, Burger H, *et al*. Biological and psychosocial factors affecting sexual functioning during the menopausal transition. In Bellino F, ed. *Biology of Menopause*. New York: Springer-Verlag, 1999:in press

20

Sexuality and breast cancer: a review

A. Graziottin and E. Castoldi

INTRODUCTION

The aim of this review is to provide physicians with an updated 'state of the art' discussion of the sexual consequences of breast cancer diagnosis and treatment. Female sexual identity, sexual function and sexual relationship may be dramatically wounded, physically and emotionally, by the many changes and challenges the woman has to face when breast cancer disrupts her life and that of her relatives[1–3].

Excellent research, both retrospective[4] and prospective[5–9], has been carried out on the many psychosocial issues facing a woman during this difficult transition of her life. Unfortunately, the majority of papers considered for this review (with a few exceptions[4,7,10,11]) address the psychological problems more than the biological ones, which are, at best, touched on only marginally.

This paper briefly reviews psychosocial issues that may affect sexuality after breast cancer diagnosis and addresses in detail the biological issues that deserve medical attention and further study.

FEMALE SEXUAL IDENTITY

Female sexual identity relies on four major dimensions[12–15]: femininity, maternity, eroticism and social role. All four dimensions of female sexual identity may be variably affected by breast cancer diagnosis and treatment.

Femininity

Femininity may suffer a major insult, for a number of biological reasons.

The breast is a prominent personal and social sign of femininity. Body image is the parameter most affected by the type of surgery performed[4,7–9,16]. Short-term impact depends on the type of surgery performed (lumpectomy versus mastectomy, with immediate or delayed reconstruction) and its cosmetic result, and on the need, or not, for adjuvant radiotherapy or chemotherapy. However, more conservative treatments do not appear to significantly modify quality of life nor female sexuality in the long term[4,7–9]. Loss of hair and worsening of its condition, secondary to chemotherapy, may contribute to damaging the inner perception of femininity and of personal beauty.

Arm lymphedema may be a major, though still underdiagnosed and undertreated, side-effect of breast cancer diagnosis and treatment[17], with an average reported incidence of 30–40%[18,19]. Disfigured body image and self-perception may severely wound the inner sense of femininity, leading to depression and avoidant coping strategies. 'Arm problems' are quoted by 43–72% of the patients, according to the different arm symptoms (pain, pins and needles, numbness, skin sensitivity, swelling) that were mentioned in Ganz and colleagues and by 26–36% in Dorval and co-workers[8,9].

Iatrogenic menopause is the third biological factor that may damage the sense of femininity and affect different dimensions of female sexual identity. Younger patients (25% of breast cancer patients are premenopausal) are more vulnerable overall to the complex impact of breast cancer diagnosis and treatment[1,2,4,6,7,13,14,20]. Estrogen also modulates the quality of brain aging and the coincident cognitive and emotional symptoms[21,22] and the quality of aging of sensory organs which are sexual targets and sexual determinants of libido[13-15,20].

Age is the fourth biological factor that may modify the outcome of diagnosis and treatment. Its importance is not limited to the potential impact of the menopause, but to the different individual and social tasks and goals of women's reproductive years, tasks that have different priorities in different decades.

Maternity

Maternity may become the core of a major identity crisis for the 25% of women diagnosed whilst still fertile[15,23]. The most relevant biological issues are discussed in the excellent review by Collichio and colleagues[11]: conception; fertility; the 'last minute baby syndrome'; risk of congenital abnormalities following chemotherapy, which fortunately does not seem to exceed normal incidence[23]; milk production, reduced in the irradiated breast; and pregnancy, with the risk it may have for the risk of recurrence of breast cancer. A number of studies deny such a risk[24-29]. However, Guinee and co-workers[30] have demonstrated a detrimental effect of pregnancy on subclinical breast cancer. Effects of the anti-estrogen tamoxifen on human pregnancies are not yet reported.

Eroticism

Breast cancer may affect sensuality, sexiness and receptiveness.

The major insult breast surgery has on breast eroticism is shown by the 44% of women with partial mastectomy and 83% of those with breast reconstruction ($p < 0.001$) who report that pleasure from breast caresses had decreased[4].

Menopausal symptoms (hot flushes, sweating, mood swings, insomnia, depression, loss of libido, arousal difficulties, orgasmic difficulties and dyspareunia), signs (wrinkles, weight gain, modified body shape, mouth dryness, vaginal dryness and overall worsened sexual response) and quality of life impairment secondary to iatrogenic (chemotherapeutic) and/or non-hormonally treatable natural menopause may dramatically devastate the woman's sense of eroticism[13,14,20,31,32]. Women who received chemotherapy tended to have desire less frequently ($p < 0.032$); had more vaginal dryness ($p < 0.001$) and dyspareunia ($p < 0.001$); had sex less frequently ($p < 0.013$); and their ability to reach orgasm through intercourse tended to be reduced ($p < 0.043$), although their ability to reach orgasm through non-coital caressing did not differ from that of other women. Coital receptiveness is therefore selectively damaged. Overall sexual satisfaction was significantly poorer ($p < 0.001$)[4].

Depression and anxiety, reactive to breast cancer, may affect self-perception and sexual function via non-hormonal pathways, and are reported on average in 17–25% of breast cancer patients[33].

Social role

Social role may represent an area relatively safe from breast cancer, particularly in well-educated women[34-36], except in the acute phase or in the more severe and aggressive cases. A strong and positive social role may reduce the impact of breast cancer on other dimensions of femininity, especially in the peri- and postmenopausal years[1,7,36,37]. However, 20% of breast cancer survivors report a reduction of energy, a decrease in recreational activities, psychological distress and cognitive problems, such as difficulties in concentrating, remembering, and thinking clearly[7]. Cognitive deficit after postoperative adjuvant chemotherapy has been described[38]. This cognitive impairment following chemotherapy was noticed in a broad domain of functioning, including attention, mental flexibility, speed of information processing, visual memory and motor function. This cognitive impairment is unaffected by anxiety, depression, fatigue and time since treatment, and is not related to the self-reported complaints of cognitive dysfunction[38].

In summary, female sexual identity may be variably affected by breast cancer diagnosis and treatment according to a number of biological factors: age at diagnosis; stage and correlated extension and type of treatment; type and cosmetic outcome of surgery; presence of lymphedema; accomplishment or not of childbearing before diagnosis; infertility; induction of a premature menopause with its cohort of symptoms and signs, including the worsening of sexual function; and biological mental damage from chemotherapy and chronic loss of estrogens. The differentiation of the relative weight of these factors with respect to psychosocial variables deserves further prospective studies, more biologically oriented.

FEMALE SEXUAL FUNCTION

Linear models (arousal, plateau, orgasm, resolution) have been widely used since the pioneering work of Masters and colleagues, recently updated[39], and Kaplan[40]. More recently, Graziottin[2,31] suggested that human sexual function can be considered as a circuit, with four main stations: libido, arousal, orgasm and satisfaction, this last dimension including both the physical phase of resolution, with its homeostatic function of returning to baseline, and the emotional evaluation of the experience (Figure 1).

This model (Figure 1), formulated by the presenting author, contributes to our immediate understanding of the frequent overlapping of sexual symptoms reported in clinical

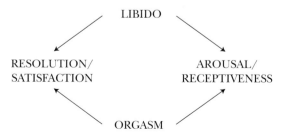

Figure 1 Cybernetic model of sexual function

practice, as different dimensions of sexual response are correlated from a physiopathological point of view, and also of the potential negative or positive feedback mechanisms operating in sexual function.

The model also addresses two critical aspects. First, the 'specificity' of receptiveness as the female characteristic of arousal. In this sense, dyspareunia could be considered not only as a pain symptom, but also as a specific receptiveness disorder. Second, the importance of the human dimension of 'satisfaction', which goes beyond the physiological phase of resolution and encompasses both physical and emotional correlates of the erotic experience.

The clinician should therefore be alerted to potential problems in any critical component of sexual function, to make appropriate differential diagnosis and suggest the best medical and/or psychosexual therapy.

LIBIDO

Libido has three major dimensions: biological, motivational-affective and cognitive[31,41], that have a complex interplay with both inhibiting and enhancing roles. A useful working definition is that 'sexual desire is normally an activated, unsatisfied mental state of variable intensity, created by external, via the sensory modalities, or internal stimuli, fantasy, memory, cognition …, that induce a feeling of a need or want to partake of sexual activity (usually with the object of desire) to satisfy the need'[42]. The three dimensions of libido may be differently affected by breast cancer diagnosis and treatment.

The biological roots of libido have been extensively discussed elsewhere[14,31,43]. In short, hormones are the necessary, but not sufficient, factors to maintain a satisfying human libido[44]. They seem to control the intensity of libido and sexual behavior, rather than its direction[41]. After breast cancer diagnosis and treatment, loss of estrogens, secondary to iatrogenic or naturally occurring menopause, may contribute to the inhibition of the sexual drive and the physical receptiveness; loss of androgens[45,46], secondary to chemotherapy or ovariectomy,

213

may further worsen the picture. Involution of sensory organs after menopause may further reduce the biological basis of libido[14,15]. Loss of libido is a multifactorial problem that may also be secondary to a number of different factors: arousal disorders, due to biological and/or psychological causes[13,14,31,47-49]; pelvic floor dysfunction[50]; psychodynamic[51], motivational, or relational causes[10,48,52]; sexual pain-related disorders[53]; orgasmic disorders[52]; and sexual dissatisfaction, physical, emotional, or both. Breast cancer diagnosis and treatment may contribute to a complex of sexual dysfunction, overlapping in different dimensions of the sexual response.

Motivational-affective and cognitive aspects of libido may further modulate the sexual scenario in breast cancer diagnosis and treatment, both with a paralysing or, less frequently, an enhancing role.

In summary, the biological components of libido deserve to be studied in patients with breast cancer, to identify the subgroups of women at higher risk of negative psychosexual adjustment, to offer better preventive and supportive cure and care. Iatrogenic menopause, dyspareunia and chemotherapy *per se* seem to be the major factors that may devastate the biological bases of libido in patients with breast cancer[1,4,16,17,49,54]. Their relative weight in comparison to psychosocial variables needs further research.

SEXUAL AROUSAL

Sexual arousal indicates a state with specific feelings, usually attached to the genitals[42]. In women, arousal difficulties may be central, non-genital peripheral and genital[55].

Estrogen and androgen loss, secondary to iatrogenic menopause, may affect all these aspects of arousal.

Biological central difficulties may be secondary to loss of sexual hormones, but they may be made worse by depression[14,15], anxiety[56], chronic stress and insomnia[50], that may also be biologically rooted and worsened by estrogen and androgen deprivation[57-60]. Reduced frequency of erotic dreams, of fantasies, of sexual daydreams and of spontaneous mental arousal

are the clinical consequences of central arousal difficulties that are anecdotally reported in patients with breast cancer.

Problems in non-genital peripheral arousal may be better described as 'touch-impaired' disorders[61].

Genital arousal is mediated by the action of vasoactive intestinal peptide, the most important neurotransmitter that 'translates' sexual drive into vaginal lubrication[55]. Without estrogen, vaginal dryness and dyspareunia are complained of by 35–50% of normal postmenopausal women[14,61,62]. Loss of estrogen is the principal biological cause of genital arousal difficulties in women and may be the critical precipitating factor that leads to dyspareunia in women with iatrogenic premature menopause[63], particularly in the 25% of breast cancer patients who were premenopausal at diagnosis. Besides estrogens, habit, that is regular and continued sexual activity (without pain!) has been found to protect against vaginal dryness[64]. Pre-existing arousal disorders may be further worsened by the menopausal loss of estrogens, leading to frank avoidance of intercourse.

Tamoxifen is the contemporary endocrine treatment most widely used in breast cancer. The drug is thought to act by blocking the estrogen receptor in the tumor cells, but alternative mechanisms of action have been proposed[65]. It also influences steroid disposition. It interacts with ovarian estrogen synthesis and elevates plasma estrogen levels in premenopausal women. In postmenopausal breast cancer patients, tamoxifen increases plasma levels of estrone sulfate ($p < 0.05$), whilst plasma estradiol is reduced ($p < 0.0005$) as well as free plasma testosterone ($p < 0.05$), due to reduced ovarian excretion of this androgen. The mechanism may be reduced gonadotropin stimulation of the ovary, as plasma follicle stimulating hormone and luteinizing hormone fell by means of 45.5 and 48.1, respectively ($p < 0.0001$ for both)[65]. Finally, it increases the liver production of sex hormone binding globulin, thus further reducing the free levels of both estradiol and testosterone[66,67]. Interestingly, one-third of patients on tamoxifen (used as an estradiol antagonist in hormone adjuvant treatment) had vaginal problems such as dryness, itching and discharge[7]. Other studies seem to confirm the negative effect of tamoxifen on sexual arousal response[49,68].

A second biological cause of arousal difficulties is vaginismus, either primary or, more frequently, secondary to vaginal dryness and dyspareunia with secondary defensive spasm of pubococcygeal muscle[50,69,70]. Secondary vaginismus may account for half the cases of postmenopausal dyspareunia. Thorough examination of the pelvic floor and perineal muscles should become part of routine gynecological examinations, as well as the attention to teach the patient an adequate rehabilitation training to normalize the muscle elasticity and tonus and to improve sexual responsiveness[70]. The attention to hypertonic conditions of the pelvic floor secondary to dyspareunia is mandatory in breast cancer patients, as teaching relaxation of levator ani muscle and encouraging self-massage with a medicated oil may rapidly cure dyspareunia and arousal disorders secondary to hypoestrogenism that may not be treated with estrogens because of breast cancer. Cure of dyspareunia removes the most important cause of avoidance of intercourse in patients with breast cancer.

Vascular problems have recently been claimed as critical factors in female arousal problems[71]. Women who smoke, who have high levels of cholesterol (which increase after the menopause, both spontaneous and iatrogenic), with diabetic vasculopathy and/or with severe atherosclerosis may have a significant reduction in their genital arousal, with reduced lubrication, increased vaginal dryness and dyspareunia. How much these vascular factors, if present, may further affect the arousal response in breast cancer patients, particularly in hypoestrogenic conditions, has not been addressed so far. This would be all the more important, as vascular causes, with persistent good libido, might have a significant clinical improvement with vasoactive drugs such as sildenafil[72] that would not be contraindicated in breast cancer patients. Considering the high prevalence of dyspareunia in patients with breast cancer, the possibility of this non-hormonal help should be urgently evaluated.

Overall, in the prospective longitudinal study of Ganz and co-workers[6], difficulty in becoming sexually aroused was reported by 61% of breast cancer patients, whilst difficulty in becoming lubricated was found in 57% of the patients. Interestingly, this study found that breast cancer survivors attain maximum recovery from the physical and psychological trauma of cancer treatment by 1 year after surgery. A number of aspects of quality of life, rehabilitation problems (mostly arm problems) and sexuality significantly worsen after that time, suggesting that some biological factors might be responsible for this unfavorable trend. According to the retrospective study by Schover and colleagues[4], women with breast cancer who received chemotherapy reported more vaginal dryness ($p < 0.001$) and dyspareunia ($p < 0.001$). Overall, postmenopausal women with breast cancer (both for natural or chemotherapy-induced menopause) were more likely to report vaginal dryness and tightness with sexual activity ($p < 0.001$) and genital pain with sexual activity ($p = 0.004$). The role of the possible worsening over time of the biological basis of the sexual response deserves to be tested in new prospective studies, analyzing biological factors from a stringent physiopathological point of view.

ORGASM

Orgasmic difficulties may be the end-point of a number of biological, as well as motivational-affective and cognitive, factors[39,40,50], particularly in breast cancer survivors. From the biological point of view, the diagnostic flow chart should look for loss of sexual hormones, with secondary libido and arousal problems, vaginal and vulvar trophism (including the clitoris) and pelvic floor status. Hypertonic conditions may cause dyspareunia, vaginismus and postcoital cystitis, thus impairing the formation of the so-called 'orgasmic platform'[39] for the negative association of fear, anxiety and pain. Hypotonic conditions, leading to vaginal hypoanesthesia, also deserve a rehabilitative approach with Kegel exercises[39,40,73].

In patients with breast cancer, difficulty in reaching orgasm is reported in 55% of patients in the prospective longitudinal study of Ganz and colleagues[7], with a significant worsening in sexual functioning over the 3 years of follow-up. In the retrospective study by Schover and associates[4], the ability to reach orgasm through intercourse tended to be significantly reduced in women who received chemotherapy ($p = 0.043$), although their ability to reach orgasm through non-coital caressing did not differ from control women. The inhibitory effect of dyspareunia on vaginal orgasm might explain this difference, together with the effect of different dominant neurochemical pathways (nitric oxide, androgen-dependent, for clitoral response; vasoactive intestinal peptide, estrogen-dependent, for the vaginal response[55]).

SATISFACTION

Satisfaction is a comprehensive and yet elusive word. It includes both physical and emotional satisfaction, which should probably be investigated as separate parameters. Pain and an overall disappointing sexual experience might also be responsible for the significantly reduced satisfaction ($p < 0.001$) reported by survivors of breast cancer in the retrospective study of Schover and colleagues[4] and in the prospective study of Dorval and colleagues[8,9], who also reported a significantly reduced satisfaction ($p < 0.003$) in breast cancer survivors, 8 years after primary treatment, in comparison to age-matched controls.

Objective parameters to quantify and qualify sexual satisfaction, both at physical and emotional levels, are still to be defined. This methodological problem must be overcome before data on the sexual satisfaction of breast cancer survivors can be fully understood.

SEXUAL RELATIONSHIP

Quality of affective bonds, and specifically of sexual relationships, both homo- or heterosexual, is a critical part of human adult satisfaction. Attachment needs have to be fulfilled, emotionally and physically to nourish the deepest roots of personal equilibrium[74–76]. A

good quality of emotional intimacy may explain why 62% of patients with breast cancer found it easier to discuss their sexual problems with their partner during their illness than with doctors and psychologists, to whom only 15% of breast cancer patients dared to express their concerns openly[49]. These figures also indicate how strong the sexual taboo still is among professionals and how long the road is to improve the quality of caring for, besides curing, cancer survivors[77].

Cancer diagnosis is a tremendous strain factor, both on the couple relationship and on the family[3,78]. Young women and couples may be particularly vulnerable from this point of view. Studies indicate that younger women experience more emotional distress than older women (see the excellent review of Northouse[10]). Younger husbands reported more problems carrying out domestic roles ($p < 0.001$) and more vulnerability to the number of life stressors they were experiencing ($p < 0.01$) in comparison to older husbands. When breast cancer is diagnosed, the demands of illness are superimposed on the normal demands of family life and this may have a different impact on the family relationships depending on the phase of the family life-cycle during which the cancer is diagnosed[79].

Focusing on the physical aspect of the problem, breast surgery may affect physical attractiveness and reduce easiness with breast foreplay, although this is difficult to admit openly as it seems rough, insensitive and/or unfeeling. It is more easily verbalized in individual consultations as part of a help request when the husband himself presents with secondary sexual symptoms. An iatrogenic premature menopause, potentially affecting different dimensions of female sexual identity and sexual function, may threaten one of the strongest bases of physical attachment, say sexual pleasure and satisfaction, and again younger husbands may be more vulnerable, mostly if sex was the 'secure basis' of the bonding. Premature menopause may diminish the male sex drive, both physically and emotionally, because of the biological loss of a woman's 'scent', which makes oral sex less pleasurable for some men, and/or because of the changes in skin texture and silkiness and in the overall perceived physical attractiveness[31]. Loss of estrogen may also make penetration more difficult because of vaginal dryness[13–15,53]. It may also precipitate an erectile deficit, when dryness itself challenges the quality of the erection or when the partner perceives vaginal dryness as a sign of refusal or somehow an indication of the 'insensitivity' of his sexual request and approach. It may impair male physical and emotional satisfaction, when the instinctive drive is arrested by physical difficulties and emotional concerns. The real impact of these specific sexual impairments has not been researched to the authors' knowledge, and it should be addressed in future studies, to give more balanced help to the partners of breast cancer survivors. This point is all the more important as husbands and couples express their relief and gratefulness when these issues, potential difficulties and/or misunderstandings are openly and spontaneously raised by the physician during the consultation and when practical suggestions are given to overcome physical and emotional problems.

CONCLUSIONS

Breast cancer may affect female sexual function, female sexual response and the couple relationship in a complex way, involving both psychosocial and biological factors. Unfortunately, whilst the first have been studied in excellent retrospective and prospective studies, the role of biological factors has been only marginally addressed. This is all the more true for women with breast cancer suffering a premature iatrogenic menopause, secondary to chemotherapy, who have to face the many biological consequences of a menopause at a younger age, when many (or all) of the goals linked to the life-cycle have not yet been fulfilled. There may be a subgroup of breast cancer survivors whose quality of life is more seriously affected by the cancer treatment.

Moreover, sex hormones contribute to biological femininity, to the basic biology of sexual function and the biological signals, leading to sexual attraction and affective bonding, that run back and forth in the couple relationship. Their action in human female sexuality is strongly context-dependent[80]. This may explain the objective methodological difficulties in asserting the relative weight of hormonal and overall physical changes on psychosexual variations in survivors of breast cancer.

Physicians, and particularly the oncologists in this specific field, should improve their skill in understanding and listening to sexual concerns and in addressing the basic biological issues that breast cancer raises for the female sexual identity. They should also at least diagnose and recommend clinical help for the most common sexual symptoms in breast cancer survivors: loss of libido, arousal disorders, dyspareunia, anorgasmia and loss of satisfaction. Best results will be obtained in sharing a 'twin competence' with a good psychosexologist or a psychiatrist with an interest in this field, to whom patients with clear psychodynamic or relational problems should be referred for specific help, after having excluded or cured the potential biological roots of the problems. Attention to the anatomy and function of the pelvic floor should become a mandatory part of a thorough clinical gynecological and sexological examination, to give breast cancer survivors the right to a full diagnosis and competent help.

Finally, the fact that overall adjustment and quality of life of survivors of breast cancer are positive in about 70–80% of cases should not mask the more painful truth: that this is true for many areas of quality of life, except for sexual function and satisfaction[4,7–9,49]. Is emotional (unconscious!) adaptive denial of the sexual cost the price of survival? And is this a reducible cost or not? This is why a new committed effort is urgently needed.

References

1. Graziottin A. La sessualità dopo la mastectomia. In Capovilla E, ed. *La Riabilitazione Psicofisica della Donna Mastectomizzata.* Padua: Lega It. Lotta Tumori Ed, 1986:65–74

2. Graziottin A. Il corpo, il piacere, l'identità sessuale. Nuove prospettive terapeutiche in psico-oncologia. In Calzavara F, ed. *Atti Convegno 'Nuove prospettive in Psico-oncologia'*, Padua, June 1987:171–3

3. Baider L, Kaufman B, Peretz T, *et al.* Mutuality of fate: adaptation and psychological distress in cancer patients and their partners. In Baider L, Cooper CL, eds. *Cancer and the Family.* Chichester: John Wiley & Sons, 1996:173–86

4. Schover LR, Yetman RJ, Tuason LJ, *et al.* Partial mastectomy and breast reconstruction. A comparison of their effects on psychosocial adjustment, body image, and sexuality. *Cancer* 1995;75: 54–64

5. Andersen BL, Anderson B, de Prosse C. Controlled prospective longitudinal study of women with cancer. I. Sexual functioning outcomes. *J Consult Clin Psychol* 1989;75:683–91

6. Ganz PA, Shag AC, Lee JJ, *et al.* Breast conservation versus mastectomy: is there a difference in psychological adjustment or quality of life in the year after surgery? *Cancer* 1992;69:1729–38

7. Ganz PA, Coscarelli A, Fred C, *et al.* Breast cancer survivors: psychosocial concerns and quality of life. *Breast Cancer Res Treat* 1996;38:183–99

8. Dorval M, Maunsell E, Deschenes L, *et al.* Long term quality of life after breast cancer: comparison of 8 years survivors with population controls. *J Clin Oncol* 1998;16:487–94

9. Dorval M, Maunsell E, Deschenes L, *et al.* Type of mastectomy and quality of life for long term breast carcinoma survivors. *Cancer* 1998;83: 2130–8

10. Northouse LL. Breast cancer in younger women: effects on interpersonal and family relations. *Monogr Natl Cancer Inst* 1994;16:183–90

11. Collichio FA, Agnello R, Staltzer J. Pregnancy after breast cancer: from psychosocial issues through conception. *Oncology (Huntingt)* 1998; 12:759–65, 769; discussion 770, 773–5

12. Baldaro Verde J, Graziottin A. Il vissuto della donna mastectomizzata. In Peirone L, ed. *L'identità Corporea in Crisi.* Milan: Collana di Psicologia Sociale e Clinica-Giuffré 1992:81–94

13. Graziottin A. Sexuality in the elderly. *European Menopause Society, IV European Congress on Menopause.* Vienna: Editions ESKA, 1998:513–22

14. Graziottin A. The biological basis of female sexuality. *Int Clin Psychopharm* 1998;13(Suppl 6): 15S–22S

15. Graziottin A. *Estrogeni, Funzioni Psichiche e Organi di Senso.* Milan: Recordati Ed, 1999:in press

16. Schover LR. Sexuality and body image in younger women with breast cancer. *J Natl Cancer Inst Monogr* 1994;16:177–82

17. Passik SD, McDonald MV. Psychosocial aspects of upper extremity lymphedema in women treated for breast carcinoma. *Cancer* 1998;83: S2817–S2820

18. Paci E, Cariddi A, Barchielli A, Bianchi S, Cardona G, Distante V. Long term sequelae of breast cancer surgery. *Tumori* 1996;82:321–4

19. Runowicz CD. Lymphedema: patients and provider education – current status and future trends. *Cancer* 1998;83:2874–6

20. Graziottin A. Sexuality and the menopause. In Studd J, ed. *Management of the Menopause–Annual Review.* Carnforth, UK: Parthenon Publishing, 1998:49–58

21. Birge SJ. The role of ovarian hormones in cognition and dementia. *Neurology* 1997;48(Suppl 7): 1S

22. Birge SJ. The role of estrogen in the treatment of Alzheimer's disease [Review]. *Neurology* 1997; 48(Suppl. 7):36S–41S

23. Lamb MA. Effects of cancer on the sexuality and fertility of women. *Semin Oncol Nurs* 1995;11: 120–7

24. Danforth D. How subsequent pregnancy affects outcome in women with a prior cancer. *Oncology* 1991;5:23–30

25. Dow KH, Harris JR, Roy C. Pregnancy after breast conserving surgery and radiation therapy for breast cancer. *Natl Cancer Inst Monogr* 1994;16: 131–7

26. Sankilar, Heinavaara S, Hakulinen T. Survival of breast cancer patients after subsequent term pregnancy: 'health mother effect'. *Am J Obstet Gynecol* 1994;170:818–23

27. Lethaby AE, O'Neill MA, Mason BH, *et al.* Overall survival from breast cancer in women pregnant or lactating at or after diagnosis. *Int J Cancer* 1996;67:75–9

28. Schoultz E, Johansson H, Wilking N, *et al.* Influence of prior and subsequent pregnancy on breast cancer prognosis. *J Clin Oncol* 1995;13: 430–4

29. Kroman N, Jensen MB, Melbyem RJ, *et al.* Should women be advised against pregnancy after breast cancer treatment? *Lancet* 1997;350:319–22

30. Guinee VF, Olsson H, Moller T, *et al.* Effect of pregnancy on prognosis for young women with breast cancer. *Lancet* 1994;343:1587–9

31. Graziottin A. Libido. In Studd J, ed. *Yearbook of the Royal College of Obstetricians and Gynaecologists.*

Carnforth, UK: Parthenon Publishing, 1996: 235–43

32. Graziottin A. Aspetti psicoemotivi del dolore. In Graziottin A, Di Benedetto P, eds. *Piacere e Dolore.* Atti Sesto Meeting della Sezione di Riabilitazione Perineale della Società Italiana di Medicina Fisica e Riabilitazione (Simfer). Trieste: Libreria Goliardica Editrice, May 1997:223–8

33. Andersen BL. Sexual functioning morbidity among cancer survivors. Current status and future research directions. *Cancer* 1985;55: 1835–42

34. Waxler-Morrison N, Hislop TG, Mears B, Kan L. Effects of social relationships on survival for women with breast cancer: a prospective study. *Soc Sci Med* 1991;33:177–83

35. Fallowfield LJ, Hall A. Psychosocial and sexual impact of diagnosis and treatment of breast cancer. *Br Med Bull* 1991;47:388–99

36. Carlsson M, Hamrin E. Psychological and psychosocial aspects of breast cancer and breast cancer treatment. A literature review. *Cancer Nurs* 1994;17:418–28

37. Ganz PA. Sexual functioning after breast cancer: a conceptual framework for future studies. *Ann Oncol* 1997;8:105–7

38. Schagen SB, van Dam FSAM, Muller MJ, Boogerd W, Lindeboom J, Bruning PF. Cognitive deficits after postoperative adjuvant chemotherapy for breast carcinoma. *Cancer* 1999;85: 640–50

39. Masters WH, Johnson VE, Kolodny RC. *Heterosexuality.* Glasgow: Harper Collins, 1994

40. Kaplan HS. *Nuove Terapie Sessuali.* 1974 Milano: Fabbri, 1974

41. Levine SB. An essay on the nature of sexual desire. *J Sex Marital Ther* 1984;10:83–96

42. Levin RJ. Human male sexuality: appetite and arousal, desire and drive. In Legg C, Boott D, eds. *Human Appetite: Neural and Behavioural Basis.* Oxford: Oxford University Press, 1994:127–64

43. Kaplan HS. A neglected issue: the sexual side effects of current treatments for breast cancer *J Sex Marital Ther* 1992;18:3–19

44. Pfaus JG, Everitt BJ. The psychopharmacology of sexual behaviour. In Bloom FE, Kupfer DJ, eds. *Psychopharmacology: the Fourth Generation of Progress.* New York: Raven Press, 1995:743–58

45. Sands R, Studd J. Exogenous androgens in postmenopausal women. *Am J Med* 1995;98:76–9

46. Plouffe L Jr. Ovaries, androgens and the menopause: practical applications. *Semin Reprod Endocrinol* 1998;16:117–20

47. Graziottin A. Soma e Psiche: strategie riabilitative della funzioni pelviche. Il punto di vista del sessuologo. In Di Benedetto, ed. *Riabilitazione Neuro-uro-ginecologica.* Arti Graf Ed Udine, 1990:224–47

48. Heiman JR, Rowland DL, Hatch JP, Gladue BA. Psychophysiological and endocrine responses to sexual arousal in women. *Arch Sex Behav* 1991;20: 171–86

49. Barni S, Mondin R. Sexual dysfunction in treated breast cancer patients. *Ann Oncol* 1997;8:149–53

50. Di Benedetto P, Graziottin A, eds. *Piacere e Dolore.* Atti del Sesto Congresso SIMFER. Trieste: Libreria Goliardica Editrice, 1997

51. Jupp JJ, McCabe M. Sexual desire, general arousability and sexual dysfunction. *Arch Sex Behav* 1989;18:509–16

52. Kaplan HS. *Disorders of Sexual Desire.* New York: Simon and Schuster, 1979

53. Graziottin A. Organic and psychological factors in vulval pain: implications for management. *Sex Marital Ther* 1998;13:329–38

54. Pressman PI. Surgical treatment and lymphedema. *Cancer* 1998;83:2782–7

55. Levin RJ. The mechanisms of human female sexual arousal. *Ann Rev Sex Res* 1992;3:1–48

56. Shear MK. Anxiety disorders in women: gender-related modulation of neurobiology and behaviour. *Semin Reprod Endocrinol* 1997;15:69–76

57. Pfaff DW. *Estrogen and Brain Function.* New York: Springer Verlag, 1980

58. Sherwin BB. Hormones, mood and cognitive functioning in postmenopausal women. *Obstet Gynecol* 1996;87:20S–26S

59. Sherwin BB. Estrogen and cognitive functioning in women. *P.S.E.B.M.* 1998;217:17–22

60. Panay N, Studd JWW. Menopause and the central nervous system. *Eur Menop J* 1996;3: 242–9

61. Sarrel PM, Whitehead MI. Sex and menopause: defining the issue. *Maturitas* 1985;7:217–24

62. Myers LS. Methodological review and meta-analysis of sexuality and menopause research. *Neurosci Biobehav Rev* 1995;19:331–41

63. Semmens JP, Wagner G. Estrogen deprivation and vaginal function in postmenopausal women. *J Am Med Assoc* 1982;248:445–8

64. Thirlaway K, Fallowfield L, Cuzick J. The sexual activity questionnaire: a measure of women's sexual functioning. *Qual Life Res* 1996; 5:81–90

65. Lonning PE, Johannessen DC, Lien EA, *et al.* Influence of tamoxifen on sex hormones, gonadotrophins and sex hormone binding globulin in postmenopausal breast cancer patients. *J Steroid Biochem Mol Biol* 1995;52:491–6

66. Sakai F, Cheix F, Clavel M, *et al.* Increases in steroid binding globulins induced by tamoxifen in patients with breast cancer. *J Endocrinol* 1978; 76:219–26

67. Geisler J, Ekse D, Hosch S, Lonning PE. Influence of treatment with the anti-oestrogen 3-hydroxytamoxifen (droloxifene) on plasma sex hormone levels in postmenopausal patients with breast cancer. *J Endocrinol* 1995;146:359–63

68. Barni S, Ardizzoia A. Tamoxifen induced sexual dysfunction in a breast cancer patient: a case report. *Tumori* 1998;84:417–18

69. Lamont J. Vaginismus. *Am J Obstet Gynecol* 1978;131:632–6

70. Baker PK. Musculoskeletal origins of chronic pelvic pain. Diagnosis and treatment. *Obstet Gynecol Clin North Am* 1993;20:719–42

71. Goldstein I, Berman J. Vasculogenic female sexual dysfunction: vaginal engorgement and clitoral erectile insufficiency syndrome. *Int J Imp Res* 1998;10(Suppl 2)S84–S90

72. Park K, Moreland RB, Goldstein I, Atala A, Traish A. Sidenafil inhibits phosphodiesterase type 5 in human clitoral corpus cavernosum smooth muscle. *Biochem Biophys Res Commun* 1998;249: 612–17

73. Kegel H. Sexual function of PC muscle. *West J Surg Obstet Gynecol* 1952;60:521–4

74. Bowlby J. *A Secure Basis*. London: Routledge, 1988

75. Carli L, ed. *Attaccamento e rapporto di Coppia*. Milan: Cortina, 1995

76. Shaver PR, Hazan C. Adult romantic attachment process: theory and evidence. In Perlman D, Jones W, eds. *Advances in Personal Relationship Outcomes*, vol. IV. London: J. Kinsey, 1995:29–70

77. Graziottin A. Codice paterno e codice materno in oncologia. In Giommi R, Perrotta M, Affront G, eds. *Eros e Thanatos*. Florence: Istituto Nazionale di Sessuologia, 1989:141–7

78. Walker BL. Adjustment of husbands and wives to breast cancer. *Cancer Pract* 1997;5:92–8

79. Haddad P, Pitceathly C, Maguire P. Psychological morbidity in the partners of cancer patients. Baider L, Cooper CL, eds. *Cancer and the Family*. Chichester: John Wiley & Sons, 1996;18:414

80. Alfonso C, Cohen MA, Levin M, *et al.* Sexual dysfunction in cancer patients: a collaborative psychooncology project. *Int J Mental Health* 1997; 26:90–8

21

Management of menopausal symptoms after breast cancer

J. A. Eden

INTRODUCTION

In Australia, breast cancer is responsible for around 4% of the deaths of women aged 55 years or more[1]. Ischemic heart disease accounts for 31% of the deaths, and stroke for 14%. Unlike most female cancers, the incidences of which rise and then plateau with age, the incidence of breast cancer continues to climb with increasing age. Since 1900, breast cancer mortality for women under the age of 40 years has remained remarkably stable, whereas for women over the age of 50, breast cancer mortality has risen dramatically, particularly in the first half of this century. Interestingly this substantial rise in breast cancer mortality in older women occurred in the era before the contraceptive pill and before hormone replacement therapy (HRT)[1]. The precise reasons for this rise remain unclear but it seems likely that the main reasons for the rise in breast cancer mortality relates to women having fewer pregnancies and starting their families at a later age, as well as to some degree of 'disease substitution'. As public health measures, such as immunization and clean water, have dramatically reduced infection, which was previously a common cause of death, so the population is more likely to die from diseases of aging such as heart disease and cancer.

The two major risk factors for breast cancer are female gender and age[1]. Other major risk factors include reproductive history, family history of breast cancer, prior history of proliferative breast disease or atypical hyperplasia, moderate alcohol consumption and the Western lifestyle and diet[2].

There are two main ways in which the menopause can have an adverse effect on women who have had breast cancer. First, for a small group, their menopausal symptoms are so severe that to ignore them would deny these women a reasonable quality of life. Also some breast cancer treatments, such as chemotherapy (by inducing premature menopause) and tamoxifen, can aggravate these symptoms. Second, estrogen deficiency can aggravate bone loss, resulting in osteoporotic fractures and perhaps an increased risk of cardiovascular disease. These two latter problems can now be prevented and treated with a number of effective non-estrogen strategies. Thus for most women and the clinicians, the question of whether or not to use HRT is focused on the relief of menopausal symptoms.

THE IMPACT OF ESTROGENS AND PROGESTOGENS ON THE BREAST

Most research in this area has implicated estrogen as the main hormonal promoter of breast cancer. In contrast, there is relatively little information about the impact of progesterone, progestogens and androgens on normal and malignant breast pathophysiology.

Estrogen

Table 1 summarizes some of the case against estrogen[1].

Henderson and colleagues[3] have suggested that it is a woman's total lifetime exposure to estrogen that determines her breast cancer risk. Early menarche and late menopause will increase a woman's exposure to endogenous estrogen and so increase her risk of developing breast cancer. Key and Pike[4] have modified this theory, postulating that not only does estrogen have an adverse effect on the breast, but having progesterone or progestogen is even worse, so that the two hormones have a synergistic adverse effect on the breast.

The impact of sex hormones on the breast is far more complex than suggested by these two hypotheses. Pregnancy is associated with markedly elevated levels of estrogen and progesterone and so the woman who has her first child early and then goes on to have many subsequent births should have the highest risk of breast cancer. In fact the converse is the case[2]. Most basic scientists now accept that there is a 'window of carcinogenesis' that remains open until the first full-term pregnancy. In other words, the immature breast is more vulnerable to carcinogens and after the first full-term pregnancy the terminal bud of the breast matures, making it less vulnerable to neoplastic changes[2].

Also, many aspects of the effect of estrogens on the breast remain unknown. The breast itself, especially breast fat and stromal tissue, is

Table 1 Estrogen and breast cancer risk

Breast cancer is much more common amongst women than men.

Estrogen stimulates the growth of some breast cancer cell lines in culture.

Estrogen stimulates proliferation of breast ductal tissue.

Breast cancer risk relates to reproductive markers such as age of menarche, first pregnancy and menopause.

Premature menopause reduces the risk of breast cancer development.

Bilateral oophorectomy is an effective palliative therapy for advanced breast cancer.

---

capable of estrogen synthesis locally[5]. The majority of breast cancers are surrounded by fat that has higher aromatase activity than fat taken from different parts of the same breast[6]. Breast tissue to plasma levels of estradiol are around 20 : 1 and this gradient is maintained both before and after the menopause[6,7]. Pasqualini's group has shown that the sulfatase pathway in the breast is between 50 and 500 times more important than the aromatase enzyme system with regard to the production of estrogens[8]. Tibolone, as well as some androgenic progestogens, can inhibit the sulfatase pathway and so may deplete the local breast production of estrogens. With the advent of selective estrogen receptor modulators (SERMs), such as raloxifene, new therapies to reduce the risk of breast cancer are likely to become feasible and increasingly popular as treatment options.

Progesterone and progestogens

The effect of progesterone and progestogens on the breast is also complex. Clinically, breast pain is common in the premenstrual phase and also during the progestogen phase in women taking sequential HRT. In general, cell culture studies suggest that most progestogens hurry cells that are already entering the S phase through the cell cycle and then arrest their growth early in G1 phase[9]. A modest increase in mitotic activity seen over the first 24 hours is followed by a profound and continued inhibition of mitotic activity as long as the progestogens are given. Interested readers are referred to the excellent review by Clarke and Sutherland[9].

HRT IN BREAST CANCER RISK

To date, all the studies examining the impact of HRT on breast cancer risk are flawed. There are no large prospective double-blind randomized trials published, although at least one is underway in the United States (The Women's Health Initiative). Most studies (e.g. refs 10 and 11) suggest that long-term use of HRT is associated with an increased incidence of breast cancer but a decreased mortality. These studies are likely to suffer from surveillance bias. HRT users need to consult a doctor to obtain a prescription and are therefore more likely to have a mammogram and/or a breast examination. It is of interest to note that high-dose progestogens (and estrogens) are an effective treatment for advanced breast cancer. High-dose progestogens have been shown to be as effective as tamoxifen when used to treat advanced breast cancer[12].

ALTERNATIVES TO HRT

For most women the two most debilitating symptoms of menopause are hot flushes, often causing insomnia, and vaginal dryness. Vaginal dryness can be managed with either non-hormonal vaginal moisturizers or poorly absorbed topical estrogens (e.g. Vagifem, Novo-Nordisk). It is probably prudent to avoid topical preparations which can be significantly absorbed from the vagina such as dienestrol and conjugated equine estrogen cream. The vulva can be moisturized with sorbolene. Soap is best avoided as this tends to dry the skin.

Menopausal flushing can be reduced by avoiding overheating, stress reduction and by avoiding aggravators such as alcohol, spicy food, coffee and tea. Clonidine has been used for the management of hot flushes but the results are conflicting[13] and side-effects are common. There is increasing interest in the use of natural therapies or a dietary approach to the management of menopausal symptoms. Two studies[14,15] have had sufficient numbers (i.e. more than 100 subjects) to demonstrate a significant improving effect of a diet high in soy and cereals on menopausal symptoms compared with placebo. Typically the effect was around 50–60% improvement in menopausal symptoms over 12 weeks compared with a placebo effect of 25–35%. A number of herbal remedies have been claimed to have a therapeutic effect on menopausal symptoms, but in most cases clinical trials have failed to confirm these claims. A double-blind, placebo-controlled randomized trial of Dong Quai[16] failed to show any effect over placebo. Similarly, a controlled trial of evening primrose oil failed to show any significant improvement on menopausal flushing when compared with placebo[17]. Komesaroff's group in Melbourne, Australia, recently examined a wild yam cream extract and once again failed to show a significant effect in a properly constructed randomized trial[18].

Moderate doses of progestogens (e.g. medroxyprogesterone acetate 20–100 mg daily or norethisterone 5–10 mg daily) have been shown to be effective in double-blind controlled trials[19,20]. When simple measures fail to control hot flushes, progestogens alone are probably the next least controversial therapy to consider.

Another commonly encountered problem is the patient who is well until she started tamoxifen. This drug commonly aggravates, or even causes, hot flushes and, after discussion with the patient's oncologist, consideration should be given to reducing or even temporarily stopping it altogether.

In a small group of patients all these measures will fail to control menopausal symptoms and so consideration should be given to HRT. Sands and colleagues recently reviewed the literature concerning HRT usage after breast cancer[21]. All the studies to date are small and case-controlled and of short duration. However, these studies do seem to suggest that short-term usage of HRT does not dramatically increase the risk of recurrence or the death rate. Our group has published one of the largest such series to date[22]. The study group comprised 1472 women who had breast cancer. A total of 167 subjects had used estrogen replacement after their treatment for breast cancer. Amongst these estrogen users 152 (91%) had also used a progestogen. Another 106 women had used a progestogen alone as a treatment for menopausal flushes. Cox regression analysis was performed using estrogen as a time-dependent covariate with disease-free interval as the outcome. The uncorrected hazard ratio for the estrogen/progestogen users was 0.67 (95% CI 0.38–1.16) and for the progestin-alone users was 0.85 (95% CI 0.44–1.65). Randomized trials are now underway, but all are having trouble recruiting subjects.

CONCLUSIONS

HRT should not be widely advocated for women who have had breast cancer because of the lack of clinical trial data. However, it would seem that continuous combined HRT used for a short time is safe. Those women with osteoporotic fractures or cardiac risk factors can be managed with a number of suitable non-estrogen treatments or strategies.

References

1. Eden JA. Estrogen replacement therapy and survivors of breast cancer – a risk–benefit assessment. *Drugs Ageing* 1996;8:127–33
2. Gail MH, Benichou J. Assessing the risk of breast cancer in individuals. *Cancer Prev* 1992;1:1–15
3. Henderson BE, Ross R, Berstein L. Oestrogens as a cause of human cancer. *Cancer Res* 1998;48:246–53
4. Key TJ, Pike MC. The role of estrogens and progestogens in the epidemiology and prevention of breast cancer. *Eur J Cancer* 1988;24:29–43
5. Bulbrook RD, Leake RE, George WD. Oestrogens in initiation and promotion of breast cancer. In Beck JS, ed. *Estrogen and the Human Breast.* Edinburgh: Royal Society of Edinburgh, 1989:67–76
6. Blankenstein MA, Szymczak J, Daroszewski J, *et al.* Oestrogens in plasma and fatty tissue from breast cancer patients in woman undergoing surgery for non-oncological reasons. *Gynecol Endocrinol* 1992;6:3–7
7. Miller WR, Mullen P. Factors influencing aromatase activity in the breast. *J Steroid Biochem Mol Biol* 1993;44:597–604
8. Chetite G, Kloosterboer HJ, Pasqualini JR. Effect of tibolone (org OD 14) and its metabolites on estrone sulfatase activity in MCF-7 and T-47D mammary cancer cells. *Anticancer Res* 1997;17:135–40
9. Clarke CL, Sutherland RL. Progestin regulation of cellular proliferation. *Endocrinol Rev* 1990;11:266–301
10. Colditz JA, Hankinson SE, Hunter DJ, *et al.* Use of estrogens and progestins and the risk of breast cancer in post menopausal women. *N Engl J Med* 1995;332:1589–93
11. Persson I, Yuen J, Bergkvist L, *et al.* Combined oestrogen–progestin replacement and breast cancer risk [Letter]. *Lancet* 1992;340:1044
12. Rose C, Mauridsen HT. Endocrine management of advanced breast cancer. *Horm Res* 1989;32 (Suppl):189–97
13. Eden JA. Oestrogen and the breast – 2. The management of the menopausal woman with breast cancer. *Med J Aust* 1992;157:247–50
14. Brzezinski A, Adlercreutz H, Shaoul R, *et al.* Short term effects of phytoestrogen-rich diet on post menopausal women. *Menopause* 1997;4:89–94
15. Albertazzi P, Pansini F, Bonaccorsi G, *et al.* The effects of dietary soy supplementation on hot flushes. *Obstet Gynecol* 1998;1:6–11
16. Hirata JD, Swiersz LM, Zell B, *et al.* Does Dong Quai have estrogenic effects in post menopausal women? A double blind, placebo controlled trial. *Fertil Steril* 1997;68:281–6
17. Chenoy R, Hussain S, Tayob Y, *et al.* Effect of oral gamolenic acid from evening primrose oil on menopausal flushing. *Br Med J* 1994;308:501–3
18. Komesaroff PA, Black CVS, Cable V. Effects of wild yam extract on menopausal symptoms and hormonal and biochemical parameters. In *Abstracts for the Australasian Menopause Congress,* 1998
19. Schiff I, Tulchinsky D, Cramer D, *et al.* Oral medroxyprogesterone in the treatment of post menopausal symptoms. *J Am Med Assoc* 1980;244:1443–5
20. Paterson MEL. A randomised double blind cross over trial into the effect of norethisterone on climacteric symptoms and biochemical profiles. *Br J Obstet Gynaecol* 1992;89:464–72
21. Sands R, Boshoff C, Jones A, *et al.* Current opinion: hormone replacement therapy after a diagnosis of breast cancer. *Menopause* 1995;2:73–80
22. Dew J, Eden J, Beller E, *et al.* A cohort study of hormone replacement therapy given to women previously treated for breast cancer. *Climacteric* 1998;1:137–42

22

Management of the menopause in women with hormone-related cancer

R. H. Sands and J. Studd

INTRODUCTION

Hormone-related cancers, such as breast and endometrial cancer, account for more than 40% of all newly diagnosed malignancies in women in developed countries. The number of women with a history of cancer is increasing and will continue to do so because of an increase in the aging population as well as improved survival due to early screening and more effective treatment. Unfortunately, the gain in longevity with modern cancer management is not necessarily complimented by an improvement in quality of life, since the majority of premenopausal women are rendered menopausal (estrogen deficient) by their primary surgery or adjuvant therapy. In one recent study, 93% of women who had received some form of ovarian suppression said that they experienced menopausal symptoms and in those treated with tamoxifen the figure was 69%[1]. This means that more time in the clinic is spent in managing problems related not only to a spontaneous menopause, but also to a premature menopause in this group of patients. The logical treatment for menopausal symptoms (hormone replacement therapy; HRT) in women with hormone-sensitive cancers has traditionally been contraindicated whether the cancer is diagnosed prior or postmenopausally. The rationale here would be that if estrogen were implicated in the causation it should not be used again because of the fear of generating a new primary cancer. The other concern has been the fear of stimulating dormant metastases and thereby increasing the risk of recurrence. This restrictive practice has been challenged by recent clinical reviews of patients where HRT has been used for controlling debilitating menopausal symptoms. The favorable results from these case-controlled studies have led now to the initiation of larger prospective randomized studies.

The knowledge that HRT is not only regarded as the comprehensive treatment for menopausal symptoms, but, over the long-term, as preventive medicine for osteoporosis, cardiovascular disease and possibly Alzheimer's disease, complicates this clinical dilemma further[2]. It would be certainly ironic if women were to survive their cancer only to succumb prematurely to disease secondary to an early menopause. This means that the impact of HRT, benefits versus risks, needs not only to be assessed for the treatment of the acute symptoms of the menopause, but also for its use over the long term.

BIOLOGY OF CANCER

The understanding of carcinogenesis is continually evolving and especially recently with insights into molecular biology (Figure 1). Cancer is a disease of misbehaved genes, usually genes that control some aspect of cell growth and division. Hundreds of genes play a role in this process, and more than 30 have been identified as

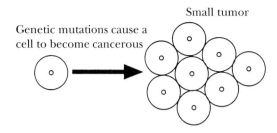

Genetic mutations cause a cell to become cancerous

Small tumor

① A constellation of genetic mutions transform a normal cell into a malignant rapidly dividing cell which grows to ± 1 cm^3. TO grow any larger it needs to recruit its own blood supply.

② Angiogenesis is triggered by a chemical signal from the malignant cell. This may take between a few months or years depending on when this new mutation occurs.

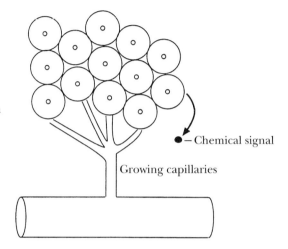

— Chemical signal

Growing capillaries

③ Capillaries now supply the important growth factors and serve as a vehicle for spread. Factors which inhibit angiogenesis or enhance immune surveillance will help contain the tumor.

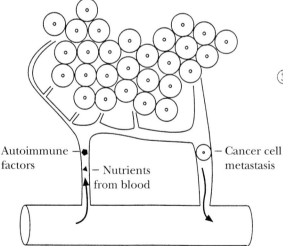

Autoimmune factors

— Nutrients from blood

— Cancer cell metastasis

Figure 1 Mechanisms of carcinogenesis

playing a role in cancer[3]. It is the right combination of mutated genes which gives cells sufficient capability to proliferate inappropriately, organize into masses, acquire neovascularization, invade and, eventually, perhaps kill the patient. Some of the genes, when amplified and overexpressed, give cells with evolving neoplastic power the potential to evade the normal response (death by apoptosis) to the acquisition of unrepairable mutations and to abnormal proliferation[4]. Cancer is caused by errors in these genes, usually multiple errors. Though some of these errors may be inherited, most are acquired during years of living. Sunlight, cigarette smoke, environmental toxins and moreover aging itself help these errors accumulate.

Estrogen and cancer

Physiological levels of estrogen have a mitogenic, and not mutagenic, effect on the endometrium and breast[5]. It is therefore unlikely that estrogens initiate breast and endometrial cancers but they may increase the number of vulnerable cells and increase the growth of existing tumors. It is also important to appreciate that carcinogenesis is a multi-stage process over 3–20 years[6] in which cell sensitivities change during progression from the normal to the metastatic stage. For example, well-differentiated breast cancers retain some of the regulatory influences of the environment in which they are growing, but, later, additional changes lead to complete autonomy[7]. Therefore, when referring to the effect of a given steroid on a cancer it needs to be related to a given stage in tumor progression. Furthermore, it is now well appreciated that the tumor–host relationship is also a dynamic process.

TUMORS WHICH ARISE IN WOMEN TAKING HRT

It is well established that the all-cause, as well as specific, mortality rates are lower in HRT users compared to non-users[8–10] (Table 1). This may be explained by the benefits of hormone therapy on the cardiovascular and skeletal systems. Another explanation could be that the tumors which arise during treatment with HRT are biologically less aggressive and this translates into an improved prognosis. The study by Bergkvist and colleagues[11] compared 261 users or former users of HRT at the time of diagnosis with 6617 women with tumors that arose during the same period who had no history of HRT use. Women who took HRT within 1 year of diagnosis of breast cancer had a greater survival compared to the controls. Survival advantage has also been demonstrated in the studies by the groups of Strickland[12] and Bonnier[13]. Increase in surveillance may be partly responsible for this phenomenon, but there are also data showing that hormone users present with slower-growing tumors of earlier stage than non-users, which suggests that the characteristics of the tumor are also a factor[14] (Table 2).

As previously mentioned, the host response to a tumor is an important consideration. It may be that some metabolites of HRT are anti-angiogenic. The formation of new blood vessels is critical for the growth of tumors and the study by Fotsis and colleagues[15] showed 2-methoxyestradiol to have anti-angiogenic activity, and suggested that it may be of therapeutic potential in cancer and other angiogenic diseases. The apparent survival advantage of HRT users may also be mediated via the immune system. It is well known that certain forms of cancer have an equal outcome in prepubescent boys and girls, but this changes after puberty in favor of girls[16]. Estrogen has been shown to help enhance the immune system by T-cell activation[17] and differentiation *in vitro*[18]. Susceptibility of breast cancer to natural killer cells is also increased *in vitro* by estrogen. Some of these changes are secondary to estrogen's effect on the enhancement of thymic factors.

Table 1 Effect of hormone replacement therapy (E/HRT) on all cancers and mortality; confidence intervals in brackets

Ref.	E/HRT	Relative risk of death: all causes	Relative risk of death: all cancers	Relative risk of death: breast cancer
9	current users	0.35 (0.10–1.22)	0.22	
8		0.56 (0.47–0.66)	0.70 (0.55–0.85)	0.76 (0.45–1.06)
10	past use			0.80 (0.60–1.07)
	current use			1.14 (0.85–1.51)
	< 5 years			0.99 (0.66–1.48)
	> 5 years			1.45 (1.01–2.09)

Table 2 Tumor characteristics and patient survival in women taking hormone replacement therapy

Ref.	Users (n)	Non-users (n)	Survival improved (p)	Comment
11	261	6617	0.02	
12	61	174	0.01	greater prevalence of lower-stage tumors in users
14	35	70	—	less virulent tumors in users
13	68	272	0.05	greater prevalence of lower-stage tumors in users

HRT AND GENITAL TRACT MALIGNANCY

Endometrial cancer

Knowledge about a hormone–tumor relationship has evolved largely from an understanding of the effect of steroid hormones on the uterus, an organ of clearly defined endocrine effects and, furthermore, easily accessible for tissue sampling. It has long been observed that conditions associated with raised endogenous estrogens, such as obesity and polycystic ovarian syndrome, are associated with an increased risk of endometrial cancer. It was noted that prolonged stimulation of the uterus by estrogen without progestational modification produced an endometrial cancer precursor, adenomatous hyperplasia[19]. In 1948, Novak and Rutledge[20] distinguished this type of hyperplasia from cystic glandular hyperplasia, and soon after Hertig and Sommers[21] confirmed this as a cancer precursor and called its extreme form carcinoma *in situ*. The development of steroid receptor science in the 1960s helped to characterize these estrogen-related tumors; namely, slow-growing, well-differentiated, relatively benign cancers sharing the biological properties of their host tissue. The central role of estrogens in the pathogenesis of endometrial cancer was further confirmed with the observation that unopposed exogenous estrogens cause an excess risk of endometrial cancer (relative risk of three to four). Evidence also suggests that long-term use and high doses further increase this risk[22]. It was then appreciated that by combining estrogen with progesterone replacement for at least 10 days per cycle could prevent the hyperplasia associated with estrogen alone.

However, current data do not show unequivocally that this increase in risk with estrogen alone is completely eliminated by added progestogen compared to the risk in non-users. The overall relative risk for endometrial cancer among women who take combined estrogen/progestogen replacement is 0.8 (95% CI 0.6–1.2)[23]. It is not surprising, therefore, that if estrogen replacement therapy is implicated in the etiology of endometrial cancer, it would be contraindicated in women cured with endometrial cancer, pre- or postmenopausal.

Although endometrial cancer is usually a disease of postmenopausal women, at least 25% of cases occur in women aged 40–50 years. About 65% of these women are cured of the disease, but all are either menopausal or rendered menopausal as a result of their treatment. With the combination of good prognosis and debilitating vasomotor symptoms not responding to non-hormonal therapies, patients and their doctors have explored the consequences of estrogen replacement therapy (ERT). Creaseman and colleagues[24] compared 47 women with Stage 1A and 1B endometrial cancer against 174 controls and found a significant survival advantage for ERT users over controls and, furthermore, found that estrogen protected against recurrence. Similar results have been reported by Lee and co-workers[25], who compared 44 women who had been given estrogen following carcinoma of the uterus with 99 women who had not been given the therapy. A more recent retrospective analysis by Chapman and colleagues[26] of 123 women treated for endometrial cancer matched with non-ERT users also demonstrated an improved disease-free interval for the ERT users. It is important to appreciate that all these studies are limited in their design and prone to confounding factors and that randomized studies are required. Pending the outcome from these randomized studies, a case could be made for recommending that patients considered cured (with early-stage and well-differentiated endometrial cancers) receive ERT and those with higher-grade, more advanced stage, disease do not. In general, there is a tendency to offer ERT to women with estrogen-receptive negative Stage 1 disease or estrogen-receptive positive Stage 1 disease associated with limited myometrial invasion and no evidence of metastatic disease in the lymph nodes or peritoneal cytology. Women who have had endometrial cancer treated in the past by surgery followed by radiotherapy or chemotherapy and have had no recurrence over 5 years may be regarded as cured even if their cellular and gland status at the time of the original surgery is unknown. This group of women could also be considered as candidates for ERT or HRT.

Progesterone leads to a decrease in estradiol receptor numbers and available intracellular estradiol[27]. They are therefore potentially capable of reversing the mitogenic activity induced by estrogen in endometrial cells. This evidence has led to the use of high doses of progestogens to inhibit the spread of endometrial cancer, although no good clinical evidence is available to confirm its effectiveness in this regard.

Sex cords/stromal tumors

Sex cord/stromal tumors (granulosa cell, Sertoli–Leydig cell) can occur in women in the reproductive years, but, in general, manifest clinically at an early stage and may be treated with conservative, fertility-preserving surgery. Women with advanced germ-cell malignancies undergo aggressive surgery followed by chemotherapy. The available evidence suggests that most sex cord/stromal tumors lack steroid hormone receptors[28] and there is no information to demonstrate that HRT following the management of sex cord/stromal tumor in a postmenopausal woman is deleterious to her health.

Uterine sarcomas

Sarcomas represent 2–6% of all uterine malignancies and leiomyosarcomas make up 20–30% of uterine sarcomas. There is a clinical tendency to avoid HRT in women with leiomyosarcomas because of the known small association of rapid growth of fibroids in some women who receive HRT. Both estrogen and progestogen receptors have been identified in uterine leiomyosarcoma specimens. There is presently little documented experience of the use of HRT following the successful treatment of uterine sarcomas[29]. Endometrial stromal sarcomas appear to behave differently and may be stimulated to grow with HRT. The use of HRT in this group of women would be contraindicated.

Ovarian cancer

Despite all the advances in diagnostic and therapeutic modalities in the management of ovarian cancer over the last 20 years, the overall 5-year survival rate has remained at about 30%. The relationship between HRT as an etiological agent is unclear. Early epidemiological studies showed an increased risk of ovarian cancer and, coupled with the knowledge that many ovarian tumor cells contain estrogen and progesterone receptors, there has been some reluctance to prescribe HRT in women treated for ovarian cancer. More recent studies have demonstrated a protective effect, with risk ratios of 0.6 to 0.9.

The traditional management of an invasive ovarian cancer has been to perform a bilateral salpingo-oophorectomy and surgical staging. Additional therapy is based upon the findings of the surgical stage. Women with Stage 1A, 1B or 1C invasive epithelial ovarian cancers can undergo conservative surgery and have their fertility preserved. As a general rule, if oophorectomy is not a routine part of the management of a malignancy in a reproductive-age woman, HRT should be safe to administer when that woman undergoes menopause. There has only been one report reviewing outcome in women who have been treated for epithelial ovarian cancers[30]. Here, 78 HRT users were compared to 295 non-users as controls. Women with well-differentiated tumors were statistically more likely to receive HRT than those who were not and younger-age women were more likely to receive HRT than older women. The overall survival for those women who received the HRT was not statistically different than that for the women who did not receive HRT.

Cervical cancer

The interplay of host–tumor defense mechanisms is partly illustrated in cancer of the cervix, since it has been established that women who are human immunodeficiency virus-positive, take immunosuppressive treatment following transplants, or smoke have an increased incidence of cervical dysplasia. Although the endocervical epithelium contains receptors for sex steroids and undergoes the changes under the influence of female sex hormones, there is no evidence to implicate these hormones or HRT in the etiology of cervical cancer. Two recent case–control studies did not demonstrate any significant correlation between HRT use and the presence of human papillomavirus and cervical cancer[31,32]. The prescription of HRT in women with cervical dysplasia or a history of cervical cancer should be no contraindication. A case could be made for their prescription, as a good proportion of these women are young and, subsequent to adjuvant therapy, experience a significant impairment of quality of life. For that group of women in whom loss of libido is still a problem despite adequate estrogen treatment, the addition of testosterone may be beneficial[33].

BREAST CANCER

There is a close link between estrogen and breast cancer (Table 3). Data would indicate that estrogen is related to breast epithelial cell proliferation and an increased exposure to estradiol is associated with increased risk of breast cancer incidence. The evidence from the latest meta-analysis would suggest that the effect of HRT on the risk of breast cancer is very modest, which would explain why there has been a lack of consensus despite more than 50 epidemiological studies and numerous meta-analyses[34]. The risk of HRT for each year of use would be equivalent to the risk associated with delaying the menopause for 1 year, although this has not been proven without doubt. It would appear that estradiol, and not progesterone, is the main hormone responsible, as the magnitude of the increase in proliferation is related to the dose of estrogen with the oral contraceptive pill. Also, in the normal human breast transplanted into nude mice, estradiol and not progesterone is the major steroid mitogen for the breast epithelium. Progestogens, on the other hand, increase proliferation over the short term, but then have a favorable effect by promoting differentiation and increasing apoptosis[35].

The three major risk factors for breast cancer are a family history of the disease, hormonal factors (e.g. an early menarche) and a breast biopsy which shows evidence of proliferation with or without atypia. The data exploring the risks of HRT in women with a family history would suggest that there is no significant difference (one out of five overviews found an increase in risk) between risk in women with and without a family history[36]. This may be because tumors in these women, BRACA 1 and 2, are not sensitive to hormone modulation. Women who have proliferative breast disease and also have a family history are at high risk of subsequent cancer development (up to

Table 3 Data suggesting an association between estrogen and breast cancer

Increased epithelial proliferation
(1) Physiological concentrations of estradiol stimulate the growth of breast cancer cell lines in culture
(2) Estradiol induces proliferation of breast ductal tissue
(3) Estradiol, but not progesterone, stimulates normal human breast tissue implanted into nude mice

Exposure to estradiol
(1) Increased risk with early menarche and late menopause
(2) Premature menopause decreases risk of breast cancer development
(3) Obesity in postmenopausal women increases risk of breast cancer

11-fold). Risk in this group of women who are taking HRT was compared with that in a similar group who were not taking HRT. This analysis showed a four-fold reduction in risk in the treated group[37]. The use of HRT in women with hormonal risk factors for breast cancer because of early menarche or late menopause is unclear. The use of HRT in women with biopsies of the breast which histologically showed early changes of neoplasia is reassuring. In an overview of five studies, Dupont[37] found that benign breast disease does not contraindicate the use of HRT and in fact may slightly reduce the risk.

The use of HRT in women with a history of breast cancer is controversial[38]. Retrospective analyses and a well-designed case–control study showed no detriment to users compared to non-users[39–43] (Table 4). Here, too, users in some studies had a survival advantage. However, these studies, due to the lack of randomization, lead to possible selection biases, but taken together they certainly justify randomized trials in patients surviving breast cancer. The issues that need to be looked at are not only the incidence of recurrence, but also the effects on mammographic detection of breast cancers and new primary cancers.

As the number of women surviving breast cancer increases, many more women will have to endure the problems of premature menopause induced by chemotherapy. It can be anticipated, therefore, that the pressure to give HRT to improve quality of life and reduce disease secondary to estrogen deficiency will grow. Until more information is available, it would

seem acceptable to offer HRT alone or in addition to tamoxifen under the following guidelines:

(1) To women who were treated for cancer premenopausally and who subsequently were stimulated by their own endogenous estrogens, without resumption of their periods, without adverse effect;

(2) Where it will improve quality of life significantly after non-hormonal methods have failed;

(3) In cases where the prognosis is good and the patient has osteoporosis or a strong family history of coronary heart disease;

(4) For patients who have strongly requested or demanded HRT after a full explanation of the available facts about benefits and side-effects.

MELANOMA

There has been concern that sex hormones are involved in the growth and spread of melanoma. This belief has been propagated by anecdotal reports relating rapid growth of melanoma in pregnancy and the alleged increased risk of melanoma in women on the oral contraceptive pill[44]. However, recent reviews have shown no evidence to implicate exogenous estrogen in the pathogenesis of melanoma. Furthermore, contradictory evidence exists[45] in that endogenous estrogen seems to have a beneficial effect, since women have a better prognosis than

Table 4 Hormone replacement therapy in women with history of breast cancer

| Ref. | n | Stage | | | | Follow-up (months) | Outcome* |
		I.S.	1	2	3		
39	50	—				24	100% NED
40	77	6	43	17	5	59	92% REL
		6					8% NED
41	35		12	14	9	43	94% NED
							6% REL
42	25	2	13	7	1	35	88% NED
		2					12% REL
43	90 versus 180 controls	—				> 72	7% REL in users versus 17% in controls

*NED, no evidence of disease; REL, relapse; I.S., *in situ* carcinoma men[46], and where melanoma is diagnosed pre-menopausally, they are more likely to meta-stasize many years later in the postmenopausal period[47]. This is supported by the data showing a significant survival advantage for premeno-pausal women with melanoma compared to postmenopausal women. Therefore, there seems no reason not to offer women with melanoma HRT under medical supervision[48].

TREATMENT OPTIONS (Table 5)

The consequence of the menopause predis-poses to four different clinical problems.

(1) The vasomotor symptoms are probably the most troublesome and intractable. HRT remains the gold standard, with no studies comparing its effectiveness with clonidine or megesterol acetate. Clonidine, a cen-trally active α_2-adrenergic agonist, may cause side-effects.

(2) Urogenital atrophy can be treated with moisturizers and lubricants in the first inst-ance or low-dose vaginal estrogen. These usually contain estriol (a low-potency estro-gen with no, or very little, systemic effect).

(3) Osteoporosis can be treated with either cal-cium and vitamin D or bisphosphonates. General recommendations to maintain skeletal integrity, such as weight-bearing exercise, a diet rich in calcium and limited in caffeine, avoidance of smoking and measures to minimize trauma, also apply.

(4) Cardiovascular disease prevention with HRT can be considered alongside primary therapy for hypertension, etc.

An approach to women with cancer; consider-ations
Recurrence risk
   histopathology
   size of tumor
   nodal involvement
   type of therapy
   time elapsed since diagnosis
Cardiovascular disease
   family history
   lifestyle
   metabolic profile
Osteoporosis
   family history
   lifestyle
   drug history
   bone mineral density
Menopausal symptoms
   vasomotor symptoms
   genitourinary symptoms
   quality of life

CANCER TREATMENT

Up until very recently, the only treatment options were surgery, radiation and chemo-therapy. Through our improvement in under-standing tumor biology and the appreciation of a disease process within an organism, new effective strategies of cancer may evolve. There are advances in chemotherapy, radiation therapy and surgical procedures, but newer approaches include anti-angiogenic, anti-metastatic and anti-oncogenic agents, gene therapy, monoclonal antibodies and vaccines (Table 6). It does seem that knowledge of the patient's and tumor's gene type will come to determine the choice of therapy in the future,

Table 5 Hormonal and non-hormonal options for the treatment of complications of the menopause

		Recurrence	CVD	Bone density	Hot flushes	Vaginitis	Other
ERT	?		decrease	increase	decrease	decrease	
Topical ERT	?		—	—		decrease	
Tsp	?		decrease	increase	decrease	decrease	
Bisphosphonates				increase			
Tamoxifen		decrease breast cancer	decrease	increase	increase	increase	other cancer
Clonidine					decrease		side-effects

CVD, cardiovascular disease; ERT, estrogen replacement therapy; Tsp, tissue-specific drugs

Table 6 Cancer treatments

Treatment	Target	Mechanism	Status
Anti-angiogenic factors	multiple	agents which block neovascularization	human tests just begun
Anti-metastatic factors	multiple	agents which inhibit ability of lytic factors	human studies; early phase
Anti-oncogenic factors	multiple	switch off oncogenes	human studies; early phase
Chemoprevention therapies	breast, head, neck	tamoxifen retinoids	studies nearing completion
Gene therapies	multiple	transfect healthy tumor-suppressor genes	human testing just begun
Chemotherapy	multiple	improved and targeted delivery	new agents introduced
Monoclonal antibodies	multiple	interfere with tumor's ability to absorb growth factors	in use
Radiation therapies	solid tumors, lymphoma	improved precision with 3-D computer images	in use
Surgical procedures	multiple	lumpectomy as opposed to mastectomy, lymphatic mapping	widely available
Vaccines	multiple	using antigens derived from tumors to activate immune system	under investigation

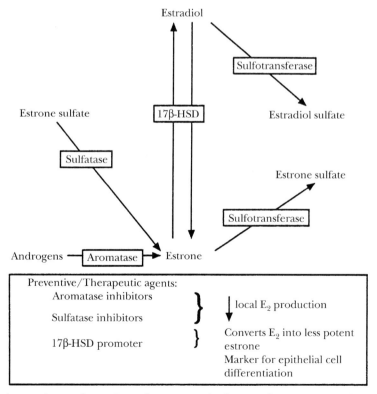

Figure 2 Formation and transformation of estrogens in human breast cancer tissue; 17β-HSD, 17β-hydroxysteroid dehydrogenase; E_2, estradiol

and insight into the tumor–host interaction will influence other avenues such as angiogenesis and metastasis.

Hormonal manipulation of estrogen/progesterone may also prove a useful avenue to prevent cancers (Figure 2). It is well known that the oral contraceptive pill is associated with a decreased risk of ovarian cancer and that a medically induced menopause with gonadotropin releasing hormone antagonists may decrease the incidence of endometrial and breast cancer[49]. Agents which have a tissue-specific action, e.g. tamoxifen, are now being evaluated as hormonal prevention agents[50].

Disclaimer

The views expressed are those of the author.

References

1. Canney PA, Hatton MQF. The prevalence of menopausal symptoms in patients treated for breast cancer. *Clin Oncol* 1994;6:297–9
2. Grady D, Rubin SM, Petitti DB, *et al.* Hormone therapy to prevent disease and prolong life in postmenopausal women. *Ann Intern Med* 1992; 117:1016–37
3. Fearon ER. Human cancer syndromes: clues to the origin and nature of cancer. *Science* 1997;278: 1043–50
4. Sherr CJ. Cancer cell cycles. *Science* 1996;274: 1672–7
5. King RJB. Oestrogen and progestin effects in human breast carcinogenesis. *Breast Cancer Res Treat* 1993;27:3–15
6. Miller AB, Howe GR, Sherman, *et al.* Mortality from breast cancer after irradiation during fluoroscopic examinations in patients being treated for tuberculosis. *N Engl J Med* 1989;321: 1285–9
7. Russo J, Tay LJ, Russo IH. Differentiation of the mammary gland and susceptibility to carcinogensis. *Breast Cancer Res Treat* 1981;2:5–73
8. Hunt K, Vessey M, McPherson K. Mortality in a cohort of long-term users of hormone replacement therapy: an updated analysis. *Br J Obstet Gynaecol* 1990;97:1080–6
9. Criqui MH, Suarez L, Barrett-Connor E, *et al.* Postmenopausal estrogen use and mortality. *Am J Epidemiol* 1988;128:606–14
10. Colditz GA, Hankinson SE, Hunter DJ, *et al.* The use of estrogens and progestins and the risk of breast cancer in postmenopausal women. *N Engl J Med* 1995;332:1589–93
11. Bergkvist L, Adami H-G, Persson I, *et al.* Prognosis after breast cancer diagnosis in women exposed to estrogen–progestogen replacement therapy. *Am J Epidemiol* 1989;130:221–8
12. Strickland DM, Gambrell RD, Butzin CA, *et al.* The relationship between breast cancer survival and prior postmenopausal estrogen use. *Obstet Gynecol* 1992;80:400–4
13. Bonnier P, Romain S, Giacalone PL, *et al.* Clinical and biological prognostic factors in breast cancer diagnosed during postmenopausal hormone replacement therapy. *Obstet Gynecol* 1995; 85:11–17
14. Squiteiri R, Tartter PI, Ahmed S, *et al.* Carcinoma of the breast in postmenopausal hormone users and non-user controls. *J Am Coll Surg* 1994;178: 167–70
15. Fotsis T, Zhang Y, Pepper MS, *et al.* The endogenous oestrogen metabolite 2-methoxyoestradiol inhibits angiogenesis and supresses tumour growth. *Nature (London)* 1994; 368:237–9
16. Adami HO, Bergstrom R, Holmberg L, *et al.* The effect of female sex hormones on cancer survival. A register-based study in patients younger than 20 years at diagnosis. *J Am Med Assoc* 1990;263: 2189–93
17. Ansar Ahmed S, Penhale WJ, Talal N. Sex hormones, immune responses and autoimmune diseases: mechanism of sex hormone action. *Am J Pathol* 1985;121:531–51
18. Kawashima I, Sakabe K, Seiki, *et al.* Hormone and immune response, with special reference to steroid hormone. 3. Sex steroid effect on T-cell differentiation. *Tokai J Exp Clin Med* 1990;15: 213–18
19. Gusberg SB. Precursors of corpus carcinoma-oestrogens and adenomatous hyperplasia. *Am J Obstet Gynecol* 1947;54:905
20. Novak E, Rutledge F. Atypical endometrial simulating adenocarcinoma. *Am J Obstet Gynecol* 1948; 55:46

21. Hertig AT, Sommers SC. Genesis of endometrial carcinoma. *Cancer* 1949;2:946
22. Smith DC, Prentice R, Thompson DJ, *et al.* Association of exogenous oestrogens and endometrial carcinoma. *N Engl J Med* 1975;293:1164–7
23. Grady D, Gebretsadik T, Kerlikowske K, *et al.* Hormone replacement therapy and endometrial cancer risk: a meta-analysis. *J Am Med Assoc* 1995; 85:304–13
24. Creaseman WT, Henderson D, Hinshaw W, *et al.* Oestrogen replacement therapy in the patient treated for endometrial cancer. *Obstet Gynecol* 1986;67:326–30
25. Lee RB, Burke TW, Park RC. Oestrogen replacement therapy following the treatment for stage 1 endometrial carcinoma. *Gynecol Oncol* 1990;36: 89–91
26. Chapman JA, Berman ML, Gillotte DL, *et al.* Oestrogen replacement therapy in surgical stage I and II endometrial cancer survivors. *Am J Obstet Gynecol* 1996;175:1195–200
27. Clarke CL, Sutherland RL. Progestin regulation of cellular proliferation. *Endocr Rev* 1990;11: 266–301
28. Schwartz PE, MacLusky N, Sakamoto H, *et al.* Steroid receptor proteins in non-epithelial malignancies of the ovary. *Gynecol Oncol* 1983; 15:305–15
29. Horowitz K, Rutherford TJ, Schwartz PE. Hormone replacement therapy in women with sarcomas. *J Gynecol Oncol* 1996;1:23–9
30. Eeles RA, Tan S, Wiltshaw E, *et al.* Hormone replacement therapy and survival after surgery for ovarian cancer. *Br Med J* 1991;302:259–62
31. Smith EM, Johnson SR, Figuerres EJ, *et al.* The frequency of human papilloma virus detection in postmenopausal women on hormone replacement therapy. *Gynecol Oncol* 1997;65:441–6
32. Ferency A, Mansour N, Franco E, *et al.* Human papilloma virus infection in postmenopausal women with and without hormone replacement therapy. *Obstet Gynecol* 1997;90:7–11
33. Sands RH, Studd JWW. Exogenous androgens in postmenopausal women. *Am J Med* 1995;98: 76–9
34. Collaborative Group on Hormonal Factors in Breast Cancer. Breast cancer and hormone replacement therapy: collaborative reanalysis of data from 51 epidemiological studies of 52 705 women with breast cancer and 108 411 women without breast cancer. *Lancet* 1997;350: 1047–59
35. Arpels JC, Nachtigall RD. Gonadal hormones and breast cancer risk: the estrogen window hypothesis revisited. *Menopause* 1994;1:49–55
36. Howell A, Baildam A, Bundred N, *et al.* 'Should I take, HRT?'. Hormone replacement therapy in women at increased risk of breast cancer and survivors of the disease. *J Br Menop Soc* 1995;1:9–17
37. Dupont WD. Influence of exogenous oestrogens, proliferative breast disease and other variables on breast cancer risk. *Cancer* 1989;63: 948–57
38. Sands RH, Studd JWW. Hormone replacement therapy for women after breast carcinoma. *Curr Opin Obstet Gynecol* 1996;8:216–20
39. Stoll BA, Parbhoo S. Treatment of menopausal symptoms in breast cancer patients. *Lancet* 1988; 1:1278–9
40. DiSaia PJ. Hormone replacement therapy in patients with breast cancer. *Cancer Suppl* 1993;71: 1490–500
41. Powles TJ, Hickish T, Casey S, *et al.* Hormone replacement therapy after breast cancer. *Lancet* 1993;341:60–1
42. Wile AG, Opfell RW, Margileth DA. Hormone replacement in previously treated breast cancer patients. *Am J Surg* 1993;165:372–5
43. Eden JA, Bush T, Nand S, *et al.* A case-controlled study of combined continuous oestrogen–progestogen replacement therapy amongst women with a personal history of breast cancer. *Menopause* 1995;2:67–72
44. Beral V, Ramcharan S, Faris R. Malignant melanoma and oral contraceptive use among women in California. *Br J Cancer* 1977;36:804–9
45. Franceshi S, Baron AE, La Vecchia C. The influence of female hormones on malignant melanoma. *Tumori* 76;439–49
46. Shaw HM, McGovern VJ, Milton GW, *et al.* Malignant melanoma: influence of site of lesion and age of patient in the female superiority in survival. *Cancer* 1980;46:2731–5
47. Raderman D, Giler S, Rothem A, *et al.* Late metastases (beyond ten years) of cutaneous malignant melanoma. *J Am Acad Dermatol* 15;374–8
48. Jatoi I, Gore ME. Sex, pregnancy, hormones and melanoma. *Br Med J* 1993;307:2–3
49. Spicer DV, Pike MC. Breast cancer prevention through modulation of endogenous hormones. *Breast Cancer Res Ther* 1993;28:179–93
50. Jones AL, Powles TJ. Chemoprevention of breast cancer. *Rev Endocrine-Related Cancer* 1993;43: 33–42

23

Progestogen and breast epithelial proliferation

G. Söderqvist and B. von Schoultz

INTRODUCTION

Breast cancer is the most common malignancy in women and constitutes about 25% of all cancer cases in Western countries. Over the past three decades, there has been a slight increase in the incidence of the disease but not in the mortality. The overall five-year survival is about 60%, with a greater range in survival between early and late stages. Estrogen receptor-positive tumors have a better prognosis and are often responsive to hormonal treatments[1-3]. More than two-thirds of all women with breast cancer are postmenopausal. The risk of developing breast cancer is related to age, heredity for breast cancer and a number of reproductive, endocrinological and hormonal factors, such as early menarche, late menopause, low parity and late age at first pregnancy. It is well established that endogenous and exogenous estrogens are involved in the etiology of breast cancer but there is much less information about the possible role of endogenous progesterone and exogenous progestogens.

All over the world, millions of women are treated with different combinations of estrogen and progestogen for the alleviation of menopausal symptoms and hormonal contraception. The possibility of an increased risk of breast cancer during such treatment is vividly discussed. A slight increase in the relative risk of breast cancer during current use of hormone replacement therapy (HRT) and hormonal contraceptives has been indicated in recent large meta- and reanalyses of epidemiological data[4,5]. In women on estrogen replacement therapy, the risk is increased during long-term treatment to a relative risk level of about 1.3–2. There are few studies on the impact of different treatment regimens and in particular on the effects of various types and doses of progestogen. However, it seems clear that the addition of a progestogen during estrogen replacement has no protective effect. In fact, one recent study suggests that progestogen addition and a continuous combined regimen may further increase breast cancer risk[6]. Elderly women may also have an increased risk level. In women on hormonal contraceptives, progestogen-only treatment was reported to give a similar risk ratio as was found in women who were on estrogen/progestogen combined hormonal contraception. The risk increase during treatment declines to reach baseline levels about 5–10 years after withdrawal of HRT and hormonal contraception. Unfortunately, the potential public health benefits of HRT have not been realized, largely because of the fear of breast cancer. Since breast cancer is such a common disease it is clear that even a small increase in relative risks will affect a considerable number of women. Women throughout the world have highly justified demands for information about exogenous hormonal treatment and an individual risk assessment.

PROLIFERATION OF THE NORMAL BREAST EPITHELIUM

An important basis of risk associated with exogenous hormonal therapy may be the regulation of cell proliferation. High rates of cell proliferation increase the risk of transformation into the neoplastic phenotype in populations of cells both *in vitro* and *in vivo*[7]. This discovery led to the development of the initiation/promotion model of carcinogenesis. According to this model, cells genetically altered by some initiating event are promoted by a second carcinogenic proliferative stimulus. In the breast, this model is supported by clinical evidence for the progression of benign proliferative breast lesions into overt breast carcinoma[8,9]. The breast is a target organ for estrogen and progesterone and a proposed mechanism for an increased cancer risk is the enhancement of the rate of cell division by sex steroids which would increase the risk that genetically damaged cells might divide and lose growth control. However, we still lack much basic understanding about the interaction between these steroids and other hormones, such as corticosteroids, prolactin and insulin, and also about hormone receptors, growth factors and their receptors, and about the interactions between stroma and epithelial cells within the breast[10]. Such information is vitally important for the interpretation of epidemiological data and for the evaluation of the potential risk of different hormonal therapy regimens.

Estrogen is a growth hormone in most target tissues; the endometrium, vagina, bone and certain aspects of liver function. In many biological systems, progestogens counteract the effect of estrogen and cause inhibition of growth. For a long time, the breast was considered to be regulated in the same way as the endometrium, where it has been established that estrogen in high doses increases proliferation and the risk of cancer and that the addition of progestogen counteracts this effect. Both progestogen-only and combined hormonal contraceptives reduce endometrial cancer risk. During the menstrual cycle, almost all glandular endometrial cells proliferate during the follicular phase, and the addition of progestogen effects during the luteal phase inhibits proliferation and causes differentiation into a secretory endometrium[11,12]. Both in breast cancer cell lines and in normal breast cells in culture, i.e. *in vitro*, it has been shown that estrogen enhances breast cell proliferation and that the addition of progestogen reduces this effect. However, *in vitro* and *in vivo* data are conflicting. Most *in vivo* studies of the normal breast have shown the proliferation of breast epithelial cells to be high during the luteal phase of the menstrual cycle[12-16]. Combined oral contraceptives are clearly shown to protect against endometrial carcinoma, but this is obviously not the case for breast cancer. During pregnancy, the combined influence of high estrogen and progesterone levels stimulates lobules and alveoli, reduces fat and connective tissue and increases the number of units apparently including a very high proliferation rate of breast epithelial cells[10,17,18]. This is clear evidence that the hormonal regulation of the normal breast is different from the endometrium. The apparent discrepancy between *in vitro* and *in vivo* findings could tentatively be explained by the fact that the breast epithelial cells are physiologically embedded in fat tissue. Breast extracellular matrix and hyaluronic acid has also been implicated in increasing breast cell proliferation. When in culture, breast cells are deprived of their surrounding milieu of fat and connective tissue and these components may exert considerable hormonal and paracrine influence via hormones as sex steroids and growth factors and their inhibitors. Furthermore, there is a downregulation of estrogen receptors in the breast during the luteal phase of the menstrual cycle while progesterone receptors remain at the same level throughout the cycle[19]. When receptor concentrations are compared between the breast and the endometrium, recent data indicate that the receptor concentrations in the breast are comparatively low. The concentrations of the progesterone receptors (0–50 fmol/mg protein) and estrogen receptors (0–10 fmol/mg protein) can be compared to levels around 600–800 and 200–300 respectively as found in the uterus. The number of positively stained cells was only 5–15% for the estrogen receptors and 15–25% for the progesterone receptors when immunohistochemical studies were performed[19,20]. This is one of the observations indicating that mechanisms other than classic receptor activation are important for the sex steroid effects in the breast.

GROWTH FACTORS AND THEIR INTERACTION WITH SEX STEROIDS

There is a constant interaction between the breast epithelium and stroma through growth factors in so-called paracrine loops[10]. Growth factors are peptide hormones acting locally, synthesized and released by one cell type to modulate neighboring cell function[21,22]. They form a system for control of cell proliferation and act through cell surface receptors which function as tyrosine and serine–threonine kinases[23,24]. Cellular internalization of the receptor is caused by ligand binding at the cell surface[25,26]. Thereafter, a cascade of steps, known as the early and late signal transduction events, is initiated. Many of these steps include phosphorylation and transduce the signal to the nucleus. The mitogen-activated protein (MAP)-kinase cascade is one of the most important of these steps, being a centre for mitogenic phosphorylation signals which phosphorylate the proto-oncogene products c-jun, c-myc and c-ets. These presumably modulate transcriptional activity[27–29]. Epidermal growth factor (EGF), insulin-like growth factors type 1 and 2 (IGF1, IGF2) and transforming growth factor-α (TGF-α), the growth factors, are stimulatory in this system. TGF-β has an inhibitory influence[10]. A cognate receptor for the growth factors TGF-α and β and EGF is the EGF-receptor (EGFR) and the receptor family includes c-erb-B_2, c-erb B_3 and c-erb-B_4. All are closely related tyrosine-kinase-linked receptors[30–32]. The IGFs have their specific receptors: IGFRs. Estrogens and progestogens can mediate transcription of the genes coding for these growth factors. For example, progestogens have been shown to augment both insulin receptor protein mRNA and IGF2 receptor protein, while they downregulated the IGF1 receptor in the breast cell line T47D[33]. Steroid hormones probably act by increasing transcription of target genes involved in the cell cycle progression. Both estrogens and progestogens have been shown to be able to increase cyclin D1 and the rate of cell cycle progression[34–36].

In most women, proliferation of normal breast epithelial cells increases from the follicular to the luteal phase of the menstrual cycle. Data from our group show a significant positive correlation between serum progesterone levels and proliferation[37]. Progestogen-only treatment induces proliferation in women on hormonal contraception[14]. Very recently we have found a significant positive correlation between the levels of levonorgestrel and proliferation in women on combined hormonal contraception (Isaksson and associates; unpublished data). Also, in some breast cancer cell lines in vitro a direct proliferative effect of progestogens has been observed in recent studies when phenol red-free media are used. Thymidine kinase, which is an enzyme of the nucleotide synthesis, is considered to be an important marker of proliferation and is stimulated by progesterone in physiological concentrations[38]. Progestogens also stimulate insulin receptor content and insulin-induced cell growth in human breast cancer cell lines[33]. These data indicate a direct stimulating action of progestogens in the breast.

APOPTOSIS

In order to achieve a more complete understanding of the turnover of normal breast epithelial cells it is necessary not only to assess proliferation but also to study programmed cell death; apoptosis. Apoptosis is important for the deletion of cells in normal tissues and also occurs in specific pathological conditions. Condensation of the cytoplasm, margination of the nuclear chromatin and production of apoptotic bodies are the major morphological characteristics. The apoptoptic bodies are phagocytosed by neighboring cells and degraded within lysosomes[39–42]. The proto-oncogene c-myc induces mitosis in serum-rich media and apoptosis in low-serum or growth factor-deprived media. In vitro it is shown that estradiol can inhibit apoptosis by increasing Bcl-2, an anti-apoptotic proto-oncogene product. Withdrawal of estrogen and progestogen stimulation is an important signal to induce apoptosis or cell cycle arrest. Interestingly, c-myc-induced apoptosis has been shown in vitro to be suppressed by IGF and platelet-derived growth factor (PDGF) irrespective of the position within the cell cycle, growth stage or whether apoptosis was triggered by low growth factors or by DNA damage[39–42].

Three large clinical studies have indicated that the prognosis of breast cancer in menstruating women may be worse if surgery is performed during the follicular phase and improved if surgery is performed during the luteal phase. While these data still need further confirmation they could possibly be related to the effect of estrogen/progestogen withdrawal in inducing apoptosis or cell cycle arrest[43–45]. Both proliferation and apoptosis have been shown to display a minimum in the follicular phase and maximum in the middle and late luteal phases[13]. The estradiol/progesterone ratio is high in the late follicular phase and low in the mid-luteal and late luteal phases. Very recently, we have found a positive correlation between the serum estradiol/progesterone ratio and the expression of IGF1 mRNA in breast tissue in women with normal menstrual cycles (Söderqvist, unpublished data). IGF1 is known to suppress apoptosis in breast cancer cells and in transgenic mice during involution of lactation[46,47].

PROLIFERATIVE EFFECTS OF ESTROGEN/PROGESTOGEN TREATMENT

In clinical practice, a variety of estrogen and progestogen combinations are used in many different therapeutic regimens by numerous women receiving hormonal replacement. It is established that the three major therapeutic principles, i.e. estrogen only, estrogen in cyclic combination with progestogen and estrogen in continuous combination with progestogen, have quite different effects in the endometrium and other target organs[11,48]. So far, there is very little basal knowledge whether and to what extent different treatment regimens may also

have different impacts on the normal mammary epithelium. Recent data from an experimental in vivo model for HRT render further support for a proliferative action of progestogens. Continuous combined treatment with conjugated equine estrogens plus medroxyprogesterone acetate in surgically postmenopausal cynomolgus macaques, induced a proliferative response in mammary epithelium. The effect of combined treatment was much more pronounced than for treatment with estrogen only. As much as 86% of monkeys treated with continuous combined therapy with conjugated equine estrogens plus medroxyprogesterone acetate showed mammary hyperplasia compared with 41% in the conjugated equine estrogen-only group[49]. Furthermore, hormonal contraception with combined or progestogen-only treatment has been reported to increase proliferation in the mammary epithelium[50]. Proliferation was also found to correlate to circulating levels of levonorgestrel in combined oral contraceptives (Isaksson and co-workers, submitted for publication). In contrast, pretreatment with progesterone was found to suppress breast epithelial cell proliferation in women undergoing breast surgery[51]. However, in comparison with earlier findings of intratissue sex steroid concentrations, the concentrations of estradiol and progesterone in that study markedly exceeded the physiological range[52]. Both estrogen and progestogen in high doses have been used in breast cancer treatment and have been found to have a growth suppressing effect[53]. The apparent increase in breast epithelial proliferation during combined estrogen/progestogen treatment found in many studies seems to occur despite a down-regulation of sex steroid receptors[19,20,54]. Hence, other mechanisms for proliferation, different from ligand binding and sex steroid receptor activation, are likely to be present. High serum concentrations of IGF1 have recently been reported as an independent risk factor for breast cancer[55]. In women on hormonal contraception we have found a correlation between IGF1 mRNA tissue levels and proliferation in breast alveoli[20].

An increasing number of reports have indicated that HRT is associated with an increased mammographic density in a significant proportion of postmenopausal women[56-58]. The mammographic picture of the breast reflects the relative amount of fat, connective and epithelial tissue. Proliferation and high amounts of connective and epithelial cells yields an increased density on the mammogram. Within the breast, epithelial and stromal cell interaction is critical for both normal and abnormal growth. Data suggest that an increase in mammographic density may be an independent risk factor for breast cancer in women and also in woman on HRT[58]. Data are also emerging of a more pronounced effect of combined estrogen/ progestogen therapy, and in particular of the continuous combined regimen[57-59]. In one small study there was a non-significant tendency for a progestogen dose-dependent increase in mammographic density[58]. However, there is a current lack of basic understanding of the histological correlates to mammographic density. It may tentatively be caused by the epithelial proliferation but also by edema, vasodilatation and fibrosis. The significance of different mammographic density patterns on cancer risks in individual women has been unclear. Mammographic screening sensitivity may be reduced by increased breast density which may hamper the diagnosis of clinically occult cancers.

It seems reasonable to assume a relationship between the given doses of sex steroid hormones and proliferation of the mammary epithelium. In the endometrium, differences between treatments associated with the progestogen component, its type, dose and duration of administration, have been clearly established. Doses required for endometrial protection during cyclic/sequential progestogen therapy have been defined. It is also known that lower doses are sufficient in the continuous combined regimen. The corresponding information about equipotency and specific differences between types of progestogens in respect to their effects on the mammary epithelium is currently lacking. However, there is experimental evidence for diverging effects of different progestogens. The hormone metabolism and biosynthesis of estrogens in peripheral target tissues can strongly influence intratissue hormone concentrations which thus may differ considerably from levels in plasma[60]. Progestogens have been found to have different effects in three important enzymatic systems relevant in this context, i.e. 17β-hydroxysteroid dehydrogenase (17-HSD), sulfatase/sulfotransferase and aromatase activity. It seems that 19-nor progestogens suppress the conversion of estrone sulfate to estrone in women on oral contraceptives while a positive correlation has been found between serum progesterone levels and the activity of this enzyme[61]. Prost-Avalet and colleagues found medroxyprogesterone acetate, quingestanol acetate, lynestrenol and progesterone increased sulfatase activity, whereas demegestone and chlormadinone acetate reduced the activity of the enzyme[62]. Expression of 17-HSD type 1 was more pronounced in women on hormonal contraception than in women with regular menstrual cycles[63]. Enhanced 17-HSD type 1 protein expression might augment the conversion of estrone to estradiol in normal mammary tissue during hormonal contraception while endogenous progesterone seems to have the opposite effect. However, the oxidating enzyme 17-HSD type 2 was not assessed, which is crucial for the achievement of total knowledge of estrogen turnover in breast tissues. There are also diverging effects of different progestogens on the aromatase enzyme responsible for the conversion of testosterone to estradiol and androstenedione to estrone. The 19-nor steroids and androgens have been shown to suppress the enzyme while 17α-hydroxysteroids and progesterone will not have this effect. Testosterone has been found to suppress proliferation in breast epithelial cells. In clinical practice, testosterone and androgenic compounds, such as danazol, are often used to relieve mastalgia and may possibly reduce proliferation[64,65].

SUMMARY

The hormonal regulation of the breast is clearly distinct from that of other target organs. In the endometrium, proliferation is stimulated by estrogen whereas progesterone inhibits mitotic activity and elicits differentiation. The content of estrogen receptors within the breast declines during the luteal phase of the menstrual cycle but progestogen receptors remain at a constant level. In most women breast epithelial proliferation is enhanced during the second half of the cycle. Virtually all superficial endometrial cells proliferate already at low estrogen concentrations but in the breast only some 10–15% of cells display cyclic variation and the majority of cells are 'resting'. The effects of progesterone and different progestogens are complex and probably mediated both via specific hormone receptors and through interaction with local growth factors and enzymes. *In vivo*, endogenous progesterone as well as exogenous progestogens have been shown to stimulate breast epithelial proliferation. In the endometrium the three major principles for HRT, estrogen alone or in cyclic or continuous combination with progestogen, have clearly different effects on proliferation. In contrast, recent data suggest that combined estrogen/progestogen treatment will enhance breast epithelial proliferation more than treatment with estrogen alone. Increased mammographic density is more frequent among women on estrogen/progestogen-combined HRT. Different progestogens display diverging effects in various enzymatic systems important for local hormone biosynthesis. The clinical importance of these data remains to be elucidated.

ACKNOWLEDGEMENTS

This work was supported by grants from the Swedish Medical Research Council (project no. 5982), the Karolinska Institute Research Funds and the Swedish Cancer Society.

References

1. Howell A, Barnes DM, Harland RNL, *et al.* Steroid-hormone receptors and survival after first relapse in breast cancer. *Lancet* 1984;i:588–91
2. Parl FF, Schmidt BP, Dupont WD, *et al.* Prognostic significance of estrogen receptor status in breast cancer in relation to tumor stage, axillary node metastasis, and histopathologic grading. *Cancer* 1984;54:2237–42
3. Alanko A, Heinonen E, Sceinin T, *et al.* Significance of estrogen and progesterone receptors, disease free interval, and site of first metastasis on survival of breast cancer patients. *Cancer* 1985;56:1696–1700
4. Collaborative Group on Hormonal Factors in Breast Cancer. Breast cancer and hormone replacement therapy: collaborative reanalysis of data from 51 epidemiological studies of 52705 women with breast cancer and 108411 women without breast cancer. *Lancet* 1997;350:1047–59
5. Collaborative Group on Hormonal Factors in Breast Cancer. Breast cancer and hormonal contraceptives: collaborative reanalysis of individual data on 53297 women with breast cancer and 100239 women without breast cancer from 54 epidemiological studies. *Lancet* 1996;347:1713–27
6. Magnusson C, Baron JA, Correia N, *et al.* Breast cancer risk following long-term oestrogen – and oestrogen-progestin-replacement therapy. *Int J Cancer* 1999;81:339–44
7. Butterworth BE, Goldsworthy TL. The role of cell proliferation in multistage carcinogenesis. *Proc Soc Exp Biol Med* 1991;198:683–7
8. London SJ, Connolly JL, Schnitt SJ, *et al.* A prospective study of benign breast disease and breast cancer. *J Am Med Assoc* 1992;267:941–4
9. Page DL, DuPont WD, Rogers LW. Ductal involvement by cells of atypical lobular hyperplasia in the breast: A long-term follow up study of cancer risk. *Hum Pathol* 1988;19:201–7
10. Dickson RB, Lippman ME. Growth factors in breast cancer. *Endocr Rev* 1995;16:559–89
11. Key TJ, Pike MC. The dose–effect relationship between 'unopposed' oestrogens and endometrial mitotic rate: its central role in explaining and predicting endometrial cancer risk. *Br J Cancer* 1988;57:205–121
12. Vogel PM, Georgiade NG, Fetter BF, *et al.* The correlation of histologic changes in the human breast with the menstrual cycle. *Am J Pathol* 1981;104:23–34

13. Anderson TJ. Ferguson DJ. Raab GM. Cell turn-over in the 'resting' human breast: influence of parity, contraceptive pill, age and laterality. *Br J Cancer* 1982;46:376–82

14. Anderson TJ, Battersby S, King RJB, *et al*. Oral contraceptive use influences breast cell proliferation. *Hum Pathol* 1989;20:1139–41

15. Longacre TA, Bartow SA. A correlative morphologic study of human breast and endometrium in the menstrual cycle. *Am J Surg Pathol* 1986;10: 382–93

16. Potten CS, Watson RJ, Williams GT, *et al*. The effect of age and menstrual cycle upon proliferative activity of the normal human breast. *Br J Cancer* 1988;58:163–70

17. Pike MC. Hormonal contraception with LHRH agonists and the prevention of breast and ovarian cancer. In: Mann RD, ed. *Oral Contraceptives and Breast Cancer*. Carnforth: Parthenon Publishing Group; 1990;323–48

18. Russo J, Gusterson BA, Rogers AE, *et al*. Comparative study of human and rat mammary tumorigenesis. *Lab Invest* 1990;62:244–78

19. Söderqvist G, von Schoultz B, Skoog L, *et al*. Estrogen and progesterone receptor content in breast epithelial cells from healthy women during the menstrual cycle. *Am J Obstet Gynecol* 1993;168:874–9

20. Isaksson E, Sahlin L, Söderqvist G, *et al*. Expression of sex steroid receptors and IGF-1 mRNA in breast tissue – effects of hormonal treatment. *J Steroid Biochem Molec Biol*. 1999; in press

21. Ullrich A, Schlessinger J. Signal transduction by receptors with tyrosine kinase activity. *Cell* 1990; 61:203–12

22. Heldin CH, Westermark B. Growth factors. Mechanism of action and relation to oncogenes. *Cell* 1984;37:9–20

23. Massague J. Epidermal growth factor-like transforming growth factor. *J Biol Chem* 1983;258: 13606–13

24. Derynck R. Transforming growth factor α. *Cell* 1988;54:593–5

25. Margolis B. Proteins with SH2 domains: transducers in the tyrosine kinase signaling pathway. *Cell Growth Diff* 1992;3:73–80

26. Feng G-S, Hui C-C, Pawson T. SH2-containing phosphotyrosine phosphatase as a target of protein tyrosine kinases. *Science* 1993;259:1607–10

27. Ransone LJ, Verma I. Nuclear proto-oncogenes FOS and JUN. *Ann Rev Cell Biol* 1990;6:539–57

28. Kato GJ, Dang CV. Function of the c-myc oncoprotein. *FASEB J* 1992;6:3065–72

29. Franklin CC, Unlap T, Adler V, Kraft AS. Multiple signal tranduction pathways mediate c-Jun protein phosphorylation. *Cell Growth Diff* 1993;4: 377–85

30. Todaro GJ, Rose TM, Spooner CE, *et al*. Cellular and viral ligands that interact with the EGF receptor. *Sem Cancer Biol* 1990;1:257–64

31. Cadena DL, Gill GN. Receptor tyrosine kinases. *FASEB J* 1992;6:2332–7

32. Plowman GD, Culouscu J-M, Whitney GS, *et al*. Ligand-specific activation of HER 4 /p180 erb B4, a fourth member of the epidermal growth factor receptor family. *Proc Natl Acad Sci* 1993; 90:1746–50

33. Goldfine ID, Papa V, Vigneri R, *et al*. Progestin regulation of insulin and insulin-like growth factor 1 receptors in cultured human breast cancer cells. *Breast Cancer Res Tr* 1992;22:69–79

34. Sutherland RL, Hamilton JA, Sweeney KJE, *et al*. Expression and regulation of cyclin genes in breast cancer. *Acta Oncol* 1995;34:651–6

35. Clarke CL, Sutherland RL. Progestin regulation of cellular proliferation. *Endocr Rev* 1990;11: 266–301

36. Truss M, Beato M. Steroid hormone receptors: interaction with deoxyribonucleic acid and transcription factors. *Endocr Rev* 1993;14:459–79

37. Söderqvist G, Isaksson E, von Schoultz B, *et al*. Proliferation of breast epithelial cells in healthy women during the menstrual cycle. *Am J Obstet Gynecol* 1997;176:123–8

38. Moore MR, Hathaway LD, Bircher JA. Progestin stimulation of thymidine kinase in the human breast cancer cell line T47D. *Biochim Biophys Acta* 1991;1096:170–4

39. Wang TTY, Phang JM. Effects of estrogen on apoptotic pathways in human breast cancer cell line MCF-7. *Cancer Res* 1995;55:2487–9

40. Kyprianu N, English H, Davidson NE, *et al*. Programmed cell death during regression of the MCF-7 human breast cancer following estrogen ablation. *Cancer Res* 1995;51:162–6

41. Kerr JFR, Winterford CM, Harmon BV. Apoptosis. Its significance in cancer and cancer therapy. *Cancer* 1994;73:2013–26

42. Evan G. The integrated control of cell proliferation and programmed cell death (apoptosis) by oncogenes. *International Symposium on the Molecular Biology of Breast Cancer*. Oslo: Institute for Cancer Research. March 1–5, 1995(abstract)

43. Senie RT, Rosen PP, Rhodes P, *et al*. Timing of breast cancer excision during the menstrual cycle influences duration of disease free survival. *Ann Intern Med* 1991;115:337–42

44. Veronesi U, Luini A, Mariani L, *et al*. Effect of menstrual phase on surgical treatment of breast cancer. *Lancet* 1994;343:1544–6

45. Badve RA, Gregory WM, Chaudary MA, *et al*. Timing of surgery during menstrual cycle and survival of premenopausal women with operable breast cancer. *Lancet* 1991;337:1261–4

46. Streuli CH, Dive C, Hickman JA, *et al.* Control of apoptosis in breast epithelium. *Endocrine Rel Cancer* 1997;4:45–53

47. Dunn SE, Hardman RA, Kari FW, *et al.* Insulin-like growth factor 1 (IGF-1) alters drug sensitivity of HBL 100 human breast cancer cells by inhibition of apoptosis induced by diverse anticancer drugs. *Cancer Res* 1997;57:2687–93

48. Vihko R, Isomaa V. Endocrine aspects of endometrial cancer. In: Voigt KD, Knabbe C, eds. *Endocrine Dependent Tumors.* New York: Raven Press, 1989:197–214

49. Cline JM, Söderqvist G, von Schoultz E, *et al.* Effects of hormone replacement therapy on the mammary gland of surgically postmenopausal macaques. *Am J Obstet Gynecol* 1996;174:93–100

50. Williams G, Anderson E, Howell A, *et al.* Oral contraceptive (OPC) use increases proliferation and decreases oestrogen receptor content of epithelial cells in the normal human breast. *Int J Cancer* 1991;48:206–210

51. Chang KJ, Lee TTY, Linares-Cruz G, *et al.* Influences of percutaneous administration of estradiol and progesterone on human breast epithelial cell cycle in vivo. *Fertil Steril* 1995;63:785–91

52. De Boever J, Verheugen C, Van Maele G, *et al.* Steroid concentrations in serum, glandular breast tissue, and breast cyst fluid of control and progesterone treated patients. In: Angeli A, ed. *Endocrinology of Cystic Breast Disease.* New York: Raven Press, 1983:93–9

53. Wren BF, Eden JA. Do progestogens reduce the risk of breast cancer? A review of the evidence. *Menopause.* 1996;3:4–12

54. Battersby S, Robertson BJ, Anderson TJ, *et al.* Influence of menstrual cycle, parity and oral contraceptive use on steroid hormone receptors in normal breast. *Br J Cancer* 1992;65:601–7

55. Hankinson SE, Willett WC, Colditz GA, *et al.* Circulating concentrations of insulin-like growth factor-I and risk of breast cancer. *Lancet* 1998; 351:1393–6

56. Kaufman Z, Garstin WIH, Hayes R, *et al.* The mammographic parenchymal patterns of women on hormonal replacement therapy. *Clin Radiol* 1991;43:389–92

57. Persson I, Thurfjell E, Holmberg L. Effect of estrogen and estrogen-progestin replacement regimens on mammographic breast parenchymal density. *J Clin Oncol* 1997;15:3201–7

58. Boyd NF, Lockwood GA, Byng JW, *et al.* Mammographic densities and breast cancer risk. *Cancer Epidemiol Biomarkers Prev* 1999;7: 1133–44

59. Greendale GA, Reboussin BA, Sie A, *et al.* Effects of estrogen and estrogen-progestin on mammographic parenchymal density. *Ann Intern Med* 1999;130:262–9

60. Poutanen M, Isomaa V, Peltoketo H, *et al.* Regulation of oestrogen action: role of 17 beta-hydroxysteroid dehydrogenases. *Ann Med* 1995; 27:675–82

61. Söderqvist G, Ohlsson H, Wilking N, *et al.* Metabolism of estrone sulphate by normal breast tissue: influence of menopausal status and oral contraceptives. *J Steroid Biochem Mol Biol* 1994;48: 221–4

62. Prost-Avalet O, Oursin J, Adessi GL. In vitro effect of synthetic progestrogens on estrone sulphatase activity in human breast carcinoma. *J Steroid Biochem Mol Biol* 1991;39:967–73

63. Söderqvist G, Poutanen M, Wickman M, *et al.* 17 beta-hydroxysteroid dehydrogenase type 1 in normal breast tissue during the menstrual cycle and hormonal contraception. *J Clin Endocrinol Metab* 1998;83:1190–3

64. Birrel SN, Bentel JM, Hicke TE, *et al.* Androgenes induce divergent proliferative responses in human breast cancer cell lines. *J Steroid Biochem Mol Biol* 1995;52:459–67

65. Pye JK, Mansel RE, Huges LE. Clinical experience of drug treatments for mastalgia. *Lancet* 1985;2:373–7

24

Do progestogens adequately protect the endometrium?

F. Wadsworth and J. Studd

INTRODUCTION

The history of hormone replacement therapy (HRT) is one of overstatement of benefits and risks. Estrogens are now offered for treatment and prevention of many conditions such as cardiovascular disease, osteoporosis and Alzheimer's disease.

The issues of hormone replacement are being increasingly widely addressed, through dedicated hospital-based menopause clinics and rising awareness in primary care, but the uptake of HRT in the United Kingdom remains disappointing. With less than 15% of women aged 40–65 years taking HRT, little impact on public health is likely[1,2]; one study showed that 20–30% of patients never even collect their prescriptions[3]. One of the main reasons women reject advice to take HRT is concern over side-effects and fear of uterine and breast cancers. Other important reasons for stopping treatment include an objection to having withdrawal bleeding and the use of an inadequate dose of estrogen, which fails to alleviate symptoms[4–6]. Ryan showed, in a group at high risk from osteoporosis, that nearly 40% of women advised to take HRT were not taking treatment at 8 months[7].

The first endogenous substance implicated in oncogenesis was estrogen[8] and there is continuing concern that exogenous estrogens are linked with endometrial hyperplasia and carcinoma of the endometrium and breast, even when opposed by progestogens. The ability of exogenous estrogen to stimulate the endometrium and progestogens to mimic the physiological endometrial opposition of progesterone has been demonstrated by Whitehead and colleagues[9].

HYPERPLASIA

There are few data available about the incidence of endometrial hyperplasia in the postmenopausal population not taking estrogens, but reports suggest it may be present in up to 5% of women[10]. Unopposed estrogen therapy has been shown to increase the incidence of hyperplasia to between 15% and 50%, dependent on dose and duration of use[11–13]. All endometrial hyperplasia is proliferative and atypical hyperplasia is a strong risk factor for subsequent endometrial carcinoma[14]. The association between carcinoma and simple hyperplasia is much weaker[15]. The exact nature of the relationship between endometrial hyperplasia and carcinoma is unclear[16].

A major issue in the diagnosis and management of hyperplasia is the difficulty in diagnosing endometrial pathology. There are arbitrary lines between hyperplasias of varying severity and between severe atypical hyperplasia and adenocarcinoma. Whitehead and Pickar reported significant differences between two expert pathologists' reports on the same specimens from patients receiving estrogen and progestogens[17].

ENDOMETRIAL CANCER

The 'unopposed estrogen hypothesis' states that the risk of endometrial cancer is increased by exposure to endogenous or exogenous estrogens not simultaneously opposed by a progestogen. The increased risk is due to mitotic promotion of the endometrium by estrogen[18]. As a result of repeated mitotic activity, the accumulation of genetic errors may ultimately produce a neoplastic phenotype. HRT represents one of the largest areas of exogenous steroid hormone use in an essentially healthy population. Endometrial cell mitotic rate during high-dose unopposed estrogen therapy equals that produced in the follicular phase of the menstrual cycle. Investigation of the mitotic rate during the menstrual phase suggests that the mitotic rate does increase with serum levels, equivalent to early follicular levels, but then reaches a plateau.

Analysis of the age–incidence curve for endometrial cancer suggests there will be lifelong effects of even a short duration of exogenous hormones. Five years of exogenous unopposed estrogen replacement will increase subsequent lifetime risk by 90%. Even 5 years of 'adequately' opposed estrogen and progesterone therapy is likely to increase subsequent lifetime risk by at least 50%[18]. Experimental evidence suggests overproduction of estrogen receptor mRNA in endometrial cancers and also the presence, in some tumors, of mutated DNA-binding domains for this RNA. Also, estrogen may lead to a disorder in the production of estrogen-inducible proteins in these tumors, promoting dedifferentiation, division and development of cancer cells[19]. *In vitro* studies have suggested that estrogen may enhance the migration potential of endometrial carcinoma through the basement membrane[20].

ENDOMETRIAL CARCINOMA

An association between adenocarcinoma and hyperplasia has been evident since 1936 when Novak and Yui published a review of over 12 000 cases, with 800 cases of endometrial hyperplasia and 100 cases of endometrial adenocarcinoma. They found numerous cases of postmenopausal hyperplasia and nearly 40% of cancerous specimens had co-existing hyperplasia. It was concluded that a relationship between the two must exist[21]. In the study by Kurmans and colleagues of endometrial hyperplasia they followed women diagnosed with endometrial hyperplasia who had not undergone hysterectomy for at least 1 year. Carcinoma occurred in 1% of hyperplasia without atypia and in 29% of women with complex atypical hyperplasia[22]. The role of exogenous estrogen in the genesis of endometrial cancer was highlighted when cancer registers in the USA showed a sharp increase in the incidence of endometrial adenocarcinoma[23]. In 1975 two retrospective case–control studies were published claiming a four- to sevenfold increase in the relative risk of endometrial cancer among estrogen users[24,25]. Many other reports followed, suggesting large relative risks associated with estrogen use. All were retrospective and many were open to methodological criticism. Jick and co-workers made a fanciful prediction of one case of endometrial cancer per 50 patients per year[26].

The wide variation in the relative risks generated by these studies was attributed to methodological differences, such as histopathological criteria for cancer, selection of cases and controls, definition of exposure and dose and duration of treatment[27]. A meta-analysis of hormone replacement and endometrial cancer risk was conducted by Grady and co-workers[28] covering 30 trials between 1970 and April 1994 (Table 1). This confirmed a relationship between estrogen and endometrial cancer that was dose and duration dependent. The overall ever-user relative risk (RR) for unopposed estrogen was 2.3 (95% CI 2.1–2.5). Even with less than a year's use the RR was 1.4 (95% CI 1.0–1.8). With unopposed short-term use of 1–5 years the RR was 2.8 (95% CI 2.3–3.5). Those on unopposed estrogen for more than 10 years had a RR of 9.5 (95% CI 7.4–12.3). Interrupted unopposed therapy was used early in the history of HRT, but the safety of this was not demonstrated by the

Table 1 Relative risk from meta-analysis: postmenopausal estrogen therapy and endometrial cancer (Adapted from reference 28)

	Relative risk	95% Confidence interval	Number of studies
Ever-users of estrogens	2.3**	2.1–2.5	29
Conjugated estrogens 0.625 mg	3.4	2.0–5.6	4
Conjugated estrogens ≥ 1.25 mg	5.8	4.5–7.5	9
Duration of use 1–5 years	2.8	2.3–3.5	12
Duration of use > 10 years	9.5*	7.4–12.3	10
Time since last use ≤ 1 year	4.1*	2.9–5.7	3
Time since last use ≥ 5 years	2.3	1.8–3.1	5
Death from endometrial cancer	2.7	0.9–8.0	3

**p homogeneity < 0.0001; *p homogeneity < 0.01

meta-analysis[28]. There was also some evidence that conjugated estrogens presented a greater risk than synthetic estrogens. The cancer risk acquired on estrogen was seen to persist after discontinuation of treatment; 5 years after treatment the RR was still 2.3. This makes past history of HRT use extremely important in the assessment of patients. It was suggested that the increase in incidence had been mirrored by a fall in mortality from endometrial cancer[29], but the meta-analysis suggested that the risk of death from endometrial cancer in estrogen users may be higher than in the rest of the population (RR 2.7, 95% CI 0.9–8.0)[28].

THE ROLE OF PROGESTOGENS

There is good evidence of the protective role of progestogen-containing contraceptives on the future risk of carcinoma of the endometrium as the incidence is reduced by about 50% among former oral contraceptive users[30]. The use of depot progestogen contraceptives has also been shown to provide protection from endometrial cancer, reducing the subsequent incidence by up to 80%[31,32]. High-dose progestogens have been shown to be effective in the treatment of some women with early-stage, well-differentiated endometrial adenocarcinoma and has been used in young women who wish to retain their fertility[33].

Cyclical therapy

The addition of progestogens to estrogen therapy is now standard practice in women with a uterus, but endometrial hyperplasia still occurs. A study of 413 patients over two and a half years suggested complex hyperplasia continued at close to the background rate[34] and that regular withdrawal bleeds did not provide reassurance of endometrial normality (see Figure 1). Earlier a large prospective study by Gambrell showed patients receiving various combinations of estrogen and progestogens had an incidence of endometrial carcinoma lower than that of an untreated population[35]. Other better designed epidemiological studies reported risk ratios of 1.3[36] and 1.8[37] for women given combined therapy as compared to no medication. However, in these retrospective studies different regimens are grouped together and progestogen non-compliance may skew results. The difficulty in obtaining data from prospective trials is illustrated by a Swedish study of more than 23 000 women. It had a total of over 100 000 patient years which still lacked the statistical power (at 90%) to detect an increased risk for endometrial cancer in users of combination therapy unless it was greater than fivefold[38].

In a population-based case–control study of over a 1000 cases of endometrial cancer by Beresford and colleagues, a higher rate of endometrial carcinoma was found in patients taking cyclical HRT than in controls. Relative to non-users, unopposed users had a four-fold increase in the risk of endometrial carcinoma[39]. Unsurprisingly the study demonstrated that progestogen given for less than 10 days reduced, but did not eliminate, the excess risk acquired by taking exogenous estrogen. When the duration of progestogen increased over 10 days a greater protective effect was demonstrated with an odds ratio of less than 1.0. However, users of combined cyclical therapy for more than 5 years had a relative risk of 2.5 when compared with non-users (Table 2)[39]. The Beresford study suggests that the current belief of the long-term safety of opposed therapy, which is not based on long-term prospective studies, may be falsely reassuring.

Endometrial supervision of these women is currently only provoked by abnormal bleeding. Padwick and associates studied the withdrawal bleeding pattern of 102 women with varying duration of estrogen therapy which was opposed for 12 days with progestogen. The timing of the bleed was correlated with endometrial histology and they found that normal endometrium was always associated with bleeding on or after 11 days of progestogen. Those women bleeding earlier all had proliferative endometrium or hyperplasia. They concluded that endometrial opposition could be demonstrated in the timing of the withdrawal bleed. This would suggest normality could be predicted in women with a regular withdrawal bleed[40].

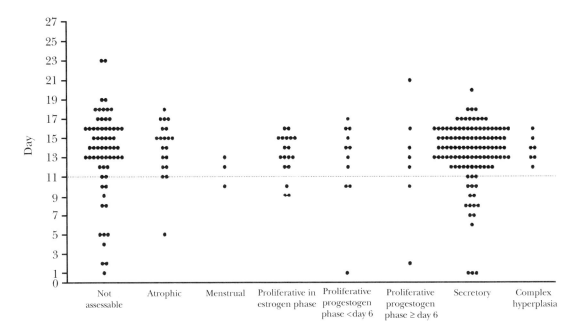

Figure 1 First bleeding day after progestogen in relation to endometrial histology in 244 women with 3 days or less of variation between cycles. (from ref. 34)

Table 2 Duration of therapy and endometrial cancer in current users of estrogen combined with cyclic progestogen (From ref. 39)

Duration of HRT	Number of cases (%)	Number of controls (%)	Odds ratio*
Never-users	87.3	89	1.0
Current users: < 10 days of progestogen per month			
6–59 months	2.8	1.7	2.2 (0.9–5.2)
> 59 months	3.6	1.2	4.8 (2.0–11.4)
Current users: > 10–21 days of progestogen per month			
6–59 months	3.1	6.2	0.7 (0.4–1.4)
> 59 months	3.1	1.9	2.7 (1.2–6.0)

*Adjusted for age, body mass index, county lived in

As a means of supervising a large population on long-term HRT, regular bleeding may be inadequate. Several studies have suggested that the timing of bleeding on HRT is an unreliable indicator of endometrial health[34]. Hyperplasia and carcinoma have been found in women with regular scheduled bleeding[12,15].

The postmenopausal estrogen/progestin interventions (PEPI) trial was a 3-year randomized double-blind placebo-controlled trial. It involved nearly 900 women and results were reassuring and consistent with current understanding. Hyperplasia both with and without atypia was commonest in the unopposed equine estrogen group and suggested a protective role of both progestogens and progesterone, reducing the incidence of hyperplasia to that of the placebo group[16].

Continuous combined therapy

Continuous combined HRT is now accepted as a safe and effective method of minimizing or avoiding vaginal bleeding on HRT. It was introduced to provide progestogenic opposition to estrogen without the need for vaginal bleeding. It was hypothesized that a lower daily progestogen dose would prevent unacceptable side-effects and the endometrial atrophy induced by continuous progestogen would prevent bleeding. By manipulating the hormones individually Magos and colleagues achieved amenorrhea in all women willing to remain in their study until conclusion (13% withdrew because of irregular bleeding) (Figure 2)[41]. Irregular bleeding has been seen to persist in those not altering treatment regimens, though the incidence does decrease with length of use[42].

The endometrial shedding produced by cyclical therapy had been hypothesized to discourage the formation of hyperplasia and therefore the development of cancer[43]. Progestogens reverse endometrial hyperplasia and reduce its occurrence on estrogen therapy, but this does not justify the assumption that progestogens completely prevent endometrial carcinoma from developing on estrogen therapy, particularly when there is no regular withdrawal bleed. Perhaps shedding of the endometrium is as

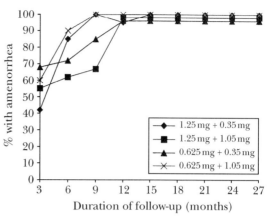

Figure 2 Amenorrhea in women starting continuous combined HRT. (Adapted from reference 41). The first dose in the inset is for conjugated estrogens (0.625–1.25 mg) and the second for norethisterone (0.35–1.05 mg)

important as the anti-proliferative effect of progestogens. Leather and colleagues reviewed 41 long-term users of continuous combined therapy after a long period of amenorrhea; only six women had experienced episodes of breakthrough bleeding, two of whom had benign endometrial polyps and two had adenocarcinoma. Both the adenocarcinomas had abnormal endometrial histology prior to diagnosis. They did not conclude that estrogen and progestogen cause carcinoma, but that previous history and bleeding after amenorrhea was like postmenopausal bleeding and required investigation with an endometrial biopsy[44].

Comerci and associates presented a set of eight cases of endometrial carcinoma occurring in patients taking continuous combined HRT. None of these patients had a previous history of unopposed estrogen use or a family history[45]. These patients were identified in a single unit over a 10-year period. Other similar observational series have also been published[46,47].

Side-effect profile and compliance

The use of progestogens in opposition to estrogen has its problems. In a study by Magos and Studd postmenopausal hysterectomized women were given norethisterone and studied for side-effects. Even the relatively low doses of progestogens used in opposition for HRT were associated with unpleasant symptoms in about 30% of patients. Significant differences were noted in concentration, behavioral change, negative affect, water retention and pain. The characteristics were typical of the premenstrual syndrome[48]. Progesterone-derived C21 progestogens, such as medroxyprogesterone, are recognized to cause side-effects including breast discomfort, nausea, irritability and water retention (again similar symptoms to premenstrual syndrome) and more rarely anaphylactoid-like reactions, psychiatric disturbance and skin reactions.

ALTERNATIVES

Progesterone has been used in opposition to estrogens. It is relatively weaker in its biological activity than the synthetic progestogens. It has been successfully used in the treatment of existing hyperplasia when given by the vaginal route[49]. The attraction of progesterone lies in its comparatively benign side-effect profile and metabolic neutrality. It has been reported that progesterone does not reduce the plasma high density lipoprotein (HDL_2) sub-fraction and therefore it should not reduce the cardioprotective effect of estrogen. There are few safety data and no long-term works on progesterone as opposition to estrogen in HRT[50].

Tibolone has been used in the treatment of the menopause; this drug is an androgen derivative which prevents bone loss[51] and controls climacteric symptoms[52]. It appears not to stimulate the endometrium[53], though changes to the lipid profile are not as attractive as is seen with estrogen[54].

Mirena and Progestasert are both intrauterine systems that have been used with estrogen replacement, particularly in women with progesterone intolerance. Respectively, they contain levonorgestrel and progesterone in slow release reservoirs. Levonorgestrel systems have been shown to be effective in controlling endometrial hypertrophy and offering adequate endometrial opposition in HRT regimens[55]. Studies are currently in progress to assess the efficacy of progesterone intrauterine systems in opposition to estrogen as HRT. The appeal of such systems is the high local concentrations of progestogen in the endometrial cavity with few systemic side-effects.

The selective estrogen receptor modulators (SERMs) may provide a future alternative to HRT for some indications. This is a group of structurally diverse compounds that act as selective agonists or antagonists to estrogen receptors in different target tissues. Raloxifene has been shown to reduce osteoporotic vertebral fractures by over 40% while causing no endometrial stimulation[56]. For patients requiring long-term therapy for osteoporosis, raloxifene provides skeletal benefit without an apparent increase in the risk of breast or endometrial cancer. These agents are new and again long-term safety data are awaited.

MONITORING THE ENDOMETRIUM

Patients on HRT who have abnormal bleeding require investigation. Traditionally such patients were managed by dilatation and curettage (D&C). However, the diagnostic accuracy of D&C is limited, with failure to diagnose in 10–25%[57,58].

Hysteroscopy and biopsy allow better assessment of the endometrium than curettage alone. It is feasible as an outpatient procedure on women taking HRT. There is a high detection rate of intrauterine abnormalities, with positive findings in around 50% of symptomatic patients[59,60]. Transvaginal ultrasound has been shown to be highly accurate at identifying focal lesions and measuring endometrial thickness, but it provides no histology. It may be a good screening tool but if symptoms persist in the presence of a normal ultrasound examination, diagnostic hysteroscopy and biopsy should be performed[61].

CONCLUSION

Progestogens have a protective effect on the endometrium when it is exposed to either endogenous or exogenous estrogen by arresting endometrial proliferation and by promoting differentiation. In regimens with a withdrawal bleed, the resulting sloughing of the endometrium reduces prolonged endometrial cell exposure to estrogen. Oral progestogens do not give complete protection from the excess risk of exogenous estrogen administration. There is also a problem in making histopathological diagnoses in a stimulated endometrium and confusing gray areas exist between hyperplasia, carcinoma in situ and well-differentiated adenocarcinoma.

Epidemiological contraceptive data suggest that exposure to exogenous progestogens in the reproductive years carries a prolonged protective effect. Progestogens are extremely clinically effective in the treatment of simple and complex endometrial hyperplasia. They reduce the incidence of endometrial hyperplasia when given in conjunction with exogenous estrogens particularly when prescribed for more than 10 days. In cyclical regimens the duration of progestogen administration is limited by symptoms. Longer courses will promote a premenstrual-like syndrome and shorter courses predispose to hyperplasia and poor cycle control. When given in a continuous fashion they induce endometrial atrophy, but protection from endometrial carcinoma has not been demonstrated in long-term studies.

Progestogenic opposition does not stop malignant transformation in the endometrium altogether as some endometrial tumors are independent of estrogen. The consequences of long-term exposure to opposed estrogen replacement are unknown and the excess risk of endometrial cancer in patients taking estrogen may not be entirely negated by the concurrent use of progestogens[39]. Long-term data suggest that the incidence of endometrial carcinoma is raised in long-term HRT users (more than 5 years) even with progestogenic opposition,

therefore some form of endometrial surveillance may be justified in asymptomatic women who have been on therapy for more than 5 years. Mortality from endometrial carcinoma also appears to be higher in ever-users of opposed HRT than never-users. This suggests that data demonstrating increased risk of endometrial adenocarcinoma represent more than histopathological over-diagnosis. There is far less information published about opposed therapy than unopposed, of which the majority concerns cyclical regimens. As it has been suggested that length of progestogen administration is more important than total dose, but that shedding may have an important role in endometrial protection, it is not possible safely to extrapolate cyclical safety data to continuous combined regimens. The long-term safety of continuous combined regimens is unknown.

The Women's Health Initiative in the US is a large, randomized, double-blind, controlled trial designed specifically to look at long-term risks and benefits of HRT. It involves 275 000 women and is due to conclude in 2007. Future prospective studies such as this are still needed to determine the dose and duration of progestogens in combination therapy and the longer-term consequences to the endometrium of HRT, as progestogens cause unpleasant side-effects and compliance remains an important issue.

Abnormal bleeding on continuous combined hormone replacement must be investigated in the same way as postmenopausal bleeding. It is also important to emphasize that normal bleeding on cyclical regimes is not reliable evidence of endometrial normality and any abnormal bleeding should be investigated if it persists.

References

1. Barlow DH, Brockie JA, Rees CMP. A study of general practice consultations and menopausal symptoms. Br Med J 1991;302:274–6

2. Wilkes HC, Meade TW. Hormone replacement therapy in general practice; a survey of doctors in the MRC's general practice framework. Br Med J 1991;302:1317–20

3. Ravnikar VA. Compliance with hormone therapy. *Am J Obstet Gynecol* 1987;156:1332–4

4. Studd JWW. Continuation rates with cyclical and continuous regimes of oral oestrogens and progestogens. *Menopause* 1996;3:181–2

5. Coope J, Marsh J. Can we improve compliance with long term hormone replacement therapy? *Maturitas* 1992;15:151–8

6. Barentson R, Groeneveld FP, Bareman FP, *et al.* Women's opinion on withdrawal bleeding with hormone replacement therapy. *Eur J Obstet Gynaecol Reprod Biol* 1993; 51:203–7

7. Ryan PJ, Harrison R, Blake G, Fogelman I. Compliance with hormone replacement therapy after screening for postmenopausal osteoporosis. *Br J Obstet Gynaecol* 1992;99:325–8

8. Stoeckel, Schröder. Nordwestdeutsch Gellerschaft für Gynakologie. *Zentralbl Gynakol* 1922;46: 193–208

9. Whitehead M, Townsend P, Pryse-Davies J, Ryder T, King R. Effects of oestrogens and progestins on the biochemistry and morphology of the post menopausal endometrium. *N Eng J Med* 305;27: 1599–1605

10. Archer DF, McIntyree-Seltman K, Wilborn WW, *et al.* Endometrial morphology in asymptomatic postmenopausal women. *Am J Obstet Gynecol* 1991;165:317–22

11. Whitehead MI The effects of oestrogens and progestogens on the postmenopausal endometrium. *Maturitas* 1987;1:87–98

12. Paterson ME, Wade-Evans T, Sturdee DW, Thom MH, Studd JW. Endometrial disease after treatment with oestrogens and progestogens in the climacteric. *Br Med J* 1980;280:822–4

13. Schiff I, Sela H, Cramer D, Tulchinsky D, Ryan K. Endometrial hyperplasia in women on cyclic or continuous oestrogen regimens. *Fertil Steril* 1982;27:79–82

14. Gusberg S, Kaplan A. Precursors of corpus cancer IV. Adenomatous hyperplasia as stage 0 carcinoma of the endometrium. *Am J Obstet Gynecol* 1963;87:662–78

15. Sturdee DW, Wade-Evans T, Paterson ME, Thom M, Studd JW. Relations between bleeding pattern, endometrial histology and treatment in menopausal women. *Br Med J* 1978;1:1575–7

16. The writing group for the PEPI trial. Effects of hormone replacement therapy on endometrial histology in postmenopausal women. *J Am Med Assoc* 1996;275:370–5

17. Whitehead MI, Pickar JH. Variation between pathologists in the reporting of endometrial histology with combination oestrogen/progestogen therapies. Presented at the British Medical Society Meeting, Exeter, UK, July 1996

18. Key TJ, Pike MC, The dose–effect relationship between unopposed oestrogens and endometrial mitotic rate: its central in explaining and predicting endometrial cancer risk. *Br J Cancer.* 1988;57:205–12

19. Fujimoto J, Hori M, Ichigo S, Nishigaki M, Itoh T, Tamaya T. Expression of aberrant oestrogen receptor mRNA in endometrial cancers in comparison with normal endometria. *Horm Res* 1994;42:116–9

20. Fujimoto J, Hori M, Ichigo S, Morishita S, Tamaya T. Oestrogen activates migration potential of endometrial cancer cells through the basement membrane. *Tumour Biol* 1996;17:48–57

21. Novak E, Yui E. Relation of endometrial hyperplasia to adenocarcinoma of the uterus. *Am J Obstet Gynecol* 1936;32:674–98

22. Kurman RJ, Kaminski PF, Norris RJ. The behaviour of endometrial hyperplasia. A long term study of untreated hyperplasia in 170 patients. *Cancer* 1985;56:403–12

23. Quint BC. Changing patterns in endometrial adenocarcinoma. *Am J Obstet Gynecol* 1975;122: 498–501

24. Smith D, Pentice R, Thompson D, Herrman W. Association of exogenous estrogen and endometrial carcinoma. *N Engl J Med* 1975;293:1164–7

25. Ziel H, Finkle W. Increased risk of endometrial carcinoma among users of conjugated oestrogens. *N Engl J Med* 1975;293:1167–70

26. Jick H, Watkins RN, Hunter JR, *et al.* Replacement oestrogens and endometrial cancer. *N Engl J Med* 1979;300:218–22

27. Hulka B. Effect of exogenous oestrogens on postmenopausal women: the epidemiologic evidence. *Obstet Gynecol Surv* 1980;35:389–99

28. Grady D, Gebretsadik T, Ernster V, Petitti D. Hormone replacement and endometrial cancer risk: a meta-analysis. *Obstet Gynecol* 1995;85:304–11

29. Studd JWW. Oestrogens as a cause of endometrial cancer. *Br Med J* (letter) 1976;i:1276

30. Grimes DA, Economy KE. Primary prevention of gynaecological cancers. *Am J Obstet Gynecol* 1995;1972:227–35

31. Cullins VE. Non-contraceptive benefits and therapeutic uses of depot medroxyprogesterone acetate. *J Reprod Med* 1996;41:428–33

32. Kaunitz AM. Depot medroxyprogesterone acetate contraception and the risk of breast and gynaecologic cancer. *J Reprod Med* 1996;41: 419–27

33. Randall TC, Kurman RJ. Progestin treatment of atypical hyperplasia and well-differentiated carcinoma of the endometrium in women under the age of 40. *Obstet Gynecol* 1997;90:434–40

34. Sturdee DW, Barlow DH, Ulrich LG, *et al.* Is the timing of withdrawal bleeding a guide to endometrial safety during sequential oestrogen/progestogen hormone replacement therapy? *Lancet* 1994;343:979–82

35. Gambrell RD. The prevention of endometrial cancer in postmenopausal women with progestagens. *Maturitas* 1978;1:107–12

36. Brinton L, Hoover R. The endometrial cancer collaborative group. Estrogen replacement therapy and risk of endometrial cancer. Remaining controversies. *Am J Obstet Gynecol* 1993;81:265–71

37. Voigt L, Weiss N, Chu J, Daling J, McKnight B, van Belle G. Progestogen supplementation of exogenous oestrogen and risk of endometrial cancer. *Lancet* 1991;338:274–7

38. Persson I, Adami HO, Bergkvist L, Lindgren A, Pattersson B. Risk of endometrial cancer after treatment with oestrogens alone or in conjunction with progestogens: results of a prospective study. *Br Med J* 1989;298:147–51

39. Beresford S, Weiss NS, LF, Voigt L, McKnight B. Risk of endometrial cancer in relation to use of oestrogen combined with cyclic progestogen therapy in postmenopausal women. *Lancet* 1997; 349:458–61

40. Padwick M, Pryse-Davies J, Whitehead M. A simple method for determining the optimal dosage of progestogen in postmenopausal women receiving oestrogens. *N Engl J Med* 1986; 15:930–4

41. Magos AL, Brincat M, Studd JW, Wardle P, Schlesinger P, O'Dowd T. Amenorrhoea and endometrial atrophy with continuous oral oestrogen and progestogen therapy in postmenopausal women. *Obstet Gynecol* 1985;4:496–9

42. Staland B. Continuous treatment with natural oestrogens and progestogens. A method to avoid endometrial stimulation. *Maturitas* 1981;3:145

43. Gambrell RD, Massey FM, Castaneda TA, Ugenas AJ, Ricci C, Wright S. Use of the progestagen challenge test to reduce the risk of endometrial cancer. *J Obstet Gynecol* 1980;55:732–8

44. Leather AT, Savvas M, Studd JWW. Endometrial histology and bleeding patterns after 8 years of continuous combined estrogen and progestogen therapy in postmenopausal women. *Obstet Gynecol* 1991;6:1008–1010

45. Comerci J, Fields A, Runowicz C, Goldberg G. Continuous low-dose combined hormone replacement therapy and the risk of endometrial cancer. *Gynecol Oncol* 1997;64:425–30

46. McGonigle K, Karlan E, Barbuto D, Leuchter R, Lagasse L, Judd H. Development of endometrial cancer in women on estrogen and progestin hormone replacement therapy. *Gynecol Oncol* 1994;55:126–32

47. Goodman L, Awwad J, Marc K, *et al.* Continuous combined hormone replacement therapy and the risk of endometrial cancer. *Menopause: J North Am Menopause Soc* 1994;1:57

48. Magos AL, Brewster E, Singh R, *et al.* The effects of norethisterone in postmenopausal women on oestrogen replacement therapy: a model for the premenstrual syndrome *Br J Obstet Gynaecol* 1986;93:1290–6

49. Affinito P, Di Carlo C, Di Mauro P, Napolitano V, Nappi C. Endometrial hyperplasia: efficacy of a new treatment with a vaginal cream containing natural micronized progesterone. *Maturitas* 1995;20:191–8

50. Casanas-Roux F, Nisolle M, Marbaix E, Smets M, Bassil S, Donnez J. Morphometric, immunohistological and three-dimensional evaluation of the endometrium of menopausal women treated by oestrogen and Crinone, a new slow-release vaginal progesterone. *Hum Reprod* 1996;11: 357–63

51. Lippuner K, Haenggi W, Birkhaeuser M, Casez J, Jaeger P. Prevention of postmenopausal bone loss using tibolone or conventional peroral or transdermal hormone replacement therapy with 17beta-estradiol and dydrogesterone. *J Bone Miner Res* 1997;12:806–12

52. Egarter C, Huber J, Leikermoser R, *et al.* Tibolone versus conjugated estrogens and sequential progestogen in the treatment of climacteric complaints. *Maturitas* 1996;23:55–62

53. Genazzani A, Benedek-Jaszmann L, Hart D, Andolsek L, Kicovic P, Tax L. Org OD 14 and the endometrium. *Maturitas* 1991;13:243–51

54. Farish E, Barnes J, Rolton H, Spowart K, Fletcher C, Hart D. Effects of tibolone on lipoprotein(a) and HDL subfractions. *Maturitas* 1994;20:215–19

55. Suhonen SP, Holmstrom T, Allonen HO. Intrauterine and subdermal progestin administration in postmenopausal hormone replacement therapy. *Fertil Steril* 1995;63:336–42

56. Delmas P, Bjarnasen N, Mitlak B, *et al.* Effects of raloxifene on bone mineral density, serum cholesterol concentrations and uterine endometrium in postmenopausal women. *N Engl J Med* 1997;337:1641–7

57. Mengart WF, Slate WG. Diagnostic dilatation and curettage as an outpatient procedure. *Am J Obstet Gynecol* 1960;79:727–31

58. Word B, Gravlee LC, Wideman GL. The fallacy of simple uterine curettage. *Obstet Gynecol* 1958;12: 642–8

59. Townsend DE, Fields G, McCausland A, Kauffman K. Diagnostic and operative hysteroscopy in the management of persistent postmenopausal bleeding. *Obstet Gynecol* 1993;82: 419–21

60. Nagele F, O'Connor H, Baskett T, Davies A, Mohammed H, Magos A. Hysteroscopy in women with abnormal uterine bleeding on hormone replacement therapy: a comparison with postmenopausal bleeding. *Fertil Steril* 1996; 65: 1145–50

61. Karlsson B, Granberg S, Hellberg P, Wikland M. Comparative study of transvaginal sonography and hysteroscopy for the detection of pathological endometrial lesions in women with postmenopausal bleeding. *J Ultrasound Med* 1994;13:757–62

25

Interpretation of endometrial pathology with hormone replacement therapy in postmenopausal women

R. C. Bentley and S. J. Robboy

INTRODUCTION

The advent of widespread hormone replacement therapy (HRT) in postmenopausal women has created a new class of endometrial biopsies that present unique problems in interpretation, both for the pathologist and for the clinician. A basic understanding of the pathological effects of HRT on the endometrium is important in managing these patients, but there has been surprisingly little literature devoted to this topic. In this chapter, we will review the wide variety of changes seen in the endometrium of patients receiving postmenopausal HRT.

EFFECTS OF ESTROGEN AND PROGESTERONE ON THE ENDOMETRIUM

At first glance, the spectrum of changes seen with postmenopausal HRT appears extremely broad, and it is certainly true that nearly any endometrial appearance can be attributed to HRT. With a basic understanding of the effects of estrogen and progesterone on the normal endometrium, however, a certain amount of order can be brought to this seemingly dizzying pathologic array. Essentially, it is possible to predict the common effects of HRT based on the known effects of the endogenous steroid hormones on normal endometrium. Several recent monographs offer excellent discussions of hor-mone effects on normal endometrium and are recommended for those interested in a more detailed discussion[1-3].

Estrogens

The basic effect of estrogens on the endometrium is to induce proliferation of the endometrial glands and stromal cells, including endothelium. The degree of proliferation can vary in proportion to the estrogenic stimulus, i.e. very low levels of estrogen or a very weak estrogen will lead to an inactive or atrophic endometrium, while intermediate estrogen levels lead to a weakly proliferative endometrium and, finally, high levels lead to a normally proliferative endometrium (Figure 1). Women who are many years postmenopause may have little response to estrogen, presumably due in part to profound endometrial atrophy.

Persistent exposure to a significant estrogenic stimulus, such as occurs in anovulation, leads to a pattern of continued, unrelieved proliferation. The endometrium cannot support such continued growth, and so histologically one sees a combination of proliferative endometrium with co-existing breakdown, or shedding, accounting for the clinical presentation of irregular bleeding (Figure 2). This pattern is also called 'anovulatory bleeding'. Because the endometrial vessels become abnormally large, bleeding can also be quite severe. Some pathologists refer to the shedding endometrium as menstrual, but it is important to distinguish this appearance from the appearance of menstrual endometrium occurring at the end of a normal cycle. In the normal menstrual endometrium, the endometrial glands will have already transformed at the time of ovulation to a secretory endometrium, and at the time bleeding begins will still show some residual changes, most commonly secretory exhaustion.

With a more prolonged estrogenic exposure, the proliferating glands tend to lose their uniformity in orientation and begin to vary in size and shape, leading to the endometrium being described as disordered proliferative endometrium. With continued, longer-term estrogen

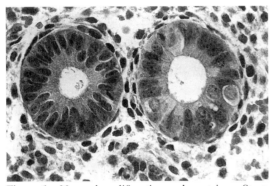

Figure 1 Normal proliferative endometrium. Stratified, mitotically active epithelium lining simple tubular glands

exposure, a high proportion of patients will ultimately develop endometrial hyperplasia. A small number will also go on to develop outright adenocarcinoma. As most women receiving HRT are under the active care of a physician, most of these cancers are caught at an early stage. Thus, these cancers are typically well differentiated and minimally invasive.

Progestins

The effect of progestins on the endometrium is dependent on 'priming' by estrogen, which induces progesterone receptors in the endometrial cells. One important feature of progestins is that they act to down-regulate estrogen and progesterone receptors; in other words, they reduce the sensitivity of the endometrium to these hormones. Prolonged exposure to progestins can thus lead to a histological picture that is paradoxically identical to the atrophy seen in a postmenopausal or hormone-suppressed patient.

In the short term, however, progestins induce secretory differentiation in endometrial glands, and predecidual change in the stroma, i.e. the classic changes of a normal secretory endometrium (Figure 3). The glands develop large glycogen vacuoles which are then secreted into the increasingly complex gland lumina. At the same time, the stromal cells become strikingly enlarged and relatively cohesive in appearance.

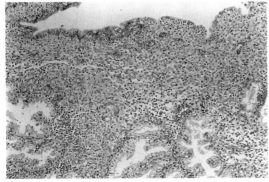

Figure 2 Normal late secretory endometrium (approximately postovulatory day 12). Complex, 'staghorn' gland outlines with stromal predecidual change

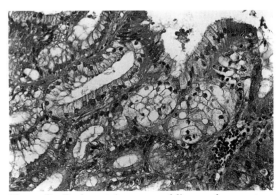

Figure 3 Endometrium resembling early secretory phase with prominent clear glycogen vacuoles in glands. The biopsy was performed 1 week after beginning high-dose progestin therapy for carcinoma

With continued exposure or repeated cycles, the receptor down-regulation causes the glands to lose their sensitivity to estrogens and they develop progressively less, such that they ultimately appear atrophic. At this stage, which only occurs after prolonged exposure or multiple cycles, the appearance is that of a massively decidualized stroma with widely dispersed atrophic glands (Figure 4). More slowly, the stroma also begins to be suppressed by the receptor down-regulation, and over months to years will also tend to become thin and atrophic, ultimately losing most of its decidual features. At this point, the appearance is identical to endometrial atrophy due to menopause or hormone suppression. The term predecidua is used to distinguish this from true decidua, which is the term given to the changes occurring during pregnancy, but, because the changes are so similar histologically, the term decidua or decidual change is often used for both pregnant and non-pregnant endometria.

COMMON TYPES OF HORMONE REPLACEMENT THERAPY

Three general types of hormone replacement therapy have been used clinically: unopposed estrogen, cyclical estrogen and progestin, and combined estrogen and progestin formulations. While the exact agents used and their dosage can vary, within each of these groups the histological findings tend to be similar, and thus they will be discussed as categories.

Unopposed estrogen

Historically, estrogen alone was given as hormone replacement for postmenopausal women, and the beneficial effects of this therapy in preventing osteoporosis and cardiovascular disease have been well documented. A series of case–control studies subsequently demonstrated a marked increase in the risk of endometrial adenocarcinoma in women using long-term unopposed estrogens, leading to the addition of progestational agents to the estrogen. With this addition, the risk of endometrial carcinoma was reduced to near control levels[4,5].

Although current practice is treatment with combined therapy, occasional patients are still treated with estrogen alone.

The endometrium from a woman being treated with unopposed estrogens will most commonly appear proliferative, and may in fact be indistinguishable from a normal proliferative endometrium in a premenopausal patient. This is especially likely if the patient is younger and immediately postmenopausal. There may also be a lesser degree of proliferation that is described as weakly proliferative, especially if the estrogen dose is low[6]. If the patient is bleeding, the endometrium will often have associated stromal breakdown with proliferative glands, a feature which specifically suggests unopposed estrogen exposure (Figure 5). It should be

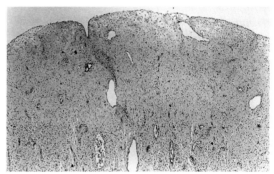

Figure 4 Completely decidualized stroma, with only rare, widely dispersed atrophic glands. The patient had received long-term oral contraceptives (Loestrin)

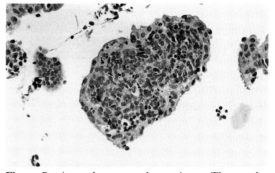

Figure 5 Anovulatory endometrium. The endometrium has a pattern of shedding with crowded, hyperchromatic stromal cells ('stromal ball') in the center, surrounded by a single layer of reactive endometrial surface epithelium. This pattern is highly suggestive of exposure to unopposed estrogens when seen in a background of proliferative endometrium

noted that the pathologist cannot distinguish the changes due to exogenous estrogens from the effects of endogenous estrogen, such as in anovulatory bleeding, or from the effects of other agents that may act as estrogenic agents in the endometrium. These include tamoxifen, various drugs and pharmaceutical agents such as digitalis or phenothiazines, and herbal preparations such as ginseng.

The full range of complications of long-term estrogen exposure can be seen, from disordered proliferative changes, to hyperplasia, to adenocarcinoma[7]. Disordered proliferative endometrium shows a basic pattern of proliferative endometrium, with the addition of irregularly dilated and focally branched glands (Figure 6). This condition is most commonly seen in women not on therapy during the perimenopause and is not felt to be pre-neoplastic.

The hallmark of endometrial hyperplasia, the earliest lesion felt to have pre-neoplastic potential, is the development of glandular crowding, to more than a 1 : 1 gland : stroma ratio. As the degree of hyperplasia increases, the severity of the cytological atypia and that of the architectural changes increase. Finally, adenocarcinomas are characterized by severe glandular crowding, with the development of cribriform or papillary architecture and at least mild nuclear atypia. As is the case for those carcinomas associated with prolonged exposure to endogenous estrogens, the tumors that develop with exogenous unopposed estrogens are usually low grade and minimally invasive, and the long-term survival rates are extremely high.

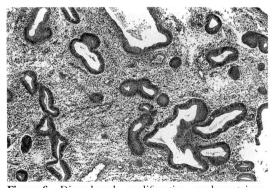

Figure 6 Disordered proliferative endometrium. The glands are variable in size, and show abnormal branching

Patients who develop adenocarcinomas usually have a minimum of 2–3 years of unopposed estrogen use, and the risk increases over time, with the highest risk in patients who have taken estrogens for 10 or more years[8].

Cyclical estrogen/progesterone

Because of the risk of endometrial adenocarcinoma with unopposed estrogens, HRT today nearly always includes a progestin (if the patient has a uterus). Cyclical or sequential HRT uses daily estrogen for the first 21–25 days of the month, with daily progestin added for the last 10–13 days. This regimen mimics to some degree the normal progression of these hormones during a menstrual cycle and typically results in a withdrawal bleed at the end of each cycle.

The pathological findings in the endometrium are somewhat, but not entirely, predictable based on our understanding of normal endometrial cycles. Not surprisingly, biopsies taken from the estrogen-only portion of the cycle typically have a proliferative or weakly proliferative appearance, and may be histologically identical to a normal proliferative endometrium. Biopsies taken after the initiation of the progestin are more variable. Most will show some degree of secretory change, beginning about 3 days after the beginning of the progestin therapy, but the changes do not follow the well-ordered daily progression seen in normal secretory endometrium and cannot be 'dated' in the same fashion[9–11]. Frequently, the glandular component develops no further than an early secretory appearance, with variably developed glycogen vacuoles persisting even late into the artificial cycle. The stroma shows a variable response to the progestin, and may develop a spotty predecidual response by the 10th day after progestin initiation (Figure 7). This is often described in pathology reports as gland–stromal dyssynchrony, and it can be caused by a variety of other factors, including intrauterine devices (IUDs), oral contraceptives, underlying mass lesions such as leiomyomas or polyps, chronic endometritis, and a variety of other hormones such as RU486, clomiphene and gonadotropins. Although this sequence of incomplete cycling is the most common picture with cyclical HRT, other patterns are not infrequent. Up to one-fifth of patients will have an atrophic or quiescent endometrium, a picture of an endometrium with some growth, but without the active signs of proliferation and development seen in a normal proliferative or secretory pattern. This group of patients generally does not experience monthly withdrawal bleeds.

A variety of other patterns are seen less frequently, but can sometimes be helpful in managing patients. For example, if biopsies show a marked predecidual change in the stroma even during the estrogen portion of the cycle, it suggests that the progestin agent is too active relative to the estrogen, and the relative doses may need to be adjusted if irregular breakthrough bleeding has been a problem. Likewise, if biopsies taken from the mid to late portion of the progestin phase of the cycle show a well-developed proliferative pattern, it suggests that the progestin dose may be too low. Finally, if the biopsies show changes consistent with atrophy, then the endometrium is not reponding at all to the hormones, and atrophy is the cause of the bleeding. This information can be helpful in trying to manage irregular bleeding in patients on cyclical HRT. Our understanding of precisely why the endometrium responds so variably to cyclical HRT is poor, but it presumably is due to a combination of host factors (age, years postmenopause, level of endogenous hormones) and medication-specific factors (precise drug, dose and duration).

Combined estrogen/progesterone

Continuous combined estrogen–progestin HRT has been shown to protect against the carcinogenic effects of unopposed estrogen. These regimens generally have a relatively predictable and uniform effect on the endometrium. As described above, the continuous long-term use of progesterone leads to down-regulation of estrogen and progesterone receptors, diminishing the responsiveness of the endometrium. This leads to the most common

appearance, namely an atrophic or inactive endometrium (Figure 8)[12,13]. There may be a weak, poorly developed predecidual change in the stromal cells, and the glandular component may show a few glycogen vacuoles suggesting a progestin effect in the glands, but these findings are variable (Figure 9). Least commonly, there is a well-developed stromal decidual change, similar to that seen with oral contraceptives (Figure 10). Metaplastic changes, such as tubal metaplasia, eosinophilic metaplasia, squamous metaplasia and papillary syncytial metaplasia, are more common with combined continuous HRT therapy[7].

As with the cyclical regimens, variations from these expected findings can sometimes be helpful in managing patients. For example, a clearly proliferative endometrial pattern would suggest an inadequate dose of the progestational agent.

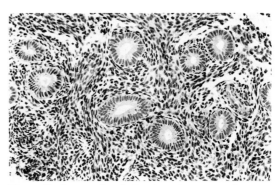

Figure 7 Incompletely developed secretory features including supranuclear clear cytoplasmic glycogen vacuoles in the glands, with little stromal predecidual change. The patient was receiving cyclical (sequential) HRT

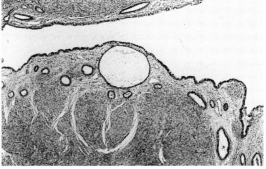

Figure 8 Atrophic endometrium. The endometrium is thin, with several scattered dilated glands

259

Other hormonal agents in postmenopausal women

Tamoxifen

Tamoxifen has been widely used in the treatment, and now the prevention, of breast cancer, functioning as an antiestrogenic agent. In the endometrium, tamoxifen is a weak estrogen agonist, i.e. a compound with estrogenic properties that competes for the estrogen receptor. In the presence of high estrogen levels, as are found in women who are in their premenopausal years, it competes for the receptor and thus blocks the effects of estrogen. In the presence of very low estrogen levels, i.e. in the postmenopausal patient, the weak estrogen-agonist activity is seen in the endometrium. While most postmenopausal women will continue to have an atrophic or inactive endometrium, a few will develop the pathological changes associated with chronic unopposed estrogen stimulation.

Multiple reports have described unusual-appearing endometrial polyps in tamoxifen-treated patients, with cystically dilated glands sometimes containing luminal secretions, a variety of metaplasias and, more rarely, decidualized stroma (Figure 11)[14,15]. Some of these changes may be dose-related. Many of the polyps are 2 cm or more in size, which is larger than seen with any other form of HRT. No studies have yet indicated why this drug alone has such a peculiar effect on the endometrial stroma[16].

Endometrial carcinomas arise at approximately the same rate as with unopposed estrogen and are indistinguishable from other endometrial malignancies. Some initial anecdotal reports and small series suggested that tamoxifen-induced carcinomas might be more frequently high grade, but larger subsequent series, including results from the National Surgical Adjuvant Breast and Bowel Project B-14 study, have shown a similar proportion of high-grade tumors as arise sporadically[17–20].

Raloxifene

Raloxifene is a new antiestrogen for the treatment of breast cancer and has been the subject of extensive recent investigations because of its selective beneficial effects on the bone and cardiovascular systems. In animal studies, it does not produce the weak estrogen-agonist activity

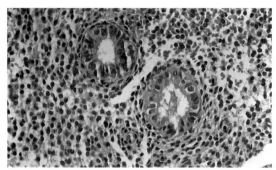

Figure 9 Inactive endometrium, with an isolated gland on lower right suggestive of secretory differentiation. The patient was receiving continuous combined HRT

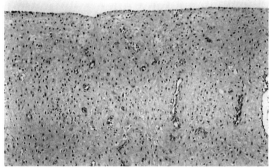

Figure 10 Diffuse, well-developed stromal decidualization, resembling oral contraceptive effect (compare to Figure 4). The patient was receiving continuous combined HRT

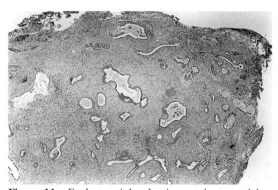

Figure 11 Endometrial polyp in a patient receiving tamoxifen. The polyp is large and has a dense stroma and cystically dilated glands

in the endometrium as seen with tamoxifen, and thus might be expected to lack any association with endometrial hyperplasia and carcinoma. Endometrial biopsies from postmenopausal women who are taking raloxifene show atrophy or inactive endometrium[21], confirming that, at least from a histological standpoint, there is essentially no estrogenic effect. Other studies have shown no increase in endometrial thickness as measured by ultrasound[22]. Whether these promising results will indeed translate to a lower rate of endometrial hyperplasia and carcinoma has not yet been determined and awaits the results of future studies.

Phytoestrogens

Phytoestrogens, a potentially new form of HRT currently being evaluated, are plant estrogens that occur naturally as constituents of many plants[23]. They have an estrogen-like effect in the body, but to a much lesser extent than the body's own estrogen. The observation of their possible effectiveness is drawn from the fact that Asian women, who are known to have a much lower incidence of endometrial carcinoma than Western women, consume much higher amounts of phytoestrogen-rich foods, such as soy and tofu. Human studies suggest that a diet high in phytoestrogens protects from endometrial adenocarcinoma[24].

The most common types of phytoestrogens in plants and foods are the isoflavones. The richest sources in nature are the leaves of the subterranean red clover, which contain levels of up to 5 g per 100 g dry weight, and soybeans, which contain levels up to 300 mg per 100 g dry weight. The most commonly studied phytoestrogens within this group are genistein and daidzein.

The only meager data available on the effects on the endometrium itself are that the thickness of the endometrium is less with phytoestrogen than without[23]. Preliminary data from research with uterine adenocarcinoma cell lines suggest that the mechanism by which genistein is effective is in the induction of cell cycle arrest and apoptosis[25].

RU486 (mifepristone)

RU486 is a derivative of norethindrone, a potent orally effective progestational agent with some estrogenic and androgenic activity, that has been used in Europe as an abortifacient. RU486 is primarily a progesterone antagonist, but has actions that are more complex. It binds to the glucocorticoid receptor and has some binding affinity for androgen receptors[26]. In postmenopausal women, in whom no progesterone is present, it also acts as a weak progesterone agonist. This drug can be used in the treatment of breast cancer and, as such, is a form of HRT and will affect the endometrium.

The drug, when given during the first half of the secretory phase of the cycle, leads to an immediate diminution of the normal glandular secretory activity. Within 3 days of the administration of the drug, the overall degeneration of the endometrium is such that bleeding begins. When given at slightly later periods during the secretory phase, the changes are not so dramatic, although dyssynchrony occurs which makes the findings difficult to interpret[12,27].

When the drug is given on a longer-term basis, the changes found are generalized and cystic and consistent with a chronic unopposed estrogen effect. In a controlled study in which women were treated for 6 months with low-dose RU486 administration, all of the women receiving the drug exhibited an abnormal endometrial morphology. The endometrial glands were irregular in size and shape. The stroma was varied but consisted predominantly of dense cellular stroma with frequent mitotic figures. A combination of epithelial types, some of which were secretory, lined the glands. No cytological atypia was seen[27].

ENDOMETRIAL HYPERPLASIA AND CARCINOMAS

The histological appearance of endometrial hyperplasias and carcinomas in patients receiving HRT is not distinctive. The full range of endometrial hyperplasias and carcinomas can be seen. Clinicians caring for patients on HRT should be familiar with these lesions. The discussion below summarizes the pathology of these neoplastic and pre-neoplastic processes. The reader is referred to several recent monographs for a more complete discussion of these entities[1,2,28,29].

Endometrial hyperplasia

Endometrial hyperplasia has been recognized as a precursor to endometrial carcinoma for most of this century. The exact rate of progression for the various types of endometrial hyperplasia is unclear, since a true study of the natural history has never been (and cannot be) performed. It is clear from numerous retrospective studies, however, that these patients are at increased risk for carcinoma, with the interval to the development of carcinoma ranging from 1 to 14 years[28].

All endometrial hyperplasias represent a poorly regulated proliferation of the endometrium. The pathological feature that reflects this is an increase in the amount of glandular epithelium relative to stroma, usually accompanied by an increase in overall endometrial thickness. The endometrial thickness can be detected by transvaginal ultrasound, which is being increasingly used, probably inappropriately[30], as a non-invasive screening test for hyperplasia. More realistically, it measures overall proliferation of the endometrium, but not the changes generally associated with pre-neoplasia. There are also a large number of cases in which the endometrium is incorrectly assessed as being thickened[30].

Many classification schemes have been proposed in an attempt to stratify patients with hyperplasia into various risk groups. Historically, no uniform system was widely adopted and by the late 1970s there were a variety of competing classification schemes using terms such as 'adenomatous hyperplasia', 'atypical adenomatous hyperplasia', 'atypical hyperplasia' and 'carcinoma *in situ*' that were used differently by different authors. The International Society of Gynecological Pathologists and the World Health Organization (WHO) have proposed a standardized classification scheme[31] that has been adopted by most pathologists. In this scheme, cytological and architectural features of the endometrium are evaluated independently. The architecture is classified as either simple or complex, and the cytological features as atypical or not atypical. In the WHO classification, adenomatous is accepted as a synonym for complex.

Simple hyperplasia

As in all endometrial hyperplasias, the defining feature of simple hyperplasia is an increase in the glandular volume relative to the stroma, often defined as exceeding a 1:1 ratio. In simple hyperplasia, the glands are not yet markedly crowded and are not yet 'back-to-back'. There is also abnormal variability in the gland size and shape, with cystically dilated glands and irregular gland outlines (Figure 12). Some examples of simple hyperplasia are composed almost entirely of cystically dilated glands lined by hyperplastic epithelium. This form of hyperplasia is often termed 'cystic hyperplasia' (Figure 13). Cystic hyperplasia needs to be distinguished from cystic atrophy, with which it was often confused in the past. The findings in simple hyperplasia are similar to those seen in disordered proliferative endometrium. The distinguishing features are the lack of true gland crowding in disordered proliferative endometrium, and the usually more diffuse nature of the findings in simple hyperplasia.

Complex hyperplasia

In complex hyperplasia, the glands show more severe crowding and appear 'back-to-back'. Usually, the glands have more markedly abnormal and complex glandular outlines than in simple hyperplasia (Figure 14). Although the glands can be severely crowded, the presence of at least a thin rim of stroma separating the glands distinguishes this lesion from adenocarcinoma.

Atypical endometrial hyperplasia

After the architecture of the hyperplasia has been classified as either simple or complex, it is then evaluated for the presence of cytological atypia. The definition of atypia in this setting has been controversial but most pathologists use the criteria of increased nuclear size, nuclear rounding, chromatin clumping and clearing, and presence of nucleoli. Another useful fea-

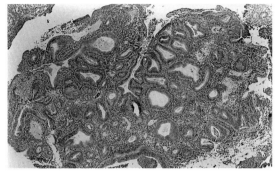

Figure 12 Simple hyperplasia. Mild endometrial gland crowding, with variation in gland size and shape

ture is the common association of these nuclear changes with marked eosinophilic change in the cytoplasm (Figure 15). Mitotic activity is not a criterion for atypia. Most examples of atypia occur in patients with complex hyperplasia; it is an unusual finding in simple hyperplasia.

The importance of atypical hyperplasias is that they allow the identification of those patients at significant risk for either having or developing an endometrial adenocarcinoma. In one series, 23% of patients with atypical hyperplasias progressed to adenocarcinoma, as compared to only 2% of the non-atypical hyperplasias[32].

Endometrial adenocarcinoma

Endometrial adenocarcinomas that occur in patients receiving HRT are not pathologically

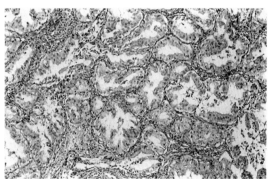

Figure 14 Complex hyperplasia. Glands are back-to-back and show markedly irregular glandular outlines

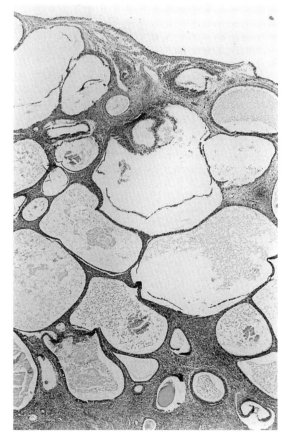

Figure 13 Cystic atrophy. Note marked cystic dilation of the glands. Cystic hyperplasia can be nearly identical in appearance at this magnification

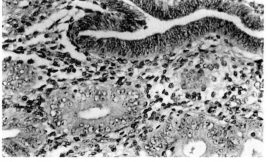

Figure 15 Atypical complex hyperplasia. The lower portion of the micrograph shows several atypical glands, with enlarged, rounded nuclei with chromatin clearing and small nucleoli. Compare with a non-atypical gland in the upper portion of the micrograph

distinct. The full range of subtypes reported includes the usual endometrioid types as well as the high-grade variants of uterine papillary serous carcinoma and clear-cell carcinoma. As mentioned above, the group of patients on unopposed estrogen therapy have a preponderance of well-differentiated, minimally invasive endometrioid adeno-carcinomas and have an excellent prognosis. When observed as a group, tumors developing in patients on HRT have an identical prognosis to tumors developing in non-HRT users, when stratified by stage and grade[33].

References

1. Zaino RJ. Interpretation of endometrial biopsies and curettings. In Silverberg SG, ed. *Biopsy Interpretation Series.* New York: Lippincott-Raven, 1996:143–73
2. Mazur MT, Kurman RJ. *Diagnosis of Endometrial Biopsies and Curettings: A Practical Approach.* New York: Springer-Verlag, 1995:109–30
3. Heller DS. Hormonal effects on the endometrium: dysfunctional uterine bleeding, iatrogenic hormone effects, and luteal phase defects. In Heller DS, ed. *The Endometrium: A Clinicopathologic Approach.* New York: Igaku-Shoin, 1994: 76–90
4. Effects of hormone replacement therapy on endometrial histology in postmenopausal women. The Postmenopausal Estrogen/Progestin Interventions (PEPI) Trial. *J Am Med Assoc* 1996;275:370–5
5. Persson I. Cancer risk in women receiving estrogen–progestin replacement therapy. *Maturitas* 1996;23:S37–45
6. Ettinger B, Bainton L, Upmalis DH, *et al.* Comparison of endometrial growth produced by unopposed conjugated estrogens or by micronized estradiol in postmenopausal women. *Am J Obstet Gynecol* 1997;176:112–17
7. Deligdisch L. Effects of hormone therapy on the endometrium. *Mod Pathol* 1993;6:94–106
8. Mazur MT, Kurman RJ. Effects of hormones. In Mazur MT, Kurman RJ, eds. *Diagnosis of Endometrial Biopsies and Curettings: A Practical Approach.* New York: Springer-Verlag, 1995: 109–30
9. Habiba MA, Bell SC, Al Azzawi F. Endometrial responses to hormone replacement therapy: histological features compared with those of late luteal phase endometrium. *Hum Reprod* 1998;13: 1674–82
10. Vandermooren MJ, Hanselaar AGJM, Borm GF, *et al.* Changes in the withdrawal bleeding pattern and endometrial histology during 17 beta-estradiol dydrogesterone therapy in postmenopausal women: a 2 year prospective study. *Maturitas* 1994;20:175–80
11. CarranzaLira S, MartinezChequer JC, Rita MTS, *et al.* Endometrial changes according to hormone replacement therapy schedule. *Menopause – North Am Menopause Soc* 1998;5:86–9
12. Ireland K, Zaino RJ. Iatrogenic patterns: what hath the physician wrought? In Zaino RJ, ed. *Interpretation of Endometrial Biopsies and Curettings.* New York: Lippincott-Raven, 1996:143–73
13. Piegsa K, Calder A, Davis JA, *et al.* Endometrial status in post-menopausal women on long-term continuous combined hormone replacement therapy (Kliofem(R)): a comparative study of endometrial biopsy, outpatient hysteroscopy and transvaginal ultrasound. *Eur J Obstet Gynecol Reprod Biol* 1997;72:175–80
14. Kennedy MM, Baigrie CF, Manek S. Tamoxifen and the endometrium: review of 102 cases and comparison with HRT-related and non-HRT-related endometrial pathology. *Int J Gynecol Pathol* 1999;18:130–7
15. Schlesinger C, Kamoi S, Ascher SM, *et al.* Endometrial polyps: a comparison study of patients receiving tamoxifen with two control groups. *Int J Gynecol Pathol* 1998;17:302–11
16. Cohen I, Perel E, Tepper R, *et al.* Dose-dependent effect of tamoxifen therapy on endometrial pathologies in postmenopausal breast cancer patients. *Breast Cancer Res Treat* 1999;53: 255–62
17. Fisher B, Costantino JP, Redmond CK, *et al.* Endometrial cancer in tamoxifen-treated breast cancer patients – findings from the national surgical adjuvant breast and bowel project (NSABP) b-14. *J Natl Cancer Inst* 1994;86:527–37
18. Dallenbach-Hellweg G, Hahn U. Mucinous and clear cell adenocarcinomas of the endometrium in patients receiving antiestrogens (tamoxifen) and gestagens. *Int J Gynecol Pathol* 1995;14:7–15

19. Silva EG, Tornos CS, Follenmitchell M. Malignant neoplasms of the uterine corpus in patients treated for breast carcinoma – the effects of tamoxifen. *Int J Gynecol Pathol* 1994;13:248–58

20. Fornander T, Hellstrom AC, Moberger B. Descriptive clinicopathologic study of 17 patients with endometrial cancer during or after adjuvant tamoxifen in early breast cancer. *J Nat Cancer Inst* 1993;85:1850–5

21. Boss SM, Huster WJ, Neild JA, *et al.* Effects of raloxifene hydrochloride on the endometrium of postmenopausal women. *Am J Obstet Gynecol* 1997;177:1458–64

22. Delmas PD, Bjarnason NH, Mitlak BH, *et al.* Effects of raloxifene on bone mineral density, serum cholesterol concentrations, and uterine endometrium in postmenopausal women. *N Engl J Med* 1997;337:1641–7

23. Hale GE, Bievre M, Hughes C. Exploring the role of progestins and phytoestrogens in menopause. *Integrative Med* 2000; in press

24. Goodman MT, Wilkens LR, Hankin JH. Association of soy and fiber consumption with the risk of endometrial cancer. *Am J Epidemiol* 1997;146:294–306

25. Muratori M, Nicoletti I, Vannelli GB, *et al.* Genistein induces a G(2)/M block and apoptosis in human uterine adenocarcinoma cell lines. *Endocr Related Cancer* 1997;4:203–18

26. Mahajan DK, London SN. Mifepristone (RU486): a review. *Fertil Steril* 1997;68:967–76

27. Murphy AA, Kettel LM, Morales AJ. Endometrial effects of long-term low-dose administration of RU486. *Fertil Steril* 1995;63:761–6

28. Bentley RC. Endometrial hyperplasias and their distinction from adenocarcinomas. In Heller DS, ed. *The Endometrium: A Clinicopathologic Approach.* New York: Igaku-Shoin, 1994:114–36

29. Anderson MC, Robboy SJ, Russell P. *Pathology of the Female Genital Tract.* London: Churchill Livingstone, 2000

30. Langer RD, Pierce JJ, O'Hanlan KA, *et al.* Transvaginal ultrasonography compared with endometrial biopsy for the detection of endometrial disease. Postmenopausal Estrogen/Progestin Interventions Trial. *N Engl J Med* 1997;337:1792–8

31. Kurman RJ, Norris HJ. Endometrial hyperplasia and related cellular changes. In Kurman RJ, ed. *Blaustein's Pathology of the Female Genital Tract.* New York: Springer-Verlag, 1994:411–38

32. Kurman RJ, Kaminski PF, Norris HJ. The behavior of endometrial hyperplasia. A long-term study of 'untreated' hyperplasia in 170 patients. *Cancer* 1985;56:403–12

33. Robboy SJ, Bradley R. Changing trends and prognostic features in endometrial cancer associated with exogenous estrogen therapy. *Obstet Gynecol* 1979;54:269–77

26

Obesity and the menopause

M. Santuz, F. Bernardi, L. Driul, L. Plaino, M. Stomati, G. Fabiani, A. R. Genazzani and F. Petraglia

INTRODUCTION

In subjects of both sexes, body weight increases with advancing age. In women, a significant rise is observed between 38 and 47 years, starting before the menopause. To explain such changes, some hypotheses have been proposed:

(1) Changes of metabolism (lipids and glycids);

(2) Hormonal changes (reduced thyroid function);

(3) Reduced physical activity;

(4) Increased food intake.

The augmented body weight approaching the menopause may be protective for female health, because fat tissue metabolizes adrenal androgens into estrogens, thus reducing the forthcoming sex steroid withdrawal syndrome typical of the climacteric period. The physiological increase of body weight in the premenopause must be distinguished from obesity.

The definition of obesity is an excessive augmentation of the body fat mass. Normally, fat tissue represents 20–25% of body mass in men and 18–25% in women. Indeed, fat tissue is an important reservoir of energy that may be utilized during pregnancy. Although it is difficult to determine the normal range of fat mass, obesity is defined as fat mass over 30% of total body mass. The body mass index (BMI) is the most widely used parameter for the description of body habitus. The BMI is closely related to fat mass, it is easy to calculate (weight/height) and

determines the severity of obesity. A BMI of > 26–27 is related to an increased risk of cardiovascular events. It should be emphasized that cardiovascular risk is related not only to the degree of obesity, but also to the distribution of fat tissue. Men tend to have an upper body (abdominal) accumulation of fat, whereas young women tend to accumulate adipose tissue in the gluteofemoral region and have more subcutaneous adipose tissue than men. Another relevant sex-related difference is the ability of women to prevent visceral accumulation of fat, while in men the visceral accumulation of fat parallels that of the other fat deposition sites[1]. It is now well established that android obesity is associated with a higher cardiovascular risk than gynoid obesity. This difference is due to the different endocrine–metabolic characteristics of adipose cells in the different districts: abdominal fat is very sensitive to catecholamine-induced lipolytic activity and therefore it can be easily mobilized, with consequently higher levels of circulating lipids and higher cardiovascular risk. Body fat mass and distribution are also influenced by biological, genetic and environmental factors. Cigarette smoking, low physical activity and stress are associated with a more pronounced upper body fat accumulation.

In the premenopausal period and in early postmenopausal years, modifications of body weight and metabolic and hormonal parameters occur (Figure 1). In particular, an

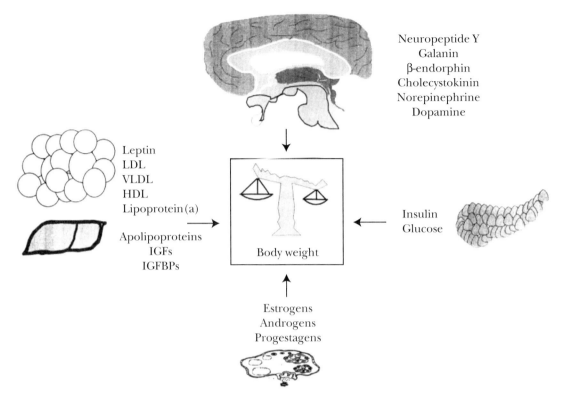

Neuropeptide Y
Galanin
β-endorphin
Cholecystokinin
Norepinephrine
Dopamine

Leptin
LDL
VLDL
HDL
Lipoprotein (a)

Apolipoproteins
IGFs
IGFBPs

Body weight

Insulin
Glucose

Estrogens
Androgens
Progestagens

Figure 1 Hormones, peptides and neuroactive transmitters involved in the regulation of body weight

association has been reported between the climacteric period and an increase in body weight, with an upper body fat distribution pattern similar to that of men. Changes of sex steroid hormones are also implicated in the regulation of body weight and of fat distribution. Sex steroid hormones, as well as the hypothalamic appetite centers, modulate metabolism. In particular, in the regulation of food intake, body weight and fat distribution, other factors, such as neurotransmitters and neuropeptides, may be involved directly or indirectly, modulated by gonadal hormones. The effect of hormone replacement therapy (HRT) on body weight changes and obesity has also been reported.

ADIPOSE TISSUE, METABOLIC FUNCTIONS AND THE MENOPAUSE

The physiological sex-related difference in body fat distribution is most probably related to the circulating levels of sex steroid hormones[1].

Typical of early menopausal years is an increase of body weight[2] and an acceleration in the rate of body weight gain in obese women. A recent survey on changes in body weight, food intake and physical activity in a group of women in the early years of the menopause reported that, in the majority of cases, weight gain occurred regardless of whether the menopause was natural or surgical and regardless of the BMI before the menopause. However, the weight gain occurred in 64% of women with a normal weight before the menopause and in 96% of those already obese before the menopause. The menopause is also associated with changes in body fat distribution, with a shift from peripheral to central fat distribution in association with a decrease in lean body mass and an increase in fat body mass[3]. Recent studies with dual-energy X-ray absorptiometry (DEXA) demonstrated that postmenopausal women had 20% more fat mass and a significantly higher proportion of upper body fat tissue than premenopausal women.

The question is how the changes of circulating sex steroid levels may affect the various metabolisms. Typical of postmenopausal women is the increase of serum total cholesterol, low-density lipoprotein (LDL)- and very-low-density lipoprotein (VLDL)-cholesterol triglycerides, lipoprotein(a) (Lp(a)) and glucose levels. In the Healthy Women's Study, a significant difference was observed between fertile women and postmenopausal women in a 4-year prospective evaluation[4]. In this study, in postmenopausal women a decrease of high-density lipoprotein (HDL)-cholesterol and an increase of LDL-cholesterol with an increase of apolipoprotein AI and AII were observed. Also, qualitative modifications of the LDL molecule were shown, with a decrease of the diameter, which is related to an increase of the atherogenicity. Estrogens affect the lipidic profile through an increase of receptor activity for LDL, and induce the hepatic production of apolipoprotein AI, which is the principal component of the HDL molecule. Moreover, estrogens promote LDL oxidation, a crucial mechanism for plaque formation. Regarding the effects of the menopause on Lp(a), a risk factor for cardiovascular disease and stroke for levels of > 25 mg/dl, there are conflicting data. Some studies showed a significant increase of Lp(a) in the postmenopausal period (data not confirmed by the Framingham study[5]). HRT exerts a favorable effect on the lipid profile, with a decrease of total cholesterol and LDL and an increase of HDL levels. HRT inhibits the enzymatic pathway for HDL metabolism, with an increase in the degradation of the enzyme lipase. The 17-OH derivatives of progestins do not modify the positive effects of estrogen, whereas the 19-nortestosterone derivatives may counteract estrogen efficacy[6]. An indicator of fat synthesis and accumulation in adipocytes is lipoprotein lipase (LPL) activity. It has been demonstrated in fertile women that LPL activity is higher in the femoral subcutaneous fat than in the abdominal fat; this phenomenon is explained by the fact that progesterone stimulates femoral LPL activity, while testosterone inhibits it. The effect of estrogens on LPL activity appears to be mediated by corticosteroid receptors. The regulation of adipose tissue metabolism by steroid hormones is related to cortisol activity. Exceedingly high levels of cortisol, as in Cushing's syndrome, lead to visceral fat accumulation[7]. Progesterone competes with glycocorticoids for the glycocorticoid receptor and may in this way protect against the effects of cortisol. This might explain why young women do not accumulate visceral fat.

Regarding the effects of the menopause and of HRT on the glycometabolic profile, few data are available. An increased risk for diabetes mellitus has been described in some reports, whereas other studies have not shown any modification of circulating glucose and insulin levels in postmenopausal women[8,9]. However, HRT induces a decrease of glucose and insulin levels; this amelioration of the glycidic profile is also decribed in women after the sixth decade of life.

ADIPOSE TISSUE, HORMONAL FUNCTIONS AND THE MENOPAUSE

Regarding the endocrine impact of the menopause, a frequently described condition in perimenopausal women is reduced thyroid activity[10]. This impairment seems to be in part related to the deregulation of the neuroendocrine systems modulating the hypothalamic–pituitary– thyroid axis. As a consequence, the state of relative hypothyroidism could be one of the factors responsible for the augmented body weight. Recently, it has been described that adipose tissue has an endocrine competence and contains a glycoprotein hormone called leptin. This hormone is directly produced by adipose cells. Because serum levels are significantly higher in obese subjects, leptin is considered a marker of the energetic reservoir of the organism. Variations of circulating leptin levels affect other endocrine systems. The reduction of leptin in serum induces a decrease in thyroid function, while it activates adrenal cortex activity and insulin secretion. The final effect is a saving of energy through a down-regulation of thermogenesis and of basal metabolism, with an increase in reactivity and anabolic function. The complex interactions between leptin, adrenal corticosteroids and insulin metabolism suggest that leptin plays a major role in the endocrine response to prolonged starving, while corticosteroids are essential in the response to stress.

Reproductive function is also influenced by serum leptin levels. The fertility of a woman has been correlated with the presence of leptin, which represents a signal of the adequacy of the energetic reserves for a possible pregnancy. The use of the adipose reserves of energy during prolonged starvation determines a reduction of leptin serum levels which switches off some non-vital functions, such as the reproductive function and thermogenesis, while enhancing corticosteroid activity and anabolic function.

The role of leptin in determining perimenopausal obesity appears unclear. Leptin is significantly higher in pre- and postmenopausal women compared to men, even after correction for differences in body mass composition. This sexual dimorphism in the relationship of leptin to fat mass is apparently due to a suppressive effect of circulating androgens on leptin[11]. On the other hand, differences in fat distribution may also play a role. In fact, subcutaneous fat expresses more leptin mRNA than does visceral fat. Therefore, central android adipose tissue may produce less leptin than gynecoid fat, accounting for the sexual dimorphism but not explaining the similar leptin levels in pre- and postmenopausal women who have a different fat distribution[12]. More details on leptin are provided in Chapter 27.

ADIPOSE TISSUE, THE GROWTH HORMONE/INSULIN-LIKE GROWTH FACTOR AXIS AND THE MENOPAUSE

Changes in body weight and fat distribution observed in postmenopausal women have also been ascribed to an altered function of the somatotropic axis[13]. The importance of growth hormone (GH) in regulating fat mass is confirmed by the observation that GH-deficient adults have an increased fat mass and reduced lean mass, and that recombinant human GH replacement therapy reverts these changes[14].

Based on the evidence that GH-deficient adults, postmenopausal women and elderly subjects undergo similar modifications in body mass composition, a hypothesis has been proposed that such modifications may depend upon the age- and menopause-related reduction in GH[15,16]. Growth hormone secretion is under the control of two hypothalamic peptides, GH releasing hormone (GHRH) (with a stimulating action) and somatostatin (with an inhibiting action). Most GH actions are mediated by insulin-like growth factors I and II (IGF-I and IGF-II), proteins with an anabolic and mitogenic action, whose bioavailability is regulated by a family of binding proteins (IGFBPs). The most important IGFBPs are IGFBP-1 and IGFBP-3: IGFBP-1 levels respond to changes in the glycometabolic state, while the levels of IGFBP-3, the main IGF carrier in the blood, are strictly dependent on GH levels. Postmenopausal women have impaired GH secretion and low IGF-1 levels compared with premenopausal women[17]. Estrogens modulate GH levels, although it is not yet clear whether they act at the hypothalamic, pituitary, or peripheral level. Recently, in a group of premenopausal and postmenopausal women aged 45–55 years, with different BMI, we observed that IGF-I levels were higher in the premenopause than in the postmenopause, independently of BMI (Figure 2). In contrast, IGF-II levels were similar in both groups. Our study also demonstrated that IGFBP-1 levels were similar in pre- and postmenopausal women, while higher levels were found in lean compared with obese subjects (Figure 2). IGFBP-3 levels are related to GH levels; however, although the postmenopause is a hyposomatotropic period, IGFBP-3 levels were not reduced, suggesting that other factors, such as age, nutritional status, thyroid, hepatic and renal function, counterbalance the effects of the GH decrease on IGFBP-3 levels.

The evidence that postmenopausal women have a reduced response of GH to GHRH, while HRT is able to restore such a response, strongly suggests a role of sex steroid hormones in the neuroendocrine control of GH release[18].

However, a similar decrease in the GH response to GHRH has also been observed in obese and elderly subjects; in these patients the administration of arginine, which inhibits the

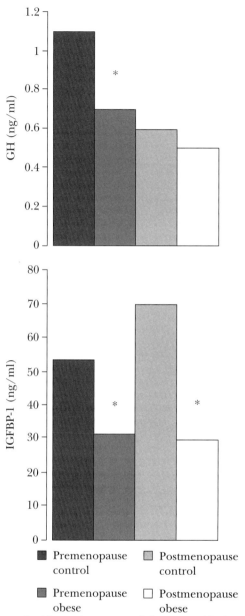

Figure 2 Mean plasma growth hormone (GH) and insulin-like growth factor binding protein (IGFBP)-1 in pre- and postmenopausal obese and control women. Modified from ref. 19

release of somatostatin in the hypothalamus, is able to restore the GH response to GHRH[15]. Recent data from our group have shown that arginine restores the GH response to GHRH in postmenopausal women, independently of BMI. It is therefore possible to hypothesize

that obesity, aging and the menopause are characterized by a common neuroendocrine modification consisting of somatostatinergic hyperactivity. In the postmenopausal period such a modification of the somatotropic axis occurs without changes in IGFBP levels[15].

It is also possible to hypothesize that the changes in body mass composition and fat distribution as well as the changes in the somatotropic axis observed in perimenopausal women may derive from an underlying glycometabolic derangement. In fact, the insulin-like activity of IGF-I and -II suggests a role for the IGF system in glucose homeostasis. Insulin is known to be the main factor modulating plasma IGFBP-1 levels, through the suppression of the hepatic synthesis of this protein. In children and young adults the fasting levels of insulin and of IGFBP-1 are inversely correlated, and an oral glucose tolerance test (OGTT) decreases serum IGFBP-1 levels by 50–60% within 2 h. Recently, we investigated whether menopausal status and BMI affect the response of GH, IGFBP-1 and IGFBP-3 to the OGTT[19]. Pre- and postmenopausal women did not differ with regard to the IGFBP-1 response to the OGTT, while overweight women showed a reduced GH response to the OGTT, compared with women of normal weight. The suppression of serum IGFBP-1 levels after oral glucose administration is ascribed mostly to the insulin-mediated inhibition of IGFBP-1 mRNA synthesis in hepatocytes. The lack of a significant difference between the four experimental groups with regard to the IGFBP-1 response to the OGTT indicates that neither postmenopausal nor overweight women show an impaired insulin-mediated hepatic regulation of IGFBP-1 synthesis. On the other hand, the absence of significant changes in IFGBP-3 levels in response to the OGTT in all groups suggests that IGFBP-3 does not respond to acute changes in the glycometabolic state and that it is regulated by other factors, such as age, nutrition, thyroid hormones and hepatic and renal function. However, these results should be evaluated cautiously, since the response of IGFBP-3 levels to the OGTT might have a latency longer than the observation time of the test. The limited impact that both BMI and menopausal condition have on the GH, IGFBP-1 and IGFBP-3 response to the OGTT seems to rule out the hypothesis that a common glycometabolic modification may influence the changes in both the body weight and the somatotropic axis observed in perimenopausal women. In conclusion, the modifications in the somatotropic axis and in body weight observed in the climacteric seem to be related to a neuroendocrine modification due to the lack of sex steroids, rather than to changes in the glycometabolic milieu.

NEUROENDOCRINE CONTROL OF FOOD INTAKE AND THE MENOPAUSE

Increased food intake is described in perimenopausal women. The mechanism causing such behavior has not yet been defined. Food intake is regulated by hypothalamic centers: the feeding and the satiety centers. Neuropeptides and neurotransmitters involved in this neuroendocrine regulation are: galanine (GAL), neuropeptide Y (NPY) and cholecystokinin (CCK), as well as endogenous opioids and norepinephrine (noradrenaline). Galanine, NPY and endogenous opioids increase appetite, while CCK is the hormone of satiety. Galanine decreases insulin secretion in experimental animals and determines the fat requirement in the daily food allowance. Immunohistochemical studies have shown that both GAL and NPY are stained in adrenergic fibers of the pancreas, and it has been proved that GAL inhibits insulin secretion more effectively than NPY[20]. In particular, NPY is an important appetite regulator and physiologically determines the carbohydrate demand: it mediates the leptin effect on food intake. Increased levels of NPY have been demonstrated in obese women, particularly in those suffering from diabetes[21]. Estrogen affects GAL and NPY. In particular, estrogens increase the NPY content in the median eminence and the synthesis of NPY and GAL, by inducing gene expression. The feeling of satiety is stimulated by CCK and estrogens enhance this effect, while progesterone has the opposite result. Among the endogenous opioid peptides, β-endorphin

modulates GAL, NPY and CCK activity and the reduction in β-endorphin observed in the postmenopause may play an etiological role in postmenopausal obesity.

Experimental and clinical studies have shown an involvement of opioid peptides in food intake behavior, obesity and glucose and lipid metabolism[22]. The injection of β-endorphin into the ventromedial hypothalamus stimulated appetite in rats and sheep, acting specifically through μ or σ receptors[23,24]. Conversely, the administration of naloxone, an opiate receptor antagonist, reduced hunger sensation and food intake in rodents[25] and in obese hirsute women[26]. Another study has reported that small doses of β-endorphin enhanced and large doses diminished feeding, while continuous infusion had no effect, and food intake stimulation in normal rats was associated with a parallel increase in β-endorphin levels[27,28]. Obese children and adults have elevated circulating β-endorphin levels with an enhanced opioidergic tone that produces an increase in pancreatic α-cell and β-cell hormonal release. A delayed response to an oral glucose load with an increase in plasma β-endorphin levels was demonstrated in obese but not in normal women[29], but other investigators reported a similar increase in both obese and non-obese subjects[30], suggesting a pancreatic origin of β-endorphin in obese subjects, modifying the metabolic balance[31]. When plasma β-endorphin level modifications in response to an OGTT were evaluated in pre- and postmenopausal women with different body weight (obese, BMI > 25; or non-obese, 20 < BMI > 24), higher basal β-endorphin levels in obese premenopausal women than in lean subjects were shown[32]. The response of plasma β-endorphin to the OGTT in the premenopausal groups was different in relation to body weight. Non-obese women had a significant increase of plasma β-endorphin after the glucose load, while no changes were shown in obese subjects, or in the OGTT in obese and non-obese postmenopausal women. These data seem to reduce the value of the correlation between an increase in β-endorphin levels and obesity. The endocrine modifications of the postmenopausal period and, in particular, the decrease of sex steroid hormones may have a major impact on the control of β-endorphin release, independently of body weight, in obese and non-obese women, with or without glucose stimulation. The opioidergic system seems to be more affected by sex steroid hormone balance than by the amount of fat tissue, thus suggesting a limited involvement of opioids in explaining the increase of body weight in the postmenopausal period.

On the other hand, norepinephrine secretion in the diencephalon is inhibited by endogenous opioid peptides: their decline at the menopause leads to an intensified sympathetic tone. However, a decrease in sympathetic tone leads to a condition of obesity, caused by the influence on food intake and energy expenditure. Catecholamines are the most potent factors regulating lipolysis: via β_2-receptors they activate lipolysis, while via α_2-receptors they inhibit it. A higher response to catecholamines in visceral adipocytes compared with subcutaneous fat adipocytes has been observed: visceral adipocytes have a low density of α_2-receptors and a high density of β-receptors. Therefore, it is possible to hypothesize that the balance between α- and β-receptors plays a role in local fat storage and that the estrogenic milieu influences the equilibrium.

BODY MASS AND HORMONAL REPLACEMENT THERAPY IN PERIMENOPAUSAL WOMEN

Conflicting data are available regarding the effects of exogenous estrogen or estrogen/progestin regimens in the postmenopause. At present, the available data suggest that weight gain in postmenopausal women is not significantly affected by HRT[33].

Inconsistent and inconclusive data have also been reported regarding the effect of HRT on body composition in the early menopause. Some studies indicate that HRT may prevent the increase in body fat observed in the menopause[34] and may increase muscular mass[35]. Conversely, other authors have not confirmed these

findings and have shown that HRT has no significant effect on total body fat stores[36]. Tonkelaar and associates initially found that the waist/hip ratio increased with age and degree of obesity and that estrogen users had a lower waist/hip ratio. However, in a later study on a larger population, they found similar waist/hip ratios in premenopausal and postmenopausal women when adjustments were made for age and obesity, and that the lesser waist/hip ratio in estrogen users was not apparent when the data were adjusted for age and degree of obesity[37]. On the other hand, a prospective placebo-controlled study of women in the early menopause with dual photon absorptiometry has demonstrated that the menopause is associated with an increase in body fat, a decline in lean body mass and an increase in the percentage of abdominal fat, but it has not provided evidence for a protective effect of HRT[38]. In an extensive review of the literature, it has been reported that the majority of interventional studies support the concept that HRT reduces the accumulation of central fat in postmenopausal women, compared with control or placebo-treated women[39]. Probably, these conflicting results stem from the different types of estrogen/progestin regimens used in these studies or from differences in the length of follow-up periods.

A recent study investigated the differential impact of conventional oral or transdermal HRT or tibolone on body composition in postmenopausal women[40]. This study showed that total body weight increased in patients treated with transdermal HRT, but decreased in women treated with oral regimens and that this reduction was due to a reduction in lean mass. No significant weight change was detected in the controls or in the tibolone-treated women. Tibolone prevents both the increase in total body fat mass and the decrease in total body lean mass. However, during tibolone treatment, an increase in trunk fat mass occurs, compensated by a decrease in fat mass of the head and extremities. These findings suggest that estrogens should be used by the oral rather than the transdermal route if an increase and centralization of body fat and weight are at risk in a particular woman. Furthermore, it has been shown that there is an increase in total body fat, central obesity and weight in women receiving transdermal HRT. The different fat mass changes in transdermally vs. orally treated women may be due to lower serum concentrations of free estradiol in the former group. It has been shown that oral estrogens appear to prevent the increase in total body fat associated with the menopause, by preserving the fat mass of the trunk; however a significant decrease in total body mass is observed, mainly due to a decrease in trunk lean mass. Transdermal estradiol appears to prevent the decrease in total lean body mass, with a significant increase of total body fat mass, mainly due to a significant increase in trunk fat mass.

Oral HRT, in contrast to transdermal HRT, increases serum levels of IGF-I[41]. There is evidence that circulating IGF-I plays an important endocrine role in the regulation of anabolic processes. It has been proposed that low IGF-I levels contribute to some of the involutional changes associated with aging, such as decreased muscle, bone and visceral mass[42].

An involvement of androgens, and in particular of dehydroepiandrosterone (DHEA), in the regulation of body weight has recently been suggested. Both DHEA and DHEA-S levels decrease in the postmenopause and this decrease is genetically determined. However, no correlation has been found between BMI and DHEA or DHEA-S circulating levels in postmenopausal women, although in obese women an increase in DHEA has been described. So far, the use of DHEA-S as an anti-obesity factor has provided conflicting results[43].

References

1. Rebuffe-Scrive M, El J, Hafstrom LO, et al. Metabolism of mammary, abdominal and femoral adipocytes in women before and after menopause. Metabolism 1986;35:792–7
2. Kuskowaska-Wolk A, Rossner S. Prevalence of obesity in Sweden: cross-sectional study of a representative adult population. J Intern Med 1990;227:241–6
3. Shimokata H, Andres R, Coon PJ, et al. Studies in the distribution of body fat. II. Longitudinal effect of change in weight. Int J Obes 1989;13:455–64
4. Matthews KA, Meilahn E, Kuller LH, et al. Menopause and risk factors for coronary heart disease. N Engl J Med 1989;321:641–6
5. Jenner JL, Ordovas JM, Lamon-Fava S, et al. Effects of age, sex and menopausal status on plasma lipoprotein (a) levels. The Framingham offspring study. Circulation 1993;87:1135–41
6. Nabulsi AA, Folsom AR, White A, et al. Association of hormone replacement therapy with various cardiovascular risk factors in postmenopausal women. N Engl J Med 1993;328:1069–75
7. Rebuffe-Scrive M. Steroid hormones and distribution of adipose tissue. Acta Med Scand (Suppl 1988;723:143–6
8. Bentsson C, Lapidus L, Lindquist O. Association between menopause and risk factors for ischemic heart diisease. In Oliver MF, Vedin A, Wilhelmsson C, eds. Myocardial Infarction in Women. Edinburgh: Churchill Livingstone, 1986:93–100
9. Barrett-Connor E, Laakso M. Ischemic heart disease risk in postmenopausal women: effects of estrogen use on glucose and insulin levels. Arteriosclerosis 1990;10:531–4
10. de Aloysio D, Altieri P, Pennacchioni P, et al. Premenopause-dependent changes. Gynecol Obstet Invest 1996;42:120–7
11. Rosenbaum M, Nicolson M, Hirsch J, et al. Effects of gender, body composition, and menopause on plasma concentrations of leptin. J Clin Endocrinol Metab 1996;81:3424–6
12. Saad MF, Damani S, Gingerich RL, et al. Sexual dimorphism in plasma leptin concentration. J Clin Endocrinol Metab 1997;82:579–84
13. Svendsen OL, Hassager C, Christiansen C. Age- and menopause-associated variations in body composition and fat distribution in healthy women as measured by dual-energy X-ray absorptiometry. Metabolism 1995;44:369–3
14. Snel YEM, Doerga ME, Brummer RJM, et al. Resting metabolic rate, body composition and related hormonal parameters in growth hormone-deficient adults before and after growth hormone replacement therapy. Eur J Endocrinol 1995;133:445–50

15. Bernardi F, Petraglia F, Seppälä M, *et al.* Somatotropic axis and body weight in premenopausal and postmenopausal women: evidence for a neuroendocrine derangement, in absence of changes of IGF BP levels. *Hum Reprod* 1998;13: 279–84

16. Rudman D. Growth hormone, body composition and aging. *J Am Geriatr Soc* 1985;33:800–7

17. Ho KY, Evans WS, Blizzard RM. Effects of sex and age on the 24-hour profile of growth hormone secretion in man: importance of endogenous estradiol concentrations. *J Clin Endocrinol Metab* 1987;64:51–8

18. Dawson-Huges B, Stern D, Goldman J, *et al.* Regulation of growth hormone and somatomedin-C secretion in postmenopausal women: effect of physiological estrogen replacement. *J Clin Endocrinol Metab* 1986;63:424–32

19. Bernardi F, Petraglia F, Seppälä M, *et al.* GH, IGFBP-1 and IGFBP-3 response to oral glucose tolerance test in perimenopausal women: no influence of body mass index. *Maturitas* 1999;in press

20. Bray G. Food intake, sympathetic activity and adrenal steroids. *Brain Res Bull* 1993;32:537–41

21. Baranowska B, Wasilewska-Dziubinska E, Radzikowska M, *et al.* Neuropeptide Y, galanin and leptin release in obese women and in women with anorexia nervosa. *Metabolism* 1997;46: 1384–9

22. Paterson SJ, Robson LE, Kosterliz HW. Classification of opioid receptors. *Br Med Bull* 1983;39: 31–6

23. Baile CA, Keim DA, Della-Fera MA, *et al.* Opiate antagonists and agonists and feeding in sheep. *Physiol Behav* 1981;26:1019

24. Grandison L, Guidotti A. Stimulation of food intake by muscimol and beta-endorphin. *Neuropharmacology* 1977;16:533

25. Margules DL, Moisset B, Lewis MJ, *et al.* Beta-endorphin is associated with overeating in genetically obese mice (ob/ob) and rats (fa/fa). *Science* 1978;202:988–91

26. Atkinson RL. Naloxone decreases food intake in obese humans. *J Clin Endocrinol Metab* 1982;55: 196–8

27. Cavagnini F, Redaelli G, Brunani A. Opioid peptides in the control of eating behaviour. In Negri M, Lotti G, Grossman A, eds. *Clinical Perspectives in Endogenous Opioid Peptides*. New York: John Wiley & Sons, 1992:275–94

28. Genazzani AR, Facchinetti F, Petraglia F, *et al.* Hyperendorphinemia in obese children and adolescents. *J Clin Endocrinol Metab* 1986;62:36–40

29. Scavo D, Facchinetti F, Barletta C, *et al.* Plasma beta-endorphin in response to oral glucose tolerance test in obese patients. *Horm Metab Res* 1987;19:204–7

30. Getto CJ, Fullerton DT, Calson IH. Plasma immunoreactive beta-endorphin response to glucose ingestion in human obesity. *Appetite* 1984;5:329–34

31. Giugliano D, Torella R, Lefebre PJ, *et al.* Opioid peptides and metabolic regulation. *Diabetologia* 1988;31:3–15

32. Stomati M, Bersi C, Bernardi F, *et al.* Beta-endorphin response to oral glucose tolerance test in obese and non obese pre and postmenopausal women. *Gynecol Endocrinol* 1998;12:35–40

33. Reubinoff BE, Wurtman J, Rojansky N, *et al.* Effects of hormone replacement therapy on weight, body composition, fat distribution, and food intake in early postmenopausal women: a prospective study. *Fertil Steril* 1995;64:963–9

34. Hassager C, Christiansen C. Estrogen/gestagen therapy changes soft tissue body composition in postmenopausal women. *Metabolism* 1989;38: 662–5

35. Jensen J, Christiansen C, Rodbro P. Estrogen/progestogen replacement therapy changes body composition in early postmenopausal women. *Maturitas* 1986;8:209–16

36. Haarbo J, Marslew U, Godfredsen A, *et al.* Postmenopausal hormone replacement therapy prevents central distribution of body fat after menopause. *Metabolism* 1991;40:1323–6

37. Tonkelaar ID, Seidel JC, van Noord PHA, *et al.* Fat distribution in relation to age, degree of obesity, smoking habits, parity and estrogen use: a cross-sectional study in 11.825 Dutch women participating in the DOM-Project. *Int J Obes* 1990;14:753–61

38. Aloia JF, Vaswani A, Russo L, *et al.* The influence of menopause and hormonal replacement therapy on body cell mass and body fat mass. *Am J Obstet Gynecol* 1995;172:896–900

39. Tchernof A, Calles-Escandon J, Sites CK, *et al.* Menopause, central body fatness, and insulin resistance: effects of HRT. *Coron Artery Dis* 1998; 9:503–11

40. Hanggi W, Lippuner K, Jaeger P, *et al.* Differential impact of conventional oral or transdermal hormone replacement therapy or tibolone on body composition in postmenopausal women. *Clin Endocr* 1998;48:691–9

41. Weissberg AJ, Ho KK, Lazatus L. Contrasting effects of oral and transdermal routes of estrogen replacement therapy on 24-hour growth hormone (GH) secretion, insulin-like growth factor 1, and GH-binding protein in postmenopausal women. *J Clin Endocrinol Metab* 1991;72:374–81

42. Rudman D, Feller AG, Nagraj HS, *et al.* Effect of human growth hormone in men over 60 years old. *N Engl J Med* 1990;323:1–6

43. Berdanier G, Parente J, McIntosch M. Is DHEA an antiobesity agent? *FASEB J* 1993;7:414–19

27

Leptin levels in the menopause

C. Di Carlo, G. A. Tommaselli and C. Nappi

INTRODUCTION

One of the main advances in the field of metabolic control of body weight and obesity treatment was the identification of the *ob* gene and its encoded protein, OB protein or leptin (from the Greek *leptòs*, meaning thin)[1–5]. Zhang and colleagues[6] were the first to identify the *ob* gene and its product, leptin, a soluble protein produced mainly by adipocytes, that circulates bound to binding proteins in concentrations positively correlated to indices of fat mass (total fat mass, per cent body fat and body mass index).

These authors gave the last evidence to a series of experiments that tended to prove the lipostatic theory: the presence of a circulating molecule, produced by adipocytes, signalling the amount of fat stores to the hypothalamic centers that regulate body weight, thus controlling eating behavior and energy expenditure (Figure 1).

Evidence supporting this theory came with the discovery of murine mutant strains, the studies on animals with lesions of the hypothalamic ventromedial nucleus and the parabiosis experiments.

The existence of mutant murine strains has been known for several years. Ingalls and co-workers[7] first identified the *obese* or *ob/ob* phenotype in mouse, characterized by a recessive defect at early onset after birth, associated with extreme obesity.

The *diabetic* or *db/db* mouse is characterized by a recessive hereditary disease associated with diabetes[8]. Both these animal strains are

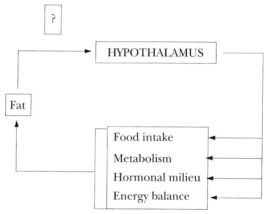

Figure 1 The lipostatic theory

obviously lacking the action of an important factor regulating body weight, the absence of which causes obesity, hyperphagia, hyperglycemia, hyperinsulinemia, insulin resistance, hypothermia and infertility[8,9], and can therefore be considered as animal models for the study of human obesity.

The aim of studying animals that have undergone lesions to the hypothalamus is to demonstrate that the destruction of the putative site of action of this lipostatic factor causes obesity. Indeed, Hervey[10] showed that lesion of the hypothalamic ventromedial nucleus causes obesity in animals. It can be therefore postulated that the circulating substance regulating body weight acts on the hypothalamus, and in particular on the ventromedial nucleus.

Parabiosis experiments consist of an arterial graft between an *ob/ob* and a *db/db* mouse, mixing the blood of the two animals together. With these experiments, Coleman's group[11,12] demonstrated that parabiotic *ob/ob* mice undergo a reduction of body weight and caloric intake, probably responding to a circulating factor produced by the *db/db* parabiotic mouse. Since no modification was observed in the *db/db* parabiotic mouse, it can be concluded that it is probably lacking the receptor for this substance (Figure 2).

THE DISCOVERY OF LEPTIN

As mentioned before, the last piece of the puzzle was positioned by Zhang and colleagues[6], when they cloned and sequenced the mouse *ob* gene and its human homolog. This gene, localized on chromosome 6 in mice and on chromosome 7q13.3 in men, encodes a 4.5 kilobase adipose tissue mRNA with a highly conserved 167 amino-acid open reading frame that yields the OB protein or leptin, which is 84% identical between mouse and human and has the structural features of a secreted protein. This protein, leptin, with a helicoid structure[13], is produced mainly, although not exclusively, by adipocytes[14], circulates in the bloodstream bound to binding protein[15] and acts on a number of receptors. Serum leptin levels were found to be approximately four-fold higher in obese human subjects in comparison to normal

subjects, and were positively correlated to indices of body fat, namely total fat mass, per cent body fat and body mass index (BMI)[16,17]. In mice, a short and a long form of leptin receptors were identified, localized on the choroid plexus and in the hypothalamus, respectively[18]. In humans, only the long form of leptin receptor has been identified as yet[18], and its amino-acid sequence is 78% identical for the extracellular domain and 71% identical for the intracellular domain to the murine long form of leptin receptor. It has been postulated that the short form of leptin receptor might act as a saturable carrier of leptin from the bloodstream into the brain[19,20]. Indeed, it has been found that obese human subjects show mean serum leptin levels 318% higher than normal subjects, while cerebrospinal fluid leptin levels are only 30% higher than normal controls[19]. These findings suggest that leptin enters the brain via a saturable transport system, i.e. the short receptor, and that this transport is saturated in obese subjects who may be 'leptin-resistant'. On the other hand, the long form may act as the real receptor in the hypothalamus which mediates the message of leptin into the hypothalamic cells.

The cloning of the murine *ob* gene allowed the identification of the causes for the *ob/ob* phenotypes: *ob/ob* mice are mutants lacking circulating leptin due to alterations in the *ob* gene, such as a single nucleotide substitution of a thymine with a cytosine in the first position of codon 105 that transforms arginine-105 into a stop codon (murine mutant strain C57BL/6J) or a mutation in the gene promoter region so that no leptin mRNA is produced (murine mutant strain SM/CkC-+Dac ob2j/ob2j). In humans, no mutations of the *ob* human homolog gene have so far been found[21], even though linkage analysis has suggested a link between the *ob* gene locus and obesity[22,23].

Thus, if the pathogenesis of obesity in mice is now clear – a gene defect – in humans it would appear that the sequence and function of the leptin gene are not primary determinants of obesity. From the data gathered up to now, it would seem that obese humans are resistant to their endogenous leptin. Indeed, these subjects

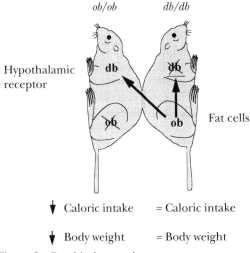

Figure 2   Parabiosis experiments

have higher leptin levels, as a reflection of their increased adipose tissue, and no differences were found in the half-life of circulating leptin between lean and obese subjects[24]. This 'resistance' to leptin is most likely to be located within the central mechanism of body weight control and is probably only in part explained by the saturable transport across the blood–brain barrier, since the saturation of this mechanism occurs at 25 ng/ml, i.e. three-fold the normal leptin concentration of lean subjects. Thus, it seems that the inability of the system to prevent hyperleptinemia before the saturation indicates that the defect is localized elsewhere in the brain. Since the hypothalamus seems to be one of the main central sites of body control, radiolabelled leptin binds to hypothalamic plasma membranes and the intraventricular administration of leptin to *ob/ob* mice causes inhibition of food intake[25], it is likely that an impairment of interactions between leptin and hypothalamic neuropeptides can lead to obesity. Recently, a consitutional defect of the adipose cell has been advocated as a major determinant of extreme obesity. Indeed, both determination of leptin mRNA expression from cultured adipocyes from massively obese subjects and *in situ* hybridization have shown an overexpression of leptin mRNA from these subjects, suggesting that mutation of the *ob* gene is likely[26,27].

LEPTIN AS A SIGNAL TO THE REPRODUCTIVE AXIS

The interest of the researchers in the field of reproductive endocrinology in the functions of leptin arose when it was evident that this peptide could have an impact on reproductive function. Indeed, the *ob/ob* mouse is infertile and shows gonadotropin levels and secretion patterns similar to those in prepubertal animals[28]. Chehab and co-workers[29] demonstrated that intraperitoneal administration of leptin to infertile *ob/ob* mice corrects the reproductive defect of these animals. Barash and colleagues[30] evaluated gonadotropin levels, reproductive organ weights and histology in *ob/ob* mice supplemented, or not, with intraperitoneal recombinant leptin and found that treated female

animals had higher luteinizing hormone (LH) levels, uterine and ovarian weight and number of primary and Graafian follicles, while treated males showed higher follicle stimulating hormone (FSH) levels, number of seminal vesicles and testis weight.

Other evidence indicating a direct influence of leptin on gonadotropin secretion was gathered by Yu and co-workers[31]. These authors demonstrated that leptin stimulated FSH and LH release by hemi-anterior pituitaries *in vitro* and the release of gonadotropin releasing hormone (GnRH) from median eminence–arcuate nuclear explants up to a concentration of $10^{-9}–10^{-11}$ M, while the release of these peptides returned to values similar to those observed in controls with higher concentrations of leptin. Furthermore, inoculation of leptin into the third ventricles of animals primed with estrogens *in vivo* caused a significant increase in LH plasma levels, while no significant differences were observed in FSH plasma levels. The authors concluded that leptin at low concentrations stimulated the release of gonadotropin and gonadotropin releasing factor *in vitro* and had a similar effect on LH, but not FSH, *in vivo*.

These results may indicate that leptin could represent the signal of the nutritional status to the reproductive axis. Whether this signal is exerted directly on the gonads or through the neuroendocrine axis is still to be determined. An important clue in determining the target of leptin on the reproductive axis was the discovery of leptin receptors in the ovary[32,33]. Nevertheless, considering the inhibitory function of leptin on hypothalamic secretion of neuropeptide Y, which also has an inhibitory function on the reproductive axis[34–38], it is tempting to hypothesize that the role of leptin on the reproductive axis is played both centrally and peripherally.

Indeed, there is a large body of evidence indicating a direct inhibition of the production and secretion of neuropeptide Y from the hypothalamus by leptin. A reduction in neuropeptide Y secretion from perfused hypothalamus has been observed following leptin administration[39]. Moreover, intraperitoneal injection of leptin in *ob/ob* mice induces a reduction of neuropeptide Y mRNA expression from the arcuate nucleus by 42.3% compared to saline-treated animals[40]. Since neuropeptide Y is both a naturally occurring appetite transducer, lowering energy expenditure and stimulating food intake[41], and may exert an inhibitory action on gonadotropin release, it is tempting to postulate that modulation of its expression may be the mechanism by which leptin affects energy metabolism and reproductive function (Figure 3).

In humans there is not much evidence that leptin may have a role in reproductive function. First, many authors have found a gender difference in serum leptin levels[17,42–48]. Indeed, a four-fold increase in women's serum leptin levels in comparison to men was observed. At the beginning, this difference was attributed to the relatively larger fat mass and fat distribution characteristic of women or to the influence of estrogens on leptin secretion[49]. However, more recently it was demonstrated that all types of female fat cells express two- to three-fold higher leptin mRNA levels than male fat cells[46]. Furthermore, this gender difference is independent of total adiposity, the association of fat distribution and leptin not being significant[45]. Moreover, it has been found that leptin mRNA expression from adipocytes of obese women is 75% higher than that from obese men[26].

Second, even though this is not direct evidence of the influence of leptin on reproductive function, amenorrheic anorectic women have serum leptin levels significantly lower than normal subjects[50–53]. Moreover, our group recently selected a subset of women with very low body mass index (< 18) who were eumenorrheic and found that their serum leptin levels, even though significantly lower than in normal subjects, were significantly higher than in anorectic women (C. Di Carlo and colleagues, unpublished data), suggesting that a certain cut-off value of leptin levels should be maintained to preserve reproductive function.

LEPTIN LEVELS DURING THE MENOPAUSE

Several authors determined serum leptin levels in postmenopausal women in order to investigate the role played by estrogens on the sexual dimorphism of serum leptin levels[47,48,54–58] (Table 1).

Havel and co-workers[47] studied 13 premenopausal and 19 postmenopausal women [11 treated with hormonal replacement therapy (HRT) and eight not treated with HRT] with similar body mass index, total and per cent body fat and reported that absolute leptin levels were independent of age, reproductive state and of replacement therapy, even after correcting for adiposity. Indeed, they found no differences in absolute and adiposity-corrected leptin levels either between premenopausal and postmenopausal women or between women receiving and not receiving HRT. The authors concluded that the discrepancies in leptin levels between men and women are unlikely to be determined by higher estrogen levels or by increased adiposity and that women needed higher leptin levels to maintain a normal weight balance.

In the study of Rosenbaum and colleagues[48], evaluating five males, nine premenopausal women and seven postmenopausal women, both absolute and fat mass-corrected leptin levels were higher in premenopausal women in comparison to postmenopausal women. These authors concluded that estrogens or progesterone have some influence on leptin levels, even though these effects cannot account for sexual dimorphism, since postmenopausal women show higher leptin levels in comparison to men. Nevertheless, this study is

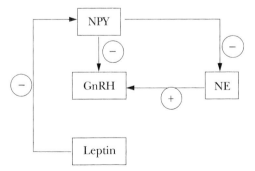

Figure 3 Effects of leptin on neuropeptide Y (NPY) and gonadotropin releasing hormone (GnRH) secretion; NE, norepinephrine

Table 1 Studies evaluating leptin levels in postmenopausal women

Study	Age (years)	BMI (kg/m²)	Fat mass (kg)	% body fat	Leptin (ng/ml)
Havel, et al. (1996)[47]					
Premenopausal	30 ± 2	23.2 ± 0.4	17.7 ± 1.0	27.2 ± 1.1	14.9 ± 1.9
Postmenopausal	60 ± 3	24.5 ± 0.6	18.3 ± 1.2	28.5 ± 1.2	16.3 ± 3.3
+HRT	60 ± 2	24.0 ± 0.5	18.4 ± 1.5	28.1 ± 1.7	17.0 ± 1.9
Rosenbaum, et al. (1996)[48]					
Premenopausal	27 ± 2	30.5 ± 2.6*	35.2 ± 6.0	38.1 ± 2.9	46.3 ± 2.1*
Postmenopausal	66 ± 2	26.0 ± 0.9	25.0 ± 1.6	37.4 ± 1.4	23 ± 3.2
Kohrt, et al. (1996)[56]					
Postmenopausal	67 ± 4	25.6 ± 3.4	28.7 ± 6.2	—	21.7 ± 7.9
+ exercise	64 ± 3	24.7 ± 4.5	24.9 ± 9.4	—	21.5 ± 23.4
+ HRT	66 ± 3	26.9 ± 5.9	29.4 ± 11.0	—	20.6 ± 11.0
+ exercise and HRT	66 ± 3	27.3 ± 4.5	31.3 ± 10.3	—	26.5 ± 17.8
Haffner, et al. (1997)[54]					
Premenopausal	45 ± 0.8	31.0 ± 1.1	—	—	27.6 ± 2.4
Postmenopausal	51.5 ± 1.1	29.8 ± 1.4	—	—	28.3 ± 3.1
+ HRT	52.2 ± 0.8	31.6 ± 1.4	—	—	27.8 ± 3.1
Shimizu, et al. (1997)[55]					
Premenopausal	41.1 ± 1.4	22.9 ± 0.5	16.5 ± 0.8	29.8 ± 0.9	10.41 ± 0.96†
Postmenopausal	60.3 ± 1.0	23.2 ± 0.5	16.5 ± 0.5	31.4 ± 1.0	7.18 ± 0.61
Moller, et al. (1998)[57]					
Young	25 ± 1	23.0 ± 0.5	18.7 ± 1.5	—	12.4 ± 2.2
Middle-age	54 ± 1	23.6 ± 0.9	24.9 ± 2.6	—	17.2 ± 2.8
Old	69 ± 1	26.5 ± 1.1	28.7 ± 2.3	—	18.8 ± 2.6
Di Carlo, et al. (1999)[59]					
Premenopausal	35.5 ± 8.5	23.09 ± 2.8	18.48 ± 3.1‡		10.12 ± 5.48‡
Postmenopausal	52 ± 4.4	24.48 ± 3.0	22.48 ± 2.76		15.82 ± 6.6
+ HRT	51.75 ± 4.2	23.8 ± 3.3	19.42 ± 3.0‡		8.14 ± 4.17‡

BMI, body mass index; *$p < 0.01$ versus postmenopausal women; †$p < 0.001$ versus postmenopausal women; ‡$p < 0.05$ versus postmenopausal women

hampered by the fact that obese and non-obese women were analyzed together, so that mean body mass index $(30.5 ± 2.6 \text{ kg/m}^2$ versus $26.0 ± 0.9 \text{ m}^2)$ and total fat mass $(35.2 ± 6.0 \text{ kg}$ versus $25.0 ± 1.6 \text{ kg})$ were higher in premenopausal in comparison to postmenopausal women.

In a prospective study, Haffner and co-workers[54], evaluated 53 premenopausal women, 28 untreated postmenopausal women and 28 postmenopausal women treated with HRT selected from the San Antonio Heart Study, a population-based study of diabetes and cardiovascular disease in Mexican Americans and non-Hispanic whites. These authors found no significant differences in serum leptin levels in the three groups, in part confirming the data of Havel's group.

Shimizu and co-workers[55] demonstrated that postmenopausal women have lower serum leptin levels in comparison to premenopausal

women and men. In the same study, the authors also demonstrated that leptin mRNA expression from white adipose tissue of rats decreased after ovariectomy in rats and that this expression was restored after estrogen supplementation. These data support a stimulatory effect of estrogens on leptin secretion.

Kohrt and co-workers[56] evaluated the impact of exercise and HRT on serum leptin levels in 61 postmenopausal women. They found that endurance exercise induces a significant reduction in serum leptin levels in older women, probably due to the loss of fat mass induced by exercise rather than exercise *per se*. On the contrary, there was no effect of HRT on leptin levels, suggesting that estrogen does not have stimulatory or inhibitory effects on leptin and that its levels are determined mainly by the amount of body fat.

Moller and colleagues[57], evaluating the correlation between plasma leptin concentrations and body fat content in subjects of different ages, demonstrated that this correlation is disrupted in older subjects of any gender. Indeed, while a strong, positive correlation between total fat mass and plasma leptin levels was observed for subjects aged 20–60 years, this correlation was lost for subjects older than 65 years of age. These data suggest an impairment of the feedback mechanism between peripheral fat tissue and the central nervous system centers that regulate appetite in elderly subjects. This dysregulation may contribute to the observed increase in the incidence of obesity with increasing age.

Nicklas and associates[58], considering the racial differences in body composition, resting energy expenditure and physical activity, evaluated serum leptin levels in African-American and Caucasian postmenopausal women and found that African-American women have 20% lower leptin levels, even after correcting for adiposity differences. These data argue in favor of differences in leptin expression and its role in the regulation of resting energy expenditure, which may play a role in the higher incidence of obesity in the African-American compared to the Caucasian population.

In a recent study from our group[59], we determined the serum leptin levels of 26 postmenopausal women, 14 untreated and 12 treated with HRT (17β-estradiol 50 μg/day plus medroxyprogesterone acetate 10 mg/day), and of 20 premenopausal controls. We demonstrated that serum leptin levels are significantly higher in untreated postmenopausal women in comparison to premenopausal women with similar body mass index (Figure 4). Moreover, women receiving transdermal HRT had lower serum leptin levels in comparison to postmenopausal women not receiving HRT.

These results are in contrast with all previously published data, even though there are some arguments that support our observation.

Indeed, all the above-mentioned studies were carried out to confirm the hypothesis that estrogens stimulate *ob* gene expression and, thus, leptin secretion and to explain sexual differences in leptin concentrations. For these reasons, all these studies concentrated on the

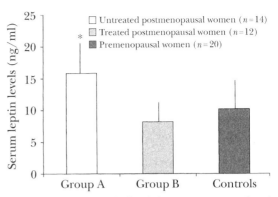

Figure 4 Serum leptin levels in premenopausal and postmenopausal women treated or untreated with HRT

correlation of leptin levels with weight parameters (body mass index, total fat mass, per cent body fat) and on fat-corrected leptin levels. In our study, on the contrary, we wanted to verify if the metabolic and hormonal changes that occur after menopause lead to an increase of total fat mass regardless of body mass index and, consequently, to increased serum leptin levels and if HRT could have an impact on these levels secondary to actions on fat storage.

For this reason, we recruited women with similar body mass indices regardless of total fat mass. Indeed, we found a lower total fat mass not only in premenopausal women than in postmenopausal women, but also in treated than in untreated women (22.48 ± 2.76 kg versus 19.42 ± 3.0 kg versus 18.48 ± 3.1 kg; $p < 0.05$). Our aim was to demonstrate that, during the years following the menopause, there is a modification of body composition with an increase of fat mass that induces an increase of leptin secretion regardless of body mass index. HRT might in part restore a premenopausal pattern of body fat that induces a reduction of leptin secretion.

Indeed, several studies have shown that, in the early postmenopausal period, there is an increase in body weight, body mass index, fat mass, per cent body fat, a decrease of lean mass and a shift toward a more central, android fat distribution[60–64]. Therefore, it is possible to hypothesize that, with the increase of fat mass, even in the absence of the stimulatory effects of estrogens, there could be an increase of serum leptin levels.

Moreover, in postmenopausal women not treated with HRT, an increase in body weight and modifications in trunk and arm fat were observed, while no modifications were present in patients on HRT[61]. These data suggest that HRT can blunt the usual postmenopausal increase in body weight and prevent the shift to a central, android fat distribution, confirming in part those reported by the PEPI trial[60], where, even though not on a significant basis, postmenopausal women displayed a higher body weight in comparison to HRT-treated subjects.

Furthermore, Hassager and Christiansen[65] demonstrated that both oral and transdermal replacement therapy prevented the increase in fat tissue observed in untreated postmenopausal women and that oral, but mainly transdermal, HRT significantly reduced forearm fat content in comparison to untreated women. The evidence that oral HRT is less effective on fat mass could in part account for the differences in the data present in literature and our data, since in most studies only oral replacement therapy was used, while our subjects were all treated with transdermal patches. It is well known that estradiol is the most potent naturally occurring estrogen[66] and that serum estradiol levels are significantly higher during transdermal HRT[67]. Thus, this trend toward a decreased fat tissue observed during transdermal therapy may explain the detectable reduction of serum leptin levels.

Since it has been widely demonstrated that HRT may prevent cadiovascular disease in postmenopausal women[68] and it has been recently shown that leptin is strongly associated with an increased risk for first-ever hemorrhagic stroke, independent of other risk markers for cardiovascular diseases[69], it is tempting to speculate that the protection played by transdermal HRT on cardiovascular disease could be mediated also by a decrease in serum leptin levels.

CONCLUSIONS

The data on serum leptin levels in postmenopausal women available at present are contradictory. This is mainly due to the selection of subjects studied, since most of the studies focused on pre- and postmenopausal women with the same amount of body fat to demonstrate a certain effect of estrogens on leptin secretion. Since it has been widely demonstrated that the major source of leptin is the adipocyte and that serum leptin levels are positively correlated to total fat mass and per cent body fat, it is obvious that women having the same amount of fat should have similar levels of circulating leptin. The role of estrogen on leptin secretion remains to be clarified. Slieker and co-workers showed a stimluatory action of 17β-estradiol on leptin, observing a two-fold increase in *ob* mRNA expression by adipocytes *in vitro*. Moreover, Casabiell and colleagues[70] found that estradiol stimulated leptin secretion from cultured female adipose tissue, being devoid of any action on leptin secretion by male specimens. Finally, as reported above, Shimizu and co-workers[55] demonstrated a stimulatory action of estrogen on circulating leptin in rats *in vivo*. All these data taken together indicate that estrogens do have a stimulatory action on leptin. However, the other studies *in vivo* on serum leptin levels in postmenopausal women argue against such an effect. This may be due either to a real lack of action of estrogens on leptin or to the existence of a complex mechanism of control of leptin levels in which estrogens play only a part.

Our results are not in contrast with the hypothesis that estrogens are stimulating agents of leptin secretion, but indicate that the major determinant of serum leptin level is the total amount of body fat, the increase of which after the menopause overcomes the reduction of estrogens, thus yielding higher levels of leptin. HRT, by restoring in part a body composition similar to that premenopause, may induce a reduction of serum leptin levels secondary to a reduction of total fat mass.

Even though differences in fat distribution between men and women (relatively larger fat mass and different fat distribution) as a determinant of sexual dimorphism in leptin levels have recently been criticized, the role of the modification toward a more android fat distribution observed during the menopause in the modification of leptin levels is still to be determined.

In conclusion, a large, longitudinal study evaluating serum leptin levels as well as body composition in treated and untreated post-menopausal women is needed to determine accurately if leptin levels during the menopause are increased, decreased, or unmodifed and to ascertain finally the distinct role played by the fat mass and estrogens.

References

1. Campfield LA, Smith FJ, Burn P. The OB protein (leptin) pathway – a link between adipose tissue mass and central neural networks. *Horm Metab Res* 1996;28:619–32

2. Considine RV, Caro JF. Leptin: genes, concepts and clinical perspective. *Horm Res* 1996;46:249–56

3. Bray GA, York DA. Leptin and clinical medicine: a new piece in the puzzle of obesity. *J Clin Endocrinol Metab* 1997;82:2771–6

4. Flier JS. What's in a name? In search of leptin's physiologic role. *J Clin Endocrinol Metab* 1998;83:1407–13

5. Kalra SP, Dube MG, Pu S, *et al.* Interacting appetite-regulating pathways in the hypothalamic regulation of body weight. *Endocr Rev* 1999;20:68–100

6. Zhang Y, Proenca R, Maffei M, *et al.* Positional cloning of the mouse obese gene and its human homologue. *Nature (London)* 1994;372:425–32

7. Ingalls AM, Dickie MD, Snell GD. Obese, new mutation in the mouse. *J Hered* 1950;41:317–18

8. Coleman DL. Obese and diabetes: two mutant genes causing diabetes–obesity syndromes in mice. *Diabetologia* 1978;14:141–8

9. Bray GA, York DA. Hypothalamic and genetic obesity in experimental animals: an autonomic and endocrine hypothesis. *Physiol Rev* 1979;59:719–809

10. Hervey GR. The effect of lesions in the hypothalamus in parabiotic rats. *J Physiol* 1958;145:336–52

11. Coleman DL, Hummel KP. The influence of genetic background on the expression of the obese (*ob*) gene in the mouse. *Diabetologia* 1973;9:287–93

12. Herberg L, Coleman DL. Laboratory animals exhibiting obesity and diabetes syndromes. *Metabolism* 1977;26:59–99

13. Madej T, Boguski MS, Buyaub SM. Threadly analysis suggests that the obese gene product may be a helical cytokine. *FEBS Lett* 1995;373:13–18

14. Masuzaki H, Ogawa Y, Isse N, *et al.* Human obese gene expression: adipocyte-specific expression and regional differences in the adipose tissue. *Diabetes* 1995;44:855–8

15. Sinha M, Opentanova I, Ohannesian JP, *et al.* Evidence of free and bound leptin in human circulation: studies in lean and obese subjects and during short-term fasting. *J Clin Invest* 1996;98:1277–82

16. Maffei M, Halaas J, Ravussin E, *et al.* Leptin levels in human and rodent: measurement of plasma leptin and *ob* RNA in obese and weight-reduced subjects. *Nature Med* 1995;1:1155–61

17. Considine RV, Sinha MK, Heiman ML, *et al.* Serum immunoreactive-leptin concentrations in normal-weight and obese human. *N Engl J Med* 1996;334:292–5

18. Tartaglia LA, Dembski M, Weng X, *et al.* Identification and expression cloning of the leptin receptor, OB-R. *Cell* 1995;83:1263–71

19. Caro JF, Kolaczynsli JW, Nyce MR, *et al.* Decreased cerebrospinal-fluid serum leptin ratio in obesity: a possible mechanism for leptin resistance. *Lancet* 1996;348:159–61

20. Schwartz MW, Peskind E, Raskind M, *et al.* Cerebrospinal fluid leptin levels: relationship to plasma levels and to adiposity in humans. *Nature Med* 1996;2:589–93

21. Considine RV, Considine EI, Williams GJ, *et al.* Mutation screening and identification of a sequence variation in the human *ob* gene coding region. *Biochem Biophys Res Commun* 1996;220:735–9

22. Clement K, Garner C, Hager J, *et al.* Indication for linkage of the human *OB* gene region with extreme obesity. *Diabetes* 1996;45:687–90

23. Reed DR, Ding Y, Xu W, *et al.* Extreme obesity may be linked to markers flanking the human *OB* gene. *Diabetes* 1996;45:691–4

24. Klein S, Coppack SW, Mohamed-Ali V, Landt M. Adipose tissue leptin production and plasma leptin kinetics in humans. *Diabetes* 1996;45:984–7

25. Wettstein JG, Earley B, Junien JL. Central nervous system pharmacology of neuropeptide Y. *Pharmacol Ther* 1995;65:397–414

26. Lonnqvist F, Arner P, Nordfors L, Schalling. Overexpression of the obese (*ob*) gene in adipose tissue of human obese subjects. *Nature Med* 1995; 9:950–3

27. Hamilton BS, Paglia D, Kwan AYM, Deitel M. Increased *obese* mRNA expression in omental fat cells from massively obese humans. *Nature Med* 1995;9:953–6

28. Swerdloff RS, Batt RA, Bray GA. Reproductive hormonal function in the genetically obese (*ob/ob*) mouse. *Endocrinology* 1994;98:1359–64

29. Chehab FF, Lim ME, Lu R. Correction of the sterility defect in homozygous obese female mice by treatment with human recombinant leptin. *Nature Genet* 1996;12:318–20

30. Barash IA, Cheung CC, Weigle DS, *et al.* Leptin is a metabolic signal to the reproductive system. *Endocrinology* 1996;137:3144–7

31. Yu WH, Walczewska A, Karanth S, McCann SM. Role of leptin in hypothalamic–pituitary function. *Proc Natl Acad Sci USA* 1997;94:1023–8

32. Cioffi JA, Shafer AW, Zupancic TJ, *et al.* Novel B219/OB receptor isoforms: possible role of leptin in hematopoiesis and reproduction. *Nature Med* 1996;2:585–9

33. Karlsson C, Lindell K, Svensson E, *et al.* Expression of functional leptin receptors in the human ovary. *J Clin Endocrinol Metab* 1997;82:4144–8

34. Clark JT, Kalra PS, Kalra SP. NPY stimulates feeding but inhibits sexual behaviour in rats. *Endocrinology* 1985;117:2435–42

35. McDonald JK, Lumpkin MD, Samson WK, McCann SMM. Neuropeptide Y suppresses pulsatile secretion of luteinizing hormone and growth hormone secretion in ovariectomized rats. *Proc Natl Acad Sci USA* 1985;82:561–4

36. McDonald JK, Lumpkin MD, DePaolo LV. Neuropeptide Y suppresses pulsatile secretion of luteinizing hormone in ovariectomized rats: possible site of action. *Endocrinology* 1989;125:186–91

37. Catzeflis C, Pierroz DD, Rohner-Jeanrenaud F, *et al.* Neuropeptide Y administered chronically into the lateral ventricle profoundly inhibits both the gonadotropic and the somatotropic axis in the intact adult female rat. *Endocrinology* 1993; 132:224–34

38. Pierroz DD, Catzeflis C, Aebi AC, *et al.* Chronic administration of neuropeptide Y into the lateral ventricle inhibits both the pituitary–testicular axis and growth hormone and insulin-like growth factor I secretion in intact adult male rats. *Endocrinology* 1996;137:3–12

39. Stephens TW, Basinski M, Bristow PK, *et al.* The role of neuropeptide Y in the antiobesity action of the *obese* gene product. *Nature (London)* 1995; 377:530–2

40. Schwartz MW, Baskin DG, Bokowski TR, *et al.* Specificity of leptin action on elevated blood glucose levels and hypothalamic neuropeptide Y gene expression in *ob/ob* mice. *Diabetes* 1996; 45:531–5

41. Kalra SP. Appetite and body weight regulation: is it all in the brain? *Neuron* 1997;227–30

42. Ma Z, Gingerich RL, Santiago JV, Klein S, Smith CH, Landt M. Radioimmunoassay of leptin in human plasma. *Clin Chem* 1996;42: 942–6

43. Haffner SM, Gingerich RL, Miettinen H, *et al.* Leptin concentration in relation to overall adiposity and regional body fat distribution in San Antonio. *Int J Obes* 1996;20:904–8

44. Hickey MS, Israel RG, Gardiener SN, *et al.* Gender differences in serum leptin levels in humans. *Biochem Mol Med* 1996;59:1–6

45. Saad MF, Damani S, Gingerich RL, *et al.* Sexual dimorphism in serum leptin concentrations. *J Clin Endocrinol Metab* 1997;82:579–84

46. Saad MF, Riad-Gabriel MG, Khan A, *et al.* Diurnal and ultradian rhythmicity of serum leptin: effects of gender and adiposity. *J Clin Endocrinol Metab* 1998;83:453–9

47. Havel PJ, Kasim-Karakas S, Dubuc GR, Mueller W, Phinney SD. Gender differences in plasma leptin concentrations. *Nature Med* 1996;2: 949–50

48. Rosenbaum M, Nicolson M, Hirsch J, *et al.* Effects of gender, body composition, and menopause on plasma concentrations of leptin. *J Clin Endocrinol Metab* 1996;81:3424–7

49. Slieker LJ, Sloop KW, Surface PL, *et al.* Regulation of expression of *ob* mRNA and protein by glucocorticoids and cAMP. *J Biol Chem* 1996;271: 5301–4

50. Hebebrand J, Van der Heyden J, Devos R, *et al.* Plasma concentration of obese protein in anorexia nervosa [Letter to the editor]. *Lancet* 1997;346:1624–5

51. Grinspoon S, Gulick T, Askaru H, *et al.* Serum leptin levels in women with anorexia nervosa. *J Clin Endocrinol Metab* 1996;81:3861–3

52. Eckert ED, Pomeroy C, Raymond N, *et al.* Leptin in anorexia nervosa. *J Clin Endocrinol Metab* 1998; 83:791–5

53. Balligand JL, Brichard SM, Brichard V, Desager JP, Lambert M. Hypoleptinemia in patients with anorexia nervosa: loss of circadian rhythm and unresponsiveness to short-term refeeding. *Eur J Endocrinol* 1998;138:415–20

54. Haffner SM, Mykkanen L, Stern MP. Leptin concentrations in the San Antonio Heart Study: effect of menopausal status and postmenopausal hormone replacement therapy. *Am J Epidemiol* 1997;146:581–5

55. Shimizu H, Shimomura Y, Nakanishi Y, *et al.* Estrogen increases *in vivo* leptin production in rats and human subjects. *J Endocrinol* 1997;154: 285–92

56. Khort WM, Landt M, Birge SJ Jr. Serum leptin levels are reduced in response to exercise training but not hormone replacement therapy, in older women. *J Clin Endocrinol Metab* 1996;81: 3980–5

57. Moller N, O'Brien P, Nair KS. Disruption of the relationship between fat content and leptin levels with aging in humans. *J Clin Endocrinol Metab* 1998;83:931–4

58. Nicklas BJ, Toth MJ, Goldberg AP, Poehlman ET. Racial differences in plasma leptin concentration in obese postmenopausal women. *J Clin Endocrinol Metab* 1997;82:315–17

59. Di Carlo C, Tommaselli GA, Pisano G, *et al.* Serum leptin levels in postmenopausal women: effects of transdermal hormonal replacement therapy. *Menopause* 1999;in press

60. The writing group for the PEPI trial. Effects of estrogen or estrogen/progestin regimens on heart disease risk factors in postmenopausal women. *J Am Med Assoc* 1995;273:199–208

61. Gambacciani M, Ciaponi M, Cappagli B, *et al.* Body weight, body fat distribution, and hormonal replacement therapy in early postmenopausal women. *J Clin Endocrinol Metab* 1997;82: 414–17

62. Burger HG, Dudley EC, Hopper JL, *et al.* The endocrinology of the menopausal transition: a cross-sectional study of a population-based sample. *J Clin Endocrinol Metab* 1995;80:3537–45

63. Forbes GB, Reina JC. Adult lean body mass declines with age: longitudinal observations. *Metabolism* 1970;19:653–63

64. Espeland MA, Stefanick MI, Kritz-Silverstein D, *et al.* Effect of postmenopausal hormone therapy on body weight and waist and hip girths. *J Clin Endocrinol Metab* 1997;82:1549–56

65. Hassager C, Christiansen C. Estrogen/gestagen therapy changes soft tissue body composition in postmenopausal women. *Metabolism* 1989;38: 662–5

66. Soules MR, Bremner WJ. The menopause and climacteric: endocrinological basis and associated symptomatology. *J Am Geriatr Soc* 1982;30: 547–61

67. Hassager C, Riis BJ, Strom V, *et al.* The long-term effect of oral and percutaneous estradiol on plasma renin substrate and blood pressure. *Circulation* 1987;76:753–8

68. Bush TL, Barrett-Connor E, Cowan LD, *et al.* Cardiovascular mortality and noncontraceptive use of estrogen in women: results from the lipid research clinics program follow-up study. *Circulation* 1987;75:1102–9

69. Soderberg S, Ahren B, Stegmayr B, *et al.* Leptin is a risk marker for first ever hemorrhagic stroke in a population-based cohort. *Stroke* 199;30: 328–37

70. Casabiell X, Pineiro V, Peinò R, *et al.* Gender differences in both spontaneous and stimulated leptin secretion by omental adipose tissue *in vitro*: dexamethasone and estradiol stimulate leptin release in women but not in men samples. *J Clin Endocrinol Metab* 1998;83:2149–55

28

The skeletal effects of estrogen depletion and replacement: histomorphometrical studies

J. Compston

INTRODUCTION

The beneficial skeletal effects of estrogen replacement at the menopause are well established but the mechanisms by which these are achieved remain only partially understood. Bone histomorphometry provides information about changes in bone remodelling and structure which cannot currently be supplied by other approaches, such as bone densitometry and biochemical markers of bone turnover. This chapter reviews normal bone remodelling and structure, the mechanisms by which bone loss or bone gain may be achieved and the effects of estrogen on these processes.

BONE STRUCTURE

Compact or cortical bone accounts for approximately 90% of the skeleton and is found predominantly in the shafts of long bones and surfaces of flat bones. Cancellous (trabecular) bone occurs mainly at the ends of long bones and inner parts of flat bones; it is composed of interconnecting plates and bars within which lies the bone marrow. The extracellular matrix of bone is composed predominantly of type I collagen, the fibers of which adopt a preferential orientation in the adult human skeleton, resulting in the formation of lamellar bone. In cortical bone, these lamellae are arranged concentrically around the Haversian systems whereas in cancellous bone they are parallel to one another.

BONE REMODELLING

In the normal adult human skeleton, the process of bone remodelling serves to maintain the mechanical strength of bone and to provide a mechanism for the transfer of calcium ions into and out of the skeleton. Remodelling is a surface-based phenomenon which occurs in bone remodelling units around Haversian systems in cortical bone and on bone surfaces in cancellous bone; it consists of the resorption, by osteoclasts, of a quantum of bone followed by the formation, within the cavity so created, of osteoid which is subsequently mineralized to form a new packet of bone (Figure 1).

The formation and mineralization of osteoid is a function of osteoblasts. The temporal sequence of events is always that of resorption followed by formation (coupling) and in the young adult skeleton the amounts of bone resorbed and formed are quantitatively similar (balance). In the human skeleton the time taken for completion of a single remodelling cycle is 3–6 months, most of which is occupied by formation.

The mineralized bone surface is prepared for resorption by a process known as activation, which involves retraction of the lining cells on the quiescent bone surface and removal of the thin membrane which covers this surface. The mechanisms by which activation is achieved have not been clearly identified, but it is believed that collagenase and possibly other metalloproteinases synthesized by osteoblasts

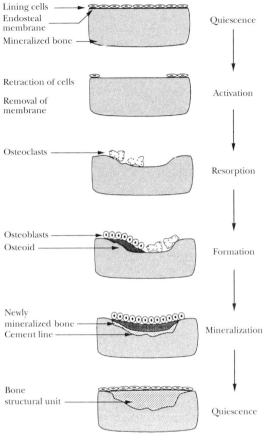

Quiescence

Activation

Resorption

Formation

Mineralization

Quiescence

Lining cells
Endosteal membrane
Mineralized bone

Retraction of cells

Removal of membrane

Osteoclasts

Osteoblasts
Osteoid

Newly mineralized bone
Cement line

Bone structural unit

Figure 1 Schematic representation of bone remodelling. Reprinted with permission from ref. 54

may be involved in removal of the endosteal membrane[1]. The sites at which new bone remodelling units are activated are unlikely to be randomly selected, but rather determined by mechanical signals acting in a site-specific manner.

MECHANISMS OF BONE LOSS

At the cellular and tissue level, there are two mechanisms of bone loss[2] (Figure 2). An increase in activation frequency results in increased bone turnover as a result of a greater number of remodelling units on the bone surface and is potentially reversible, since the resorption cavities formed will eventually be filled in with new bone. Increased activation frequency or bone turnover is quantitatively the most important mechanism of bone loss in osteoporosis. Remodelling imbalance describes changes within individual bone remodelling units, in which the amount of bone formed is less than that resorbed, due to an increase in the amount resorbed, a decrease in the amount formed or a combination of these two. This form of bone loss is irreversible once the remodelling cycle has been completed. In practice, these two forms of bone loss commonly co-exist.

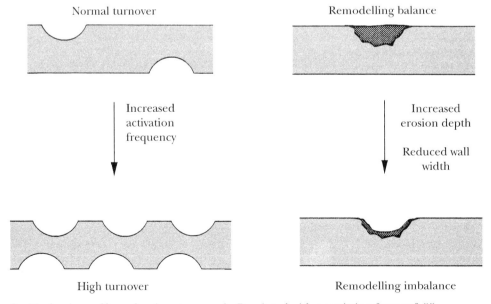

Normal turnover

Increased activation frequency

High turnover

Remodelling balance

Increased erosion depth

Reduced wall width

Remodelling imbalance

Figure 2 Mechanisms of bone loss in osteoporosis. Reprinted with permission from ref. 55

STRUCTURAL CONSEQUENCES OF BONE LOSS

The architectural changes in cancellous bone are determined by the underlying cellular and tissue mechanisms of bone loss[3]. Increased bone turnover, particularly if associated with an increase in the depth of resorption cavities, favors trabecular penetration and erosion, resulting in reduced connectivity of the cancellous bone structure. Remodelling imbalance caused by decreased bone formation leads to trabecular thinning which, as it progresses, will be associated with an increasing risk of trabecular penetration. These two structural changes, namely trabecular penetration and thinning, are thus to some extent interdependent; for any given bone mass, trabecular penetration is associated with greater adverse mechanical consequences than is trabecular thinning.

In cortical bone, loss may occur as a consequence of cortical thinning or increased cortical porosity. Cortical thinning is usually caused by changes on the endosteal surface of the cortex; in contrast, under normal circumstances, periosteal appositional growth continues throughout life.

HISTOMORPHOMETRIC ASSESSMENT OF BONE REMODELLING

Changes in bone remodelling, turnover and structure can be quantitatively assessed on histological sections of bone using well-established histomorphometric techniques[4]. *In vivo*, biopsies are obtained from the iliac crest; a trans-iliac approach is most commonly used, so that the biopsy contains both inner and outer cortical plates and intervening cancellous bone. These biopsies are usually performed on an outpatient basis, using mild sedation and local anesthetic.

Some limitations of bone histomorphometry should be recognized. These reflect both imperfections in the measurement techniques and variations in bone remodelling and structure throughout the skeleton. Measurement variance associated with bone histomorphometry is considerable and is due to a number of factors, including inter- and intra-observer variation,

sampling variation and methodological issues[5]. Estimation of some of the key processes in bone remodelling, particularly activation frequency, can only be made indirectly and relies on a number of assumptions about bone remodelling which may not always be tenable[2]. Accurate assessment of remodelling balance is also problematic, largely because of difficulties associated with measurement of completed resorption depth.

ASSESSMENT OF BONE TURNOVER

Administration of two, time-spaced doses of tetracycline prior to bone biopsy enables dynamic indices of bone formation to be measured directly and also provides the basis for calculation of activation frequency[6]. Tetracycline binds to calcium at actively forming bone surfaces and fluoresces when viewed under blue light on unstained sections. Measurement of the separation and surface extent of the tetracycline labels provides information about bone formation both at cellular and tissue level and forms the basis for calculation of all dynamic indices related to bone formation and resorption[7].

In the absence of tetracycline labelling assessment of bone turnover can only be made from the surface extent of osteoid (formation) and of resorption. The latter may be unreliable since the presence of resorption cavities does not necessarily indicate active resorption but may instead reflect the failure of osteoblasts to form new bone within these cavities[8].

ASSESSMENT OF REMODELLING BALANCE

The accurate assessment of remodelling balance requires measurement both of the amount of bone resorbed and formed within individual remodelling units. The amount of bone formed is termed wall width and can be measured after identification of completed bone remodelling units under polarized light or using stains such as toluidine blue or thionin[9,10]. It is important to recognize that recently formed bone structural units cannot be differentiated from those formed previously and that changes in wall width induced either by disease or its treatment may only be detectable after some years because of the long life-span of the bone remodelling unit, most of which is occupied by bone formation[11].

There are also problems associated with assessment of the other component of remodelling balance, namely the depth of resorption cavities. Identification of resorption cavities is to some extent subjective and it is also often not possible to differentiate between cavities in which resorption has been completed and those in which resorption has become arrested (a phenomenon which may be permanent). Approaches to the measurement of resorption depth include the counting of eroded lamellae at the edges of the cavity, with or without morphological identification of cells associated with the different stages of resorption[12,13] and measurement of the mean depth of cavities after computerized or manual reconstruction of the eroded bone surface[14]. Neither of these approaches is ideal; the latter approach provides information about cavities at all stages of resorption rather than generating a value for completed resorption depth.

ASSESSMENT OF BONE STRUCTURE

A number of methods for the histomorphometric assessment of cancellous bone structure have been described and provide information about trabecular size, shape, connectivity and anisotropy[15]. Two-dimensional approaches which can be applied to histological sections include the measurement or calculation of trabecular width, number and separation[16], strut analysis[17], star volume[18] and trabecular bone pattern factor[19]. These provide only indirect information about connectivity, which is a three-dimensional quality, although there is evidence that they reflect three-dimensional structure. Cortical structure can be assessed by measurements of cortical width and porosity; however, it should be noted that cortical width in iliac crest biopsies is significantly affected by the site and angle at which the biopsy is taken.

THE EFFECTS OF ESTROGEN DEFICIENCY ON BONE REMODELLING AND STRUCTURE

Histomorphometric data on the skeletal changes associated with menopausal bone loss are sparse and restricted to cross-sectional studies in relatively small numbers of women. Some of these studies have provided evidence for an increase in bone turnover during the menopause, both in cortical and cancellous bone[20–22], although this finding has not been universal[23]. These somewhat conflicting data contrast with results obtained from kinetic and biochemical measurements of bone turnover, which have invariably demonstrated an increase in bone turnover during the menopause[24,25]. Furthermore, estrogen replacement therapy is associated with a return to premenopausal values of biochemical markers of bone resorption and formation. The failure of histomorphometric studies to demonstrate unequivocally an increase in bone turnover in association with the menopause is likely to be attributable to several factors including the small numbers studied, lack of prospective data and the large measurement variance associated with bone histomorphometry.

A consistent finding in postmenopausal women has been a reduction in wall width, indicating reduced bone formation at the cellular level and hence a reduction in osteoblast activity[9,20]. Whether this change is specifically related to estrogen deficiency is uncertain; similar changes occur in men and conventional estrogen replacement at the menopause has not been demonstrated to reverse this change. In women, an age-related decrease in wall width has also been reported in cortical bone in some, but not all, studies[22,26,27]. Measurement of resorption depth has demonstrated a small decrease or no change in postmenopausal women, suggesting that the negative remodelling balance is primarily due to reduced bone formation[28,29]. However, studies of acute estrogen deficiency in premenopausal women, induced by administration of gonadotropin releasing hormone analogs, suggest that there may be a transient increase in resorption depth[30]. In these women, rapid and significant disruption of cancellous bone architecture was observed after 6 months of therapy; these changes are unlikely to be due solely to increased bone turnover and would be consistent with an early and transient increase in osteoclastic activity, resulting in increased cavity depth and trabecular penetration and erosion. Furthermore, in cortical bone an increase in resorption depth within Haversian systems was demonstrated in these patients[31]. This hypothesis is also supported by the greater age-related disruption of cancellous bone architecture in women than in men[32,33].

EFFECTS OF ESTROGEN DEFICIENCY ON CANCELLOUS BONE STRUCTURE

Qualitative and quantitative studies of cancellous bone structure in women have clearly demonstrated a reduction in trabecular continuity after the menopause and loss of whole trabeculae. Whether there is significant trabecular thinning is less certain; some studies have reported significant or non-significant decreases in trabecular width whereas others have found no change[33–37]. The increase in trabecular separation which has consistently been demonstrated in postmenopausal women may thus mainly reflect loss of whole trabeculae rather than trabecular thinning. It is also possible that there is preferential erosion of thin trabeculae, so that the contribution of trabecular thinning to bone loss is underestimated.

THE EFFECTS OF ESTROGEN REPLACEMENT THERAPY ON BONE REMODELLING AND STRUCTURE

There have been relatively few bone histomorphometric studies of the effects of hormone replacement therapy. Kinetic and biochemical data have demonstrated a reduction in bone turnover following hormone replacement at the menopause but more subtle changes in bone remodelling balance and cancellous bone structure can only be assessed by bone histomorphometry. In the following section the effects both of hormone replacement therapy

used in 'conventional' doses and of high-dose estrogen therapy administered in the form of estradiol, are considered.

Histomorphometric evidence that hormone replacement reduces bone turnover was first reported by Riggs and colleagues in 1972[38]. In a prospective study of 17 women with established osteoporosis, bone biopsies were obtained before and either 2.5–4 months (short-term) or 26–42 months (long-term) after treatment with premarin. The dose, 2.5 mg daily, was then considered to be a 'physiological replacement dose' although it would now be considered a high dose. Using microradiographs of iliac crest biopsies, active bone resorption and formation surfaces were quantitatively assessed. Prior to treatment, bone resorbing surfaces were significantly increased in the majority of women (13/17), indicating increased bone turnover. After 2.5–4 months, there had been a significant reduction in bone-resorbing but not in bone-forming surfaces; in contrast, after 26–42 months there was a significant reduction in both resorbing and forming surfaces. These data thus indicate that estrogen replacement reduces bone turnover, a suppressive effect on bone resorption being followed by a later decrease in bone formation.

A more detailed histomorphometric analysis of the effects of hormone replacement therapy on bone remodelling was later reported in a study of postmenopausal women with established osteoporosis[39]. These women were randomized to treatment with either oral cyclic estrogen/progestin or oral calcium, 2 g daily. The hormone replacement formulation was Trisequens (2 mg estradiol + 1 mg estriol for 12 days, 1 mg norethisterone + 2 mg estradiol + 1 mg estriol for 10 days and 1 mg estradiol + 0.5 mg estriol for 6 days). Iliac crest biopsies were obtained before, and 12 months after, hormone replacement in 10 patients. Bone formation rate at tissue level and activation frequency, both indices of bone turnover, were significantly decreased at 1 year, to approximately 50% of the pre-treatment value. No significant changes were observed in resorption depth or wall width, suggesting that remodelling balance was unchanged, although the treatment period of 1 year in this study was insufficient to assess changes in wall width and the number of patients studied may have been too small to detect changes in resorption depth.

Similar changes in bone turnover have been reported after transdermal estradiol therapy. In a double-blind, randomized controlled trial of dermal patches delivering 0.1 mg 17β-estradiol for days 1–21 and oral medroxyprogesterone acetate 10 mg daily from days 11–21, bone biopsies were obtained from postmenopausal osteoporotic women at baseline and after 1 year of treatment[40]. Activation frequency and bone formation rate were both significantly lower in the post-treatment biopsies, bone turnover being suppressed to well below pretreatment values. Indices of remodelling balance were not reported in this study.

The effects of estradiol implants, 75 mg monthly, were examined in a prospective 1-year study of 16 postmenopausal women with low bone mineral density[41]. There was a reduction in activation frequency which just attained statistical significance, indicating reduced bone turnover, although the bone formation rate showed a non-significant increase. Cavity depth was not assessed but no significant change in wall width was seen over the course of the study.

In a long-term, prospective study of 22 women with postmenopausal osteoporosis, bone biopsies were obtained before and a mean of 2 years after treatment with oral or transdermal hormone replacement therapy[42]. As in previous studies, a significant reduction in bone turnover was seen; post-treatment values were approximately one-half those encountered prior to treatment and were similar to those found in normal premenopausal women. Assessment of resorption cavity characteristics demonstrated a trend towards decreased cavity size after treatment, consistent with suppression of osteoclastic activity by hormone replacement therapy. There was also a small, but statistically significant, reduction in wall width after treatment, possibly reflecting compensatory changes in response to the reduction in resorption cavity size. These data thus indicate that long-term hormone replacement

therapy, at least in the doses used in this study, does not result in any significant improvement in remodelling balance.

In the above cohort, changes in cancellous bone structure were also investigated using strut analysis, marrow star volume and trabecular bone pattern factor, all of which provide quantitative information related to connectivity[43]. There were no significant changes in any of the structural indices assessed during the 2-year study period, indicating that hormone replacement therapy preserves existing bone microstructure but does not reverse previously induced structural disruption.

Taken together, these studies provide strong evidence that hormone replacement therapy, whether given as estrogen alone or combined with a progestin, preserves bone mass predominantly by reducing bone turnover. The relative contribution to this action of effects on the process of activation *per se* and those on osteoclast number and activity have not been established; a role for the latter mechanism is supported by the well-documented effects of estrogen on osteoclast proliferation, differentiation and activity demonstrated *in vitro*. The effects of estrogen administration on remodelling balance remain to be fully elucidated but there is no evidence from existing studies that, when given in conventional doses, estrogens increase bone formation at the cellular level. This contention is supported by a recently reported study in which very early changes in bone remodelling were investigated in 10 postmenopausal women treated with estradiol valerate 2 mg/day and dydrogesterone 5 mg/day given as a continuous combined regimen; during the first 4 weeks of treatment, no stimulatory effects on bone formation at the cellular or tissue level could be demonstrated[44]. It is therefore possible that the age-related decrease in wall width may be an estrogen-independent phenomenon. Conversely, there is some evidence that estrogen replacement reduces resorption cavity size and hence improves this component of remodelling imbalance. Quantitatively, however, suppression of bone turnover is by far the most important mechanism by which estrogen replacement preserves bone mass and is reflected in the transient increase in bone mineral density seen during the first 1–2 years of treatment.

SKELETAL EFFECTS OF HIGH-DOSE ESTROGEN THERAPY

Evidence from animal studies indicates that high doses of estrogens have anabolic skeletal effects[45,46], but until recently it was unknown whether similar effects occur in the human skeleton. Percutaneous estrogen implant therapy has been reported to be associated with higher bone mineral density levels than oral or transdermal hormone replacement, an observation which may be related to the higher serum estradiol concentrations associated with this form of treatment[47–50]. Many of these studies, however, were cross-sectional and involved the co-administration of testosterone implants, thus providing only indirect evidence for an anabolic skeletal effect.

Recently Wahab and co-workers[51] reported high bone mineral density values in a cohort of women who had received high-dose estradiol implant therapy, without testosterone, for more than 15 years. These women had undergone hysterectomy and bilateral salpingo-oophorectomy for benign diseases and estradiol implant therapy was started immediately postoperatively. The mean Z score in the lumbar spine was + 3.36 and in the femoral neck, + 2.27, providing further evidence that estrogen, in high doses, has anabolic skeletal effects. Direct evidence to support this contention and exploration of potential mechanisms have recently been provided by a histomorphometric study of bone biopsies obtained from this cohort[52]. In this study, iliac crest bone biopsies were obtained from 12 women with a mean age of 58 years who had been treated with estradiol implants, 100 mg approximately 6-monthly for a minimum of 14 years, although the last 2–3 years the dose had been reduced to an average of 50 mg every 6 months. Comparison of histomorphometric indices was made with a group of premenopausal women, based on the rationale that significant age-related bone loss had not occurred in the patient group prior to estradiol

replacement and that any differences between the two groups would therefore reflect effects of high-dose as opposed to physiological estrogen replacement. The results of this study demonstrated a highly significant increase in wall width in the implant-treated group (Figure 3), providing direct histological evidence that high-dose estrogens produce anabolic skeletal effects in postmenopausal women and indicating that these are achieved by stimulation of osteoblastic activity resulting in increased bone formation at cellular level, hence improving remodelling balance.

These findings have been confirmed in a recent prospective study of women undergoing treatment with estradiol implant therapy[53]. In this study, not only was a significant increase in wall width observed but changes indicative of increased connectivity of cancellous bone structure were also demonstrated. This raises the interesting possibility that the anabolic skeletal effects associated with high-dose estrogen therapy in postmenopausal women may result not only from improvement in remodelling balance but also de novo bone formation; the latter mechanism is well documented in mice but further studies are required to investigate its potential contribution to the observed changes in the human skeleton.

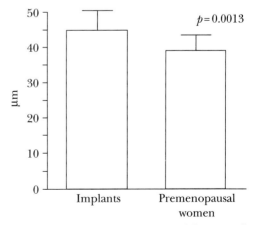

Figure 3 Wall width in women receiving estradiol implants and normal premenopausal women. Data is shown as the mean +1 standard deviation.

CONCLUSIONS

Estrogen plays an essential role in maintaining the integrity of the female skeleton throughout life. The application of bone histomorphometric techniques to bone biopsies has provided novel information about the mechanisms by which estrogen deficiency and repletion affect bone remodelling and structure (Figure 4). Acute estrogen deficiency in premenopausal women is associated with increased bone turnover and rapid disruption of cancellous bone structure; indirect evidence suggests that in the early stages of estrogen deficiency there is also an increase in osteoclastic activity. Bone loss associated with the menopause is due predominantly to increased bone turnover; remodelling imbalance is also seen, although whether this is estrogen dependent remains to be established. Prevention of menopausal bone loss by estrogen replacement in conventional doses is associated with a reduction in bone turnover but no demonstrable improvement in remodelling

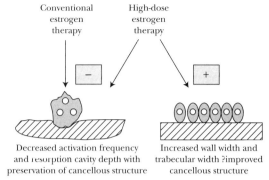

Figure 4 Summary of the effects of estrogen on bone remodelling and structure

balance. However, recent studies have demonstrated the potential for high doses of estrogens to exert anabolic effects in the female skeleton, with an increase in bone formation at the cellular level. The mechanism by which this is achieved has important implications for the development of new therapeutic interventions aimed at increasing bone mass.

References

1. Bord S, Horner A, Hembry RM, *et al.* Production of collagenase by human osteoblasts and osteoclasts in vivo. *Bone* 1996;19:35–40
2. Compston JE, Croucher PI. Histomorphometric assessment of trabecular bone remodelling in osteoporosis. *Bone Miner* 1991;14:91–102
3. Compston JE, Mellish RWE, Croucher PI, *et al.* Structural mechanisms of trabecular bone loss in man. *Bone Miner* 1989;6:339–50
4. Compston JE. Bone Histomorphometry. In: Feldman D, Glorieux FH, Pike JW, eds. *Vitamin D.* San Diego: Academic Press Inc, 1997:573–86
5. Wright CDP, Vedi S, Garrahan NJ, *et al.* Combined inter-observer and intermethod variation in bone histomorphometry. *Bone* 1992;13:205–8
6. Frost HM. Tetracycline-based histological analysis of bone remodeling. *Calcif Tissue Res* 1969;3:211–37
7. Parfitt AM, Drezner MK, Glorieux FH, *et al.* Bone histomorphometry: standardisation of nomenclature, symbols and units. *J Bone Miner Res* 1987;2:595–610
8. Croucher PI, Gilks W, Compston JE. Evidence for interrupted bone resorption in human iliac cancellous bone. *J Bone Miner Res* 1995;10:1537–43
9. Lips P, Courpron P, Meunier PJ. Mean wall thickness of trabecular bone packets in the human iliac crest: changes with age. *Calcif Tissue Int* 1978;26:13–17
10. Derkz P, Birkenhager-Frenkel DH. A thionin stain for visualizing bone cells, mineralizing fronts and cement lines in undecalcified bone sections. *Biotech Histochem* 1995;70:70–4
11. Kragstrup J, Melsen F, Mosekilde L. Thickness of bone formed at remodeling sites in normal human iliac trabecular bone: variations with age and sex. *Metab Bone Dis Rel Res* 1983;5:17–21
12. Eriksen EF, Melsen F, Mosekilde L. Reconstruction of the resorptive site in iliac trabecular bone: a kinetic model for bone resorption in 20 normal individuals. *Metab Bone Dis Rel Res* 1984;5:235–42
13. Palle S, Chappard D, Vico L, *et al.* Evaluation of osteoclastic population in iliac crest biopsies

from 36 normal subjects: a histoenzymologic and histomorphometric study. *J Bone Miner Res* 1989; 4:501–6

14. Garrahan NJ, Croucher PI, Compston JE. A computerised technique for the quantitative assesment of resorption cavities in bone. *Bone* 1990;11:241–6

15. Compston JE. Connectivity of cancellous bone: assessment and mechanical implications. *Bone* 1994;15:436–66

16. Parfitt AM, Mathews CHE, Villanueva AR, *et al.* Relationships between surface volume and thickness of iliac trabecular bone in ageing and in osteoporosis. Implications for the micro-anatomic and cellular mechanisms of bone loss. *J Clin Invest* 1983;72:1396–409

17. Garrahan NJ, Mellish RWE, Compston JE. A new method for the two-dimensional analysis of bone structure in human iliac crest biopsies. *J Microsc* 1986;142:341–9

18. Vesterby A. Star volume of marrow space and trabeculae in iliac crest: sampling procedure and correlation to star volume of first lumbar vertebra. *Bone* 1990;11:149–55

19. Hahn M, Vogel M, Pompesius-Kempa M, *et al.* Trabecular bone pattern factor – a new parameter for simple quantification of bone microarchitecture. *Bone* 1992;13:327–30

20. Vedi S, Compston JE, Webb A, *et al.* Histomorphometric analysis of dynamic parameters of trabecular bone formation in the iliac crest of normal British subjects. *Metab Bone Dis Rel Res* 1983;5:69–74

21. Eastell R, Delmas PD, Hodgson SF, *et al.* Bone formation rate in older normal women; concurrent assessment with bone histomorphometry, calcium kinetics and biochemical markers. *J Clin Endocrinol Metab* 1988;67:741–8

22. Brockstedt H, Kassem M, Eriksen EF, *et al.* Age- and sex-related changes in iliac cortical bone mass and remodeling. *Bone* 1993;14:681–91

23. Melsen F, Mosekilde L. Tetracycline double-labelling of iliac trabecular bone in 41 normal adults. *Calcif Tissue Res* 1978;26:99–102

24. Heaney RP, Recker RR, Saville PD. Menopausal changes in bone remodelling. *J Lab Clin Med* 1978;92:964–70

25. Uebelhart D, Schlemmer A, Johansen JS, *et al.* Effect of menopause and hormone replacement therapy on the urinary excretion of pyridinium cross-links. *J Clin Endocrinol Metab* 1991;72: 367–73

26. Frost HM. Mean formation time of human osteons. *Can J Biochem Physiol* 1963;41:1307–10

27. Jett S, Wu K, Frost HM. Tetracycline-based histological measurement of cortical endosteal bone formation in normal and osteoporotic rib. *Henry Ford Hosp Med J* 1967;15:325–44

28. Eriksen EF, Mosekilde L, Melsen F. Trabecular bone resorption depth decreases with age: differences between normal males and females. *Bone* 1985;6:141–6

29. Croucher PI, Garrahan NJ, Mellish RWE, *et al.* Age-related changes in resorption cavity characteristics in human trabecular bone. *Osteoporosis Int* 1991;1:257–61

30. Compston JE, Yamaguchi K, Croucher PI, *et al.* The effects of gonadotrophin-releasing hormone agonists on iliac crest cancellous bone structure in women with endometriosis. *Bone* 1995;16:261–7

31. Bell KL, Loveridge N, Lindsay PC, *et al.* Cortical remodelling following suppression of endogenous estrogen with analogs of gonadotrophin releasing hormone. *J Bone Miner Res* 1997;12: 1231–40

32. Mellish RWE, Garrahan NJ, Compston JE. Age-related changes in trabecular width and spacing in human iliac crest biopsies. *Bone Miner* 1989;6: 331–8

33. Compston JE, Mellish RWE, Garrahan NJ. Age-related changes in iliac crest trabecular microanatomic bone structure in man. *Bone* 1987;8:289–92

34. Wakamatsu E, Sissons HA. The cancellous bone of the iliac crest. *Calcif Tissue Res* 1969;4:147–61

35. Aaron JE, Makins NB, Sagreiya K. The microanatomy of trabecular bone loss in normal ageing men and women. *Clin Orthop Rel Res* 1987;215:260–71

36. Weinstein RS, Hutson MS. Decreased trabecular width and increased trabecular spacing contribute to bone loss with aging. *Bone* 1987;8:127–42

37. Birkenhager-Frenkel DH, Courpron P, Hupscher EA, *et al.* Age-related changes in cancellous bone structure. A two-dimensional study in the transiliac and iliac crest biopsy sites. *Bone Miner* 1988;4:197–216

38. Riggs BL, Jowsey J, Goldsmith RS, *et al.* Short- and long-term effects of estrogen and synthetic anabolic hormone in postmenopausal osteoporosis. *J Clin Invest* 1972;51:1659–63

39. Steiniche T, Hasling C, Charles P, *et al.* A randomised study of the effects of estrogen/gestagen or high dose oral calcium on trabecular bone remodelling in postmenopausal osteoporosis. *Bone* 1989;10:313–20

40. Lufkin EG, Wahner HW, O'Fallon WM, *et al.* Treatment of postmenopausal osteoporosis with transdermal estrogen. *Ann Intern Med* 1992;117: 1–9

41. Holland EFN, Chow JWM, Studd JWW, *et al.* Histomorphometric changes in the skeleton of postmenopausal women with low bone mineral density treated with percutaneous implants. *Obstet Gynecol* 1994;83:387–91

42. Vedi S, Skingle SJ, Compston JE. The effects of long-term hormone replacement therapy on bone remodelling in postmenopausal women. *Bone* 1996;19:535–9

43. Vedi S, Croucher PI, Garrahan NJ, *et al.* Effects of hormone replacement therapy on cancellous bone microstructure in postmenopausal women. *Bone* 1996;19:69–72

44. Patel S, Pazianas M, Tobias J, *et al.* Early effects of hormone replacement therapy on bone. *Bone* 1999;24:245–8

45. Edwards MW, Bain SD, Bailey MC, *et al.* 17beta estradiol stimulation of endosteal bone formation in the ovariectomised mouse: an animal model for the evaluation of bone-targeted estrogens. *Bone* 1992;13:29–34

46. Tobias JH, Compston JE. Does estrogen stimulate osteoblast activity in postmenopausal women? *Bone* 1999;24:121–30

47. Savvas M, Studd JWW, Fogelman I, *et al.* Skeletal effects of oral oestrogen compared with subcutaneous oestrogen and testosterone in postmenopausal women. *Br Med J* 1988;297:331–31

48. Studd JWW, Savvas M, Fogelman I, *et al.* The relationship between plasma estradiol and the increase in bone density in women following treatment with subcutaneous hormone implants. *Am J Obstet Gynecol* 1990;163:1474–9

49. Garnett T, Studd J, Watson N, *et al.* A cross-sectional study of the effects of long-term percutaneous hormone replacement therapy on bone density. *Obstet Gynecol* 1991;78:1002–7

50. Ryde SJS, Bowen-Simpkins K, Bowen-Simpkins P, *et al.* The effect of oestradiol implants on regional and total bone mass: a three year longitudinal study. *Clin Endocrinol* 1994;40:33–8

51. Wahab M, Ballard P, Purdie DW, *et al.* The effect of long-term oestradiol implantation on bone mineral density in postmenopausal women who have undergone hysterectomy and bilateral oophorectomy. *Br J Obstet Gynaecol* 1997;104:728–31

52. Vedi S, Compston JE, Ballard P, *et al.* Bone remodelling and structure in postmenopausal women treated with long-term, high-dose oestrogen therapy. *Osteoporosis Int* 1999;10:52–8

53. Khastgir G, Studd J, Holland N, *et al.* Anabolic effect of estrogen in bone: histological evidence in a longitudinal follow-up study of women with established osteoporosis. *Bone* 1998;23:S495

54. Compston JE. Bone morphology: quality quantity and strength. In Shaw RW, ed. *Advances in Reproductive Endocrinology*, Vol. 8, *Oestrogen deficiency: causes and consequences*. Carnforth: Parthenon Publishing Group 1996:63–84

55. Compston JE. Bone physiology and the pathogenesis of osteoporosis. In: *Report on Osteoporosis in the European Community*. Luxembourg: European Commission, 1998:31–7

29

Bisphosphonates

J.-Y. Reginster, I. Paul, G. Fraikin and O. Bruyère

INTRODUCTION

The historical background of bisphosphonates, previously called diphosphonates, is closely linked to the history of inorganic pyrophosphates. Inorganic pyrophosphate is the simplest polyphosphate, a family of compounds characterized by the existence of at least one phosphorus–oxygen–phosphorus (POP) bridge. Polyphosphates prevent precipitation of calcium carbonate in solution, which is the main reason for their long-lasting marketing as additives that prevent calcium carbonate scaling in salt water[1]. Noticing the interest of the physicochemical properties of pyrophosphates, Russell and Fleisch, starting in 1970, searched for analogs that were stable *in vivo*, and resisted enzymatic hydrolysis: bisphosphonates, in which a stable phosphorus–carbon–phosphorus (PCP) bridge replaced the former POP bridge[2]. Bisphosphonates, *in vitro*, prevent the precipitation of calcium and phosphorus in solution, block transformation of amorphous calcium phosphates in hydroxyapatite and inhibit aggregation of hydroxyapatite crystals[3]. Bisphosphonates are extremely potent inhibitors of bone resorption[4]. They interfere with several stages of the osteoresorption process. Different mechanisms of action, acting simultaneously and synergistically, are likely to be involved, including an acute phenomenon, mainly physicochemical, and a cellular and/or biochemical effect, which has a longer latency[5]. The relative contribution of each of them depends on the nature of the respective bisphosphonate. The antiresorptive action of bisphosphonates has been widely used in human patients. Several bisphosphonates were tested in various clinical situations related to an increase of osteoclastic resorption, including Paget's disease of bone, tumor- and non-tumor-induced hypercalcemia, primary hyperthyroidism, osteoporosis of hypodynamism, glucocorticoid-induced osteoporosis, juvenile idiopathic osteoporosis, or primary involutional osteoporosis[6]. Postmenopausal osteoporosis is a disorder characterized by an increase in bone resorption relative to bone formation, consistently linked to an increased rate of bone turnover[7]. Therefore, it was logical to consider bisphosphonates, which are selective inhibitors of osteoclastic bone resorption, as a potential preventive and therapeutic approach to postmenopausal osteoporosis[8].

ETIDRONATE

Etidronate has been widely investigated as a monotherapy for postmenopausal osteoporosis given either continuously[9] or intermittently[10]. This bisphosphonate has already been used in several protocols based on the concept of a 'coherence therapy' of osteoporosis[11,12]. Discrepant outcomes resulted from the various therapeutic regimens[9,12,13]. Storm and colleagues[10], when giving etidronate intermittently, 400 mg/day for 14 days every 4 months over 3 years, to osteoporotic women, observed a significant increase (1.8% per year) in bone mineral density at the spine without any concomitant loss of cortical bone. Nevertheless, the rate of new vertebral fractures observed in the treated group during the 3 years of the trial was not significantly different to that observed in the control group (treated with the placebo). A separate analysis of the second and third years (excluding the first year) of treatment was the only way to show a significant ($p = 0.023$) reduction of the fracture incidence in the group treated with etidronate. In a multicenter North American trial[11] during which etidronate was administered after a similar regimen (400 mg/day for 14 days every 3 months for 2 years), although in half of the patients this was after the administration over 3 days of 1 g/day phosphorus, patients who received etidronate had a significant increase in spinal bone density (2.6% and 2.1%/year for etidronate/phosphorus and etidronate/ placebo, respectively) with no cortical loss. The incidence of new fractures was identical in the four groups involved in the trial (etidronate/ phosphorus, etidronate/placebo, phosphorus/ placebo, placebo/placebo). However, when pooling patients treated with etidronate, independent of their former intake of phosphorus, the authors reported a slightly significant reduction in the incidence of vertebral fractures ($p = 0.043$) compared with the two other therapeutic groups. The follow-up of this trial for another year revealed an increase in the rate of vertebral fractures in the group treated with etidronate. At the end of the global period of 3 years, there was no more significant difference in the overall population between patients treated with placebo and those treated with etidronate. A *post hoc* analysis revealed, however, that patients whose spinal bone mineral density was below the *50th* percentile of the distribution of bone mineral density in osteoporotic patients and who concomitantly had more than two prevalent fractures at the start of the trial (17% of the population) experienced a significant reduction in the rate of vertebral fractures when treated with etidronate compared with those treated with the placebo. These results suggested a plausible role for etidronate in the treatment of severe osteoporosis[14]. No effect of etidronate on non-vertebral fracture rates was demonstrated in a prospective

controlled trial. In a study collecting information from 550 general practices in the UK that provide a medical record to the general practice research database, a total of 7977 patients taking cyclical etidronate treatment and 7977 age- and practice-matched control patients with a diagnosis of osteoporosis were analyzed. People taking cyclical etidronate have a significantly reduced risk of non-vertebral fracture (by 20%) and of hip fracture (34%) relative to the osteoporosis control patients. Once fracture incidence rates were compared between the two groups, the rate of non-vertebral, hip and wrist fractures decreased significantly with increasing etidronate exposure[15]. Intermittent administration of etidronate at the previously mentioned doses for 2–3 years appears to be related to an increased prevalence of histological abnormalities, characterized by histological osteomalacia and mineralization impairments[16,17], but these abnormalities have not been shown to have clinical significance[16–18]. The absence of a relation between these histological changes and the clinical pattern of patients treated with cyclical etidronate is in accordance with further results which show normal histological features and an absence of and increase in vertebral fracture incidence when cyclical administration of etidronate was prolonged for 4 or 5 years[19,20].

In a subset of osteoporotic women treated for up to 7 years with cyclical etidronate, results from transiliac crest bone biopsy samples suggested that, after 3 years of treatment, bone turnover returned towards baseline levels whereas bone mineralization remained within normal limits by histological and histomorphometric assessment[21].

CLODRONATE

Clodronate has been exhaustively investigated and prescribed in several disorders characterized by enhanced bone resorption[22]. However, limited data are available concerning the use of this bisphosphonate in osteoporosis. Administration of intermittent oral clodronate (200–600 mg/day for 3 months followed by a similar washout period) to a small cohort of patients with osteoporosis yielded a significant increase in total body calcium (8%) after 20 months[23]. Oral clodronate (400 mg daily for 30 days every 3 months) with or without concomitant calcitriol was also associated with a significant increase in lumbar bone density (+3.88% and +3.21% respectively without and with calcitriol) after 12 months while untreated patients lost 2.34% of their spinal bone during the same period[24]. Monthly intravenous infusion of 200 mg clodronate to women with low lumbar bone mineral density, for 2 years, prevented further bone loss to a similar extent to transdermal 17β-estradiol (50 μg/24 hours)[25]. In a long-term study evaluating the effects of intravenous infusion of 200 mg of clodronate every 3 weeks for 6 years to osteoporotic patients (T-score < -2.5 for spinal bone mineral density), lumbar bone mineral density increased significantly and the upward trend persisted for all 6 years of therapy (5.69%) versus controls (-1.47%)[26]. In a subset of patients monitored for 3 years, clodronate was reported to reduce, borderline significantly ($p = 0.067$), the number of patients experiencing new vertebral fractures, while the total number of vertebral fractures was significantly reduced ($p = 0.0013$)[27]. However, studies evaluating the effect of clodronate in osteoporosis have been conducted either with too few patients or with inadequate methodology to convincingly demonstrate the efficacy of this bisphosphonate in postmenopausal osteoporosis.

AMINOBISPHOSPHONATES

Aminobisphosphonates currently developed and/or marketed for osteoporosis management mainly comprise pamidronate, alendronate, neridronate and ibandronate.

Pamidronate

Administration of 150 mg/day of pamidronate for 2 weeks was reported to normalize calcium balance while such a treatment given for up to 6.2 years (mean 3.7 years) was associated with a significant and sustained 3% annual increase in lumbar bone mineral density[28].

However, this study had major methodological flaws, precluding the drawing of any significant conclusions.

More recently, a similar regimen (150 mg/day continuously) was investigated in a prospective, double-blind, placebo-controlled study where 48 postmenopausal women with established osteoporosis were followed for 2 years. Significant increases in bone mineral density were observed in patients treated with pamidronate, for total body (+1.9%), lumbar spine (+7%) and femoral trochanter (+5.4%), while the significant decrease observed for the placebo group at the femoral neck and Ward's triangle did not occur in the pamidronate group. Vertebral fracture rates were non-significantly ($p = 0.07$) reduced in the pamidronate group[29].

However, the development of the oral form of pamidronate was jeopardized by the report of erosive esophagitis, which seems to be a common feature of all aminobisphosphonates[30], while its intravenous administration yielded only transient positive results in terms of bone mineral density[31].

Alendronate

Exhaustive preclinical assessment of alendronate evaluated the effects of this bisphosphonate on the biomechanical properties of the skeleton. Globally, results obtained both in rats[32] and baboons[33] concluded that alendronate significantly improves both bone mineral content and biomechanical resistance of trabecular and cortical bone.

In women in early postmenopause, 2.5 or 5 mg/day of alendronate prevented cortical and trabecular bone loss, over 2 years, in a similar way to conjugated equine estrogens (0.625 mg/day) and medroxyprogesterone acetate (5 mg/day) or 17β-estradiol (1–2 mg/day) and norethisterone acetate (0–1 mg/day). The 5 mg/day dose gave better results than the 2.5 mg/day dose at all measured sites including spine (+3.46% versus +2.28%), total hip (+1.85% versus +1.06%) and total body (+0.67% versus −0.03%)[34]. Dose-dependent effects of alendronate to reduce bone turnover and increase spinal bone mass were reported in postmenopausal women with low bone mineral density. In this population, the 10 mg/day dose, suggested to correspond to the best risk–benefit ratio for treatment of osteoporosis, induced significant increases in bone mineral density after 2 and 3 years[35,36]. In the 2-year study, mean changes in bone mineral density with 10 mg/day alendronate were +7.21% at the spine, +5.27% at total hip and +2.53% for total body, while biochemical markers of bone remodeling declined by about 50% after 3 months for resorption markers and 6 months for formation markers[35].

The 3-year study shows similar results with increases of 2.4%, 5.5% and 7.2% for lumbar spine, femoral neck and trochanter bone mineral density, respectively[36]. The results obtained from two studies where three doses of alendronate were given for 3 years (5 mg/day, 10 mg/day and 20 mg/day for 2 years followed by 5 mg/day for 1 year) to women with low bone mineral density (including a 20% subset with prevalent fractures) were pooled[37]. Compared to the placebo group, a significant reduction in the proportion of women with new vertebral fractures (3.2% versus 6.2%; $p = 0.03$) and a decreased progression of vertebral deformities (33% versus 41%; $p = 0.028$) were observed. Significant reduction of the relative risk (RR) of vertebral (RR = 0.54), hip (RR = 0.49), wrist (RR = 0.56) and all clinical fractures (RR = 0.72) was also reported in the Fracture Intervention Trial, among women who had low bone mineral density and vertebral fractures[38]. In women with low bone mineral density but without vertebral fracture, 4 years of alendronate safely increased bone mineral density and decreased the risk of vertebral deformity. This anti-fracture efficacy was only documented in women whose baseline bone mineral density T-score at the femoral neck was less than 2.5 standard deviations below the normal young adult mean[39].

Other aminobisphosphonates

Ibandronate is a new bisphosphonate which is 2, 10, 50 and 500 times more potent than risedronate, alendronate, pamidronate and clodronate, respectively, as inhibitor of the retinoid-induced bone resorption in the thyro-parathyroidectomized rat model[40]. Both oral and intravenous routes of administration of ibandronate have currently been investigated in postmenopausal osteoporosis. Continuous daily oral intake of 2.5 mg ibandronate for 12 months induced a recorded bone mineral density increase of 4.8% (spine), 2.0–3.3% (hip), 2.0% (total skeleton) and 0.9% (forearm)[41]. In a population with postmenopausal osteoporosis, intravenous ibandronate was investigated in a randomized, partly double-blinded, placebo-controlled study. Women received either a placebo or ibandronate (0.25, 0.5, 1, or 2 mg) every 3 months. Lumbar spine bone mineral density did not change in the placebo group, but increased by 2.4%, 3.5%, 3.7% and 5.2% at 12 months for dose-ranging groups. The increase was statistically significantly different from placebo for the 0.5 mg, 1 mg and 2 mg groups whereas with 0.25 mg no significant differences occurred. After 1 year, total hip and trochanter bone mineral density increased significantly by 1.8% and 2.9% for total hip and 2.7% and 4.2% for trochanter in the 1 and 2 mg groups, respectively. There was no significant difference in the overall number of adverse events in the ibandronate groups compared with the placebo group. Considering specific adverse events, no dose dependency or difference to placebo could be observed apart from acute reactions that occurred in 7% of the patients[42].

If these extremely promising results are confirmed, in terms of antifracture efficacy, intermittent parenteral administration of ibandronate should become a first-choice alternative to solve the problem linked to poor compliance or tolerance of oral medications of the bisphophonates family.

Neridronate was recently shown to suppress selectively peptide-bound deoxypyridinoline excretion in postmenopausal women with low bone mineral density[43]. Further investigations of the effects and mechanisms of action of this bisphosphonate are required and are in progress.

Tiludronate

Preclinical studies evaluating the effects of tiludronate on skeletal metabolism were of particular interest. They demonstrated a dose-dependent inhibition of osteoclastic resorption in several models of rodent[44] or non-rodent[45] mammals (in accordance with results obtained with other bisphosphonates) and they confirmed the harmlessness of this compound on the biomechanical resistance of trabecular and cortical bone[45]. The most original features of these investigations were the observation of an increase in the mineralization rate and an improvement of bone mechanical properties in a callus from dogs having been exposed to hemi-osteotomy of the ulna[46]. These results were in agreement with previous reports of the efficacy of tiludronate in Paget's disease of the bone[47,48] where the proportion of responders to tiludronate was twice as high as that for etidronate. Tiludronate, given for 6 months to healthy early postmenopausal women, prevented spinal bone loss for up to 12 months compared with women who received placebo for the same duration[49]. This early report was later confirmed in a multicenter trial where women treated with oral tiludronate 200 mg/day, continuously for 6 months, lost significantly ($p = 0.016$) less femoral bone after 18 months than those receiving a placebo (-1% versus -2.8%). Results at the level of the lumbar spine show a similar trend, borderline significant ($p = 0.065$)[50,51].

However, the results of two large, prospective, double-blind, randomized controlled trials, evaluating the effect of tiludronate in the treatment of established osteoporosis, including either women with low bone mineral density or with prevalent vertebral fractures, failed to demonstrate any significant anti-fracture effect. This negative conclusion is likely to be related to the use of a largely suboptimal dose of tiludronate, i.e. 200 mg daily for 7 days per month[52,53].

Risedronate

In rats, subcutaneous injection of risedronate 5 µg/kg/day significantly reduced histological parameters reflecting osteoclastic resorption without interaction with bone formation or mineralization[54]. Similarly, the biochemical properties of vertebrae and femoral neck obtained from dogs treated with risedronate for 2 years at doses from 0.2 mg/kg/day to 2 mg/kg/day were not significantly modified. In women with breast cancer and chemotherapy-induced menopause, risedronate was given intermittently (10–30 mg/day for 2 weeks every 3 months) for 2–3 years[55]. These doses of risedronate prevented the bone loss observed in the control population. A dose of 5 mg risedronate, given either continuously or intermittently (2 weeks of risedronate followed by 2 weeks of placebo) for 2 years was evaluated in early postmenopausal women with normal bone mass. At the end of the trial, a significant difference ($p < 0.0001$) appeared among the three groups in the evolution of lumbar spine bone mass. At the trochanteric level, bone mass increased ($+2.3\%$) in the group treated with the continuous regimen, was maintained ($+0.5\%$) with the intermittent regimen and decreased (-1%) in the placebo arm[56]. This effect was mediated by a decreased bone resorption, as confirmed by a drastic reduction in urinary deoxypyridinoline (-31% and -15% for continuous and intermittent risedronate regimen respectively)[56]. Paired bone biopsies obtained before and after 1 year of treatment revealed no signs of osteomalacia[57].

In severe osteoporosis (low bone mass and prevalent fractures), risedronate (two periods of 20 mg/day for 7 days each, followed by 14 days of calcium) decreased urinary excretion of collagen cross-links significantly by more than half and for up to 3 months[58]. Daily administration of 2.5 mg risedronate to osteoporotic women with prevalent spinal fractures at baseline resulted in a significant trend toward an increased bone mass at the spine and trochanter but no reduction of new vertebral fractures[59]. More recently, 3-year administration of risedronate (5 mg/day) to women with established postmenopausal osteoporosis (prevalent vertebral fractures and low bone mineral density) resulted in a significant decrease in the incidence of new vertebral fractures (risk reduction of 41–49%), with bone biopsy samples indicating that risedronate produced moderate (50%) suppression of bone turnover and that bone formed during risedronate treatment was of normal structure and mineralization[60-62].

However, since the prolonged use of risedronate in women with established osteoporosis was recently linked to a statistically significant increase in the occurrence of pulmonary cancer, the use of risedronate in the treatment of postmenopausal osteoporosis will have to be assessed on the basis of a large and extensive review of its risk–benefit ratio.

References

1. Fleisch H. *Bisphosphonates in Bone Disease. From the Laboratory to the Patient.* Carnforth: Parthenon Publishing, 1995

2. Russell RGG, Fleisch H. Inorganic pyrophosphate and pyrophosphatases in calcification and calcium homeostasis. *Clin Orthop* 1970;69: 101–7

3. Fleisch H. Diphosphonates: history and mechanisms of action. *Metab Bone Dis Rel Res* 1981;3: 279–88

4. Treschel U, Stutrer A, Fleisch H. Hypercalcaemia induced with an arotinoid in thyroparathyroidectomized rats. New model to study bone resorption in vivo. *J Clin Invest* 1986;80: 1979–86

5. Fleisch H. Experimental basis for the use of bisphosphonates in Paget's disease of bone. *Clin Orthop Rel Res* 1987;217:72–8

6. Reginster J-Y. *Ostéoporose Postménopausique. Traitement Prophylactique.* Paris: Masson, 1993.

7. Riggs BL, Melton LJ. Involution osteoporosis. *Am J Med* 1986;314:1676–84

8. Reginster J-Y. Les bisphosphonates constituent-ils un réel progrès thérapeutique dans l'ostéoporose? *Méd Hyg* 1996;54:1497–501

9. Heaney RP, Saville PD. Etidronate disodium in postmenopausal osteoporosis. *Clin Pharm Therap* 1976;20:593–604

10. Storm T, Thamsborg G, Steinich T, Genant HK, Sorense OH. Effect of intermittent cyclical etidronate therapy on bone mass and fracture rate in women with postmenopausal osteoporosis. *N Engl J Med,* 1990;322:1265–71

11. Watts NB, Harris ST, Genant HK, *et al.* Intermittent cyclical etidronate treatment of postmenopausal osteoporosis. *N Engl J Med* 1990;323:73–91

12. Pacifici R, MacMurtry C, Vered I, Rupich R, Avioli LV. Coherence therapy does not prevent axial bone loss in osteoporotic women: a preliminary comparative study. *J Clin Endocrinol Metab* 1988;66:747–53

13. Smith ML, Fogelman I, Hart DM, Scotte E, Bevan I, Leggate I. Effect of etidronate disodium on bone turnover following surgical menopause. *Calcif Tissue Int* 1989;44:74–9

14. Harris ST, Watts NB, Jackson RD *et al.* Four years of intermittent cyclical etidronate treatment of postmenopausal osteoporosis: Three years of blinded therapy followed by one year of open therapy. *Am J Med* 1993;95:557–67

15. Van Staa TP, Abenhaim L, Cooper C. Use of cyclical etidronate and prevention of non-vertebral fractures. *Br J Rheumatol* 1998;37:1253–4

16. Axelrod DW, Teitelbaum SL. Results of long-term cyclical etidronate therapy: bone histomorphometry and clinical correlates. *J Bone Miner Res* 1994;9S1:136S

17. Thomas T, Lafage MH, Alexandre C. Atypical osteomalacia after 2 years etidronate intermittent cyclic administration in osteoporosis. *J Rheum* 1995;22:11

18. Storm T, Thamsborg G, Kollerup G, Sorensen HA. Five years of intermittent cyclical etidronate therapy increases bone mass and reduces vertebral fracture rates in postmenopausal osteoporosis. *Bone Miner* 1992;17S1:24S

19. Jackson RD, Harris ST, Genant HK, *et al.* Cyclical etidronate treatment of postmenopausal osteoporosis: 4-year experience. *Bone Miner* 1992: 17S1:154

20. Miller P, Huffer W, MacIntyre D, *et al.* Bone histomorphometry after long-term treatment with cyclical phosphorus and etidronate. *Bone Miner* 1992;17S1:S23

21. Storm T, Sorensen HA, Thamsborg G, *et al.* Bone histomorphometric changes after up to seven years of cyclical etidronate treatment. *J Bone Miner Res* 1996;11S1:S151

22. Plosker GL, Goa KL. Clodronate. A review of its pharmacological properties and therapeutic efficacy in resorptive bone disease. *Drugs*, Adis International Limited, Auckland, New Zealand, 1994;47:945–82

23. Chesnut CH. Synthetic calcitonin, diphosphonates and anabolic steroids in the treatment of postmenopausal osteoporosis. In Christiansen C, Arnaud CD, Nordin BEC, *et al.*, eds. *Osteoporosis*. Copenhagen: Osteopress, 1984:594–655

24. Giannini S, D'Angelo A, Malvasi L, *et al.* Effects of one-year cyclical treatment with clodronate on postmenopausal bone loss. *Bone* 1993;14:137–41

25. Filipponi P, Pedetti M, Fedell L, *et al.* Cyclical clodronate is effective in preventing postmenopausal bone loss: a comparative study with transcutaneous hormone replacement therapy. *J Bone Miner Res* 1995;10:697–703

26. Filipponi P, Cristallini S, Rizello E, *et al.* Cyclical intravenous clodronate in postmenopausal osteoporosis: results of a long-term clinical trial. *Bone* 1996;18:179–84

27. Filipponi P, Cristallini S, Rizzello E, Policani G, Gregorio F, Boldrini S. 6-year cyclical intravenous clodronate in postmenopausal osteoporosis effect on bone mass and vertebral fractures. *Osteoporosis Int* 1996; 6:260

28. Valkema R, Vismans FJE, Papapoulos SE, Pauwels EKJ, Bijvoet OLM. Maintained improvement in calcium balance and bone mineral content in patients with osteoporosis treated with the bisphosphonate APD. *Bone Miner* 1989;5:183–92

29. Reid IR, Wattie DJ, Evans MC, Gamble GD, Stapleton JP, Cornish J. Continuous therapy with pamidronate, a potent bisphosphonate, in postmenopausal osteoporosis. *J Clin Endocrinol Metab* 1994;79:1595–9

30. Lufkin EG, Argueta R, Whitaker MD, *et al.* Pamidronate: an unrecognized problem in gastrointestinal tolerability. *Osteoporosis Int* 1994; 4:320–2

31. Devogelaer JP, Esselinckx W, Nagant de Deuxchaisnes CA. A randomized, controlled trial of APD (disodium pamidronate) given intravenously with and without sodium fluoride in involutional osteoporosis. *J Bone Miner Res* 1992;5:252S

32. Toolan BC, Shea M, Myers ER, *et al.* Effects of 4-amino-1-hydroxybutylidene bisphosphonate on bone biomechanisms in rats. *J Bone Miner Res* 1992;7:1399–406

33. Balena R, Toolan BC, Shea M, *et al.* The effects of 2-year treatment with the aminobisphosphonate alendronate on bone metabolism, bone histomorphometry, and bone strength in ovariectomized non human primates. *J Clin Invest* 1993; 92:2577–86

34. Hosking DJ, McClung MR, Ravn P, *et al.* Alendronate in the prevention of osteoporosis: EPIC study two-year results. *J Bone Miner Res* 1996;11:S133

35. Chesnut CH, McClung MR, Ensrud KE, *et al.* Alendronate treatment of the postmenopausal osteoporotic woman: effect of multiple dosages on bone mass and bone remodeling. *Am J Med* 1995;99:144–52

36. Devogelaer JP, Broll H, Correa-Rotter R, *et al.* Oral alendronate induces progressive increases in bone mass of the spine, hip, and total body over 3 years in postmenopausal women with osteoporosis. *Bone* 1996;18:141–50

37. Liberman U, Weiss SR, Broll J, *et al.* Effect of oral alendronate on bone mineral density and the incidence of fractures in postmenopausal osteoporosis. *N Engl J Med* 1995;333:1437–43

38. Black DM, Cummings SR, Thompson D. Alendronate reduces the risk of vertebral and clinical fractures in women with existing vertebral fractures: results of the fracture intervention trial. *Lancet* 1996;348:1535–41

39. Cummings SR, Black DM, Thompson EE, *et al.* Effect of alendronate on risk of fracture in women with low bone density but without vertebral fractures. *JAMA* 1998;280:2077–82

40. Muhlbauer RC, Bauss F, Schenk R, *et al.* Ibandronate, a potent new bisphosphonate to inhibit bone resorption. *J Bone Miner Res* 1991;6: 1003–11

41. Ravn P, Clemmesen B, Riis J, Christiansen C. The effect on bone mass and bone markers of different doses of ibandronate – a new bisphosphonate for prevention and treatment of postmenopausal osteoporosis. A 1-year, randomized, double-blind, placebo-controlled dose-finding study. *Osteoporosis Int* 1996;6:301.

42. Thiebaud D, Burckhardt P, Kriegbaum H, *et al.* Three monthly intravenous injections of ibandronate in the treatment of postmenopausal osteoporois. *Am J Med* 1997;103:298–307

43. Tobias JH, Laversuch CV, Wilson N, Robins P. Neridronate preferentially suppresses the urinary excretion of peptide-bound deoxypyridinoline in postmenopausal women. *Calcif Tiss Int* 1996;55:407–9

44. Ammann P, Rizzoli R, Caverzasio J, *et al.* Effects of the bisphosphonate tiludronate on bone resorption, calcium balance, and bone mineral density. *J Bone Miner Res* 1993;8:1491–8

45. Geusens P, Nijs J, Van der Perre G, *et al.* Longitudinal effect of tiludronate on bone mineral density, resonant frequency, and strength in monkeys. *J Bone Miner Res* 1992;7:599–609

46. Chastagnier D, Barbier A, de Vernejoul MC, Geusens P, Lacheretz F. Effects of two bisphosphonates (tiludronate and etidronate) on bone healing. *J Bone Miner Res* 1993;8:2365

47. Reginster J-Y, Colson F, Morlock G, Combe B, Ethgen D, Geusens P. Evaluation of the efficacy

and safety of oral tiludronate in Paget's disease of bone. A double-blind, multiple-dosage, placebo-controlled study. *Arthritis Rheum* 1992;35:967–74

48. Roux C, Gennari C, Farrerons J, *et al.* Comparative, prospective, double-blind, multicenter study of the efficacy of tiludronate and etidronate in Paget's disease of bone. *Arthritis Rheum* 1995;38:851–8

49. Reginster J-Y, Lecart MP, Deroisy R, *et al.* Prevention of postmenopausal bone loss by tiludronate. *Lancet* 1989;ii:1469–71

50. Roux C, Deroisy R, Basse-Cathalinat B, *et al.* Prevention of early postmenopausal bone loss with oral tiludronate. *Osteoporosis Int* 1996;6:(S1)–249

51. Chappard D, Miner P, Privat C, *et al.* Effects of tiludronate on bone loss in paraplegic patients. *J Bone Miner Res* 1995;10:112–8

52. Reginster J-Y, Roux C, Christiansen C, Rouillon A, Tou C. Intermittent cyclical low dose tiludronate in treatment of postmenopausal osteoporosis. Report of two phase III European studies (2305 patients). *Bone* 1998;23:S594

53. Genant HK, Chestnut CH, Eisman JA, *et al.* Chronic intermittent cyclical administration of tiludronate in postmenopausal osteoporosis: report of two multicenter studies in 2316 patients. *Bone* 1998;23:S175

54. Wronski TJ, Yen CF, Scott KS. Estrogen and disphosphonate treatment provide long-term protection against osteopenia in ovariectomized rats. *J Bone Miner Res* 1991;6:387–94

55. Ettinger B, Genant H, Bekker P, Shen I, Axelrod D. A pilot three-year of risedronate in women with breast cancer and chemotherapy-induced menopause. *J Bone Miner Res* 1995;10:(S1)S198

56. Mortensen L, Charles P, Bekker P, Digennaro J, Johnston C. Risedronate increases bone mass in an early postmenopausal population: two years of treatment plus one year of follow up. *J Clin Endocrinol Metab* 1998;83:396–402

57. Langdahl B, Eriksen EF, Mortensen L, Charles P, Bekker P, Axelrod D. Histomorphometry from a three-year risedronate bone loss prevention study. *J Bone Miner Res* 1995;10:S199

58. Zegels B, Balena R, Eastell R, Russell RGG, Pack SE, Reginster J-Y. Effect of risedronate on collagen cross links in postmenopausal osteoporosis. *J Bone Miner Res* 1995;10:S455

59. Clemmensen B, Ravin P, Zegels B, Taquet AN, Christiansen C, Reginster J-Y. A two-year phase II study with 1-year of follow-up of risedronate (NE58095) in postmenopausal osteoporosis. *Osteoporosis Int* 1997;7:488–95

60. Watts NI, Hangartner C, Chesnut C, *et al.* Risedronate treatment prevents vertebral and non-vertebral fractures in women with postmenopausal osteoporosis. *Calcif Tissue Int* 1999;(64)S98

61. Eastell R, Minner H, Sorensen O, *et al.* Risedronate reduces fracture risk in women with established postmenopausal osteoporosis. *Calcif Tissue Int* 1999;(64)S99

30

The role of initiating hormone replacement therapy to prevent and treat osteoporosis in the older postmenopausal woman

A. Vashisht, G. Khastgir and J. Studd

INTRODUCTION

Osteoporosis is characterized by an increased bone turnover, whereby bone resorption exceeds bone formation, leading to a progressive thinning of bone and increased susceptibility to fracture. This is a particular problem for menopausal women. Estrogen has been long proven as an effective treatment to combat postmenopausal bone loss[1–5]. Additionally, it has the benefits of controlling climacteric symptoms[6], improving cardiovascular health[7,8], urogenital complaints[9,10], mood disorders[11] and reducing the incidence of Alzheimer's disease[12,13]. Unfortunately, however, many women either do not start estrogen replacement therapy, or stop taking estrogen prematurely[14]. Certainly the incidence of hormone replacement therapy (HRT) use in the elderly is low[15]. Ironically, this is at a time when women are at most risk of sustaining an osteoporotic fracture. Many may fear initiating estrogen due to concern over breast cancer, or the unwanted recommencement of menses. Furthermore, physicians may mistakenly believe that osteoporosis is inevitable beyond a certain age or, even worse, that estrogen therapy is ineffective in the elderly.

INCIDENCE

The incidence of postmenopausal fracture increases with age[16–20]. Over the age of 60, 25% of white women have radiological evidence of vertebral crush fractures[21]. For a 50-year-old white woman the lifetime risk of sustaining a fracture has been estimated at 32% at the vertebra and 15.6% at the hip[22]. Fracture of the hip rises exponentially beyond the age of 50[20,23,24] (Figure 1). Within the first year of sustaining a fracture the mortality rate is between 20 and 40%[17,25]. Only 50% return to their pre-injury ambulatory or functional status[25,26]. The number of osteoporotic fractures is expected to rise appreciably over the next 50 years as a result of the increasing population growth and higher life expectancy[27]. Even accounting for an increase in the elderly population, a study in

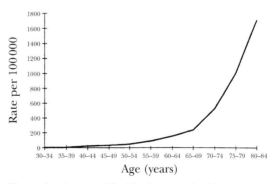

Figure 1 Age-specific hip fracture incidence rates for women by 5-year age intervals, National Hospital Discharge Survey, 1974–79. Adapted from reference 20

Oxford recorded a doubling in the cases of fracture of the proximal femur[19]. Recent estimates of cost calculations reveal the vast expenditure incurred. In the UK, the annual cost of fractures occurring in women over the age of 50 has been estimated at between £740 and £1000 million[28].

METABOLIC CHANGES IN THE ELDERLY

The elderly exhibit altered metabolic dynamics compared to the younger, even perimenopausal, woman. There is a rise in parathyroid hormone levels[29], decreased levels of vitamin D[30,31] and a decreased intestinal absorption of calcium[32,33]. These factors, coupled with years of postmenopausal bone loss, result in a considerably thinned and weakened bone[34], exposing the elderly as sitting ducks for an osteoporotic fracture.

ESTROGEN'S MECHANISM OF ACTION ON BONE

General effects

Numerous studies unequivocally show that estrogen therapy arrests early postmenopausal bone loss[1,35]. This manifests itself with a lowered fracture rate[2,36-39]. The precise mechanism by which estrogens act on osteoblasts and osteoclasts to protect the skeleton are unclear. It is known that there are receptors on osteoblasts, although reports of the effects of estrogen on cell proliferation and function are variable[40,41]. Estrogen treatment leads to an increased production of transforming growth factor-β by osteoclasts[42] which may induce osteoclast cell death and thus inhibit bone resorption[43]. Others have suggested alterations in the balance of cytokines[44]. In fact, the action of estrogen on bone may well be mediated via a large number of growth factors and cytokines; the relative contributions of each require further elucidation.

The bone remodelling cycle consists of bone resorption and formation. In osteoporosis, resorption outpaces formation. Cyclical estrogen/gestogen has been shown to decrease the activation frequency of remodelling cycles in trabecular bone to around 50% of the pretreatment value[45]. The activation of new remodelling cycles involves the perforation of the trabecular network which can impair bone strength and hence increase susceptibility to fracture. By reducing the frequency of these cycles, not only does estrogen improve bone mineral content, but also decreases the number of potentially dangerous perforations[45].

Prolonged therapy

The bone remodelling space is comprised of the amount of bone resorbed by the osteoclasts, but not yet formed by the osteoblasts. This represents around 6–8% of the skeletal volume[46]. It has been proposed that estrogen therapy will be most pronounced in the first year or two after treatment as this remodelling space is closed down, and that there is a finite time span for effective treatment. However, Garnett and colleagues, in a cross-sectional study, demonstrated that bone density apparently increased with duration of implant use up to 8 years[47]. In another cross-sectional study using low-dose estradiol implants, Naeseen and co-workers demonstrated even beyond 8 years the persistence of bone-preserving effects during long-term treatment (mean period of 16 years)[48] (Figure 2). Amongst the implant users, regression analysis revealed no significant relationship between age and bone mineral density, contrasting with non-users who showed an inverse relationship between age and bone mineral density. Furthermore, increases of a median 12.6% at the lumbar spine have been demonstrated using implant therapy[49], so clearly closing the bone remodelling space does not fully account for estrogen's role on the skeleton. Indeed, Khastgir and colleagues have shown histomorphometric evidence for an anabolic effect of estrogen, irrespective of the age at which therapy is commenced[50]. These findings all suggest that it is estrogen deficiency rather than age that is the predominant cause of bone loss after the menopause.

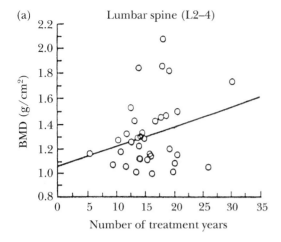

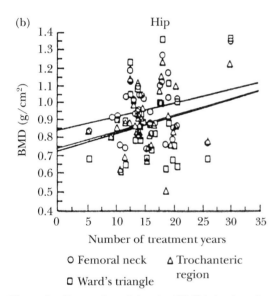

○ Femoral neck   △ Trochanteric
□ Ward's triangle   region

Figure 2   Bone mineral density (BMD), by duration of treatment (years) at the spine (a) and hip (b) in women with estradiol implants. Best-fit regression lines are shown. From reference 48

BONE LOSS AND THE ELDERLY

Early studies suggested that bone loss slows or arrests in the elderly[51–53]. Unfortunately, they involved small numbers of patients in older age groups, and did not take into account factors that confounded and frequently underestimated the rate of bone loss with age[23,54]. This gave rise to a perception that, beyond the age of 70, women had lost most of the bone they were going to lose. Estrogen was thought to be of little

benefit to them[18,55]. Larger-scale studies have shown that bone loss in fact continues, and that the inverse relationship between age and bone mass persists into the ninth decade[23,56–59].

Each standard deviation reduction in bone density correlates with a relative risk for fracture of about $2^{60–62}$. The value of bone density to predict non-spinal fractures remains even in the very elderly[63]. Since bone loss continues into late age, and bone mass remains a good predictor for fracture risk, it would suggest that active intervention in the elderly might be useful in lowering fracture rates.

ESTROGEN REPLACEMENT IN THE ELDERLY

One of the first prospective studies to evaluate the potential benefit of later initiation of estrogen was by Quigley and co-workers[51]. They found that women who had started estrogen therapy after the age of 65 had significantly greater protection against bone loss compared with never users. Others similarly concluded that starting estrogen treatment after the age of 60 did in fact lead to substantial increases in bone density[64–67]. Ettinger and Grady predicted the difference in bone density at the age of 85 between women who use estrogen continuously starting at the menopause or at 65 to be only between 2 and 6%[68]. Table 1 highlights the differences in bone density and subsequent osteoporotic fracture risk reduction in women who start estrogen therapy at the time of the menopause and continue its use lifelong, those who start at the menopause and stop at the age of 65, those who commence therapy at 65, and those who never start hormone replacement therapy. The risk reduction in osteoporotic fracture is most marked in the former group of women (73%), although women who initiate therapy at the age of 65 have almost as much protection (between 57 and 69% risk reduction, depending on whether the gain in bone mass at the time hormone therapy is started is 5% or 10%).

In another study, Lindsay and Tohme[69] looked at the effects of oral estrogen therapy in older females with established osteoporosis. The average age of the women in the treatment group was 62.3 years, and they were an average 14.6 years from the menopause. Vertebral bone mass increased significantly over the 2-year treatment course. The most pronounced increase in bone mass in response to estrogen intervention was noted in those women furthest from the menopause (and consequently with the lowest initial bone mass). The authors concluded that women with postmenopausal osteoporosis can benefit from the introduction of estrogen therapy at least up to 35 years after the menopause.

There tends to be a positive relationship between duration of estrogen use and subsequent bone density[70,71]. This is clinically manifested by a reduced fracture incidence[72,73]. Felson and colleagues[70] found the most significant benefits in terms of increased bone density were noted in those women who were younger than 75 years, and who had taken estrogen for 7 or more years. Even 10 or more years of estrogen use amongst women 75 years and older did not have a significant effect on bone density[70]. However, the majority of these women had stopped therapy many years previously, and this factor was not separately analyzed. This is an important omission, as studies that have differentiated past and current use have found very contrasting results[24,74].

Cauley and co-workers found, in a population of women 65 years and older, only current users of estrogen to have a reduced risk of non-spinal fractures[74]. In the Rancho Bernardo cohort[75], involving 740 women aged 60–98, women were stratified according to age at initiation of estrogen therapy and according to past or current use. There was no significant difference in bone mineral density between women who had commenced estrogen replacement at the time of the menopause, or at the age of 60. The most important factor in this study and others[71] is current estrogen use; past use provided little benefit for the preservation of bone density (Figure 3).

Many have suggested that, once a woman commences estrogen therapy, it should be continued indefinitely[51,55,75], since discontinuing

Table 1 Predicted difference in mean bone density and relative risk for fracture between ages 75 and 85 among women who never used estrogen (never users), those who used continuously, beginning at the menopause (always users), those who began use at menopause and stopped at age 65 (early users), and those who used continuously starting at age 65 (late users)[68]

	Difference in bone density (%)	Relative risk for osteoporotic fracture
Never users	0	1.0 (referent)
Always users	22	0.27
Early users	8	0.77
Late users		
5% gain	14	0.43
10% gain	19	0.31

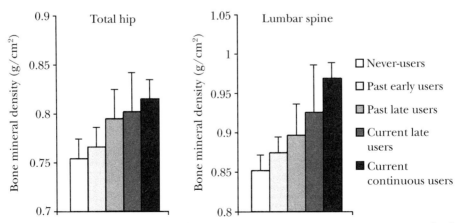

Figure 3 Mean bone mineral density (95% confidence interval) by estrogen use groups in the Rancho Bernardo Study. From reference 75

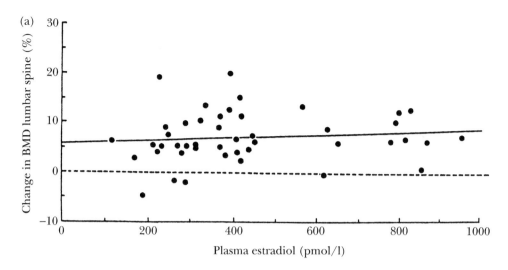

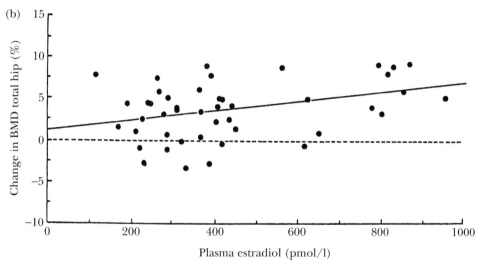

Figure 4 The relationship between post-treatment estradiol levels and the increase in bone mineral density (BMD) at the (a) lumbar spine ($r = 0.26$; $p < 0.05$) and (b) proximal hip ($r = 0.25$; $p < 0.05$). From reference 79

therapy leads to an accelerated bone loss[76,77]. Early postmenopausal use and subsequent premature discontinuation of estrogen thus may not be osteoprotective in later years. In women who have stopped estrogen therapy, bone mineral density has been shown to be inversely associated with the number of years since discontinuation of therapy[71,75].

ACHIEVING PHYSIOLOGICAL LEVELS OF ESTRADIOL IN THE OLDER WOMAN

The percutaneous route of estrogen administration avoids the enterohepatic circulation and is associated with physiological plasma levels of estradiol and estrone. High levels of treatment continuation can be achieved[48,49]; Studd and colleagues found significant correlations between the estradiol level and increased bone density[49,78,79] (Figure 4). Furthermore, the increases in bone density seen at the lumbar spine were greatest in older women furthest from the menopause[79].

Addressing the specific issue of implant therapy in an elderly population, Holland and co-workers[49] used 75 mg estradiol implants in 30 women who were 60 years and above, and who had an initial low bone mineral density.

After 1 year of treatment, they found a 12.6% median increase in lumbar spine bone density, and 5.2% at the hip. Histomorphometric analysis revealed a significant reduction in osteoid volume, osteoid surface and activation frequency[80]. After 6 years of implant therapy, there was a rise in cancellous bone volume, mean wall thickness, trabecular thickness and trabecular number, suggesting an anabolic effect of estrogen[50]. Neither the age nor the interval since menopause at the beginning of treatment influenced the histomorphometric variables.

PREVALENCE OF HRT USE IN THE ELDERLY

Few studies have looked at the prevalence of estrogen use in the elderly. In a population of community-dwelling women aged over 65, a 6.1% usage of estrogen was reported[15]. Women in the highest income group were over four times more likely to use estrogen than women in the lowest income group. Estrogen use was negatively associated with age, decreasing by 12% with each year of life. More worryingly, estrogen use was less likely amongst thinner women or women who smoked.

Cauley and colleagues reported a 13.7% current use of oral hormone replacement therapy in women 65 years and older. A diagnosis of osteoporosis was the major determinant of continued estrogen use, but only 24% of women with a diagnosis of osteoporosis used estrogen replacement therapy[81].

Increased awareness of the potential benefits of hormone replacement therapy improves the likelihood of starting therapy. More than three-quarters of women who initiated estrogen at the age of 60 or above agreed with the statement 'HRT can reduce the risk of fractures', compared with a fifth of women who did not initiate therapy[82].

COMPLIANCE

Compliance with taking estrogen is a recognized problem. Of those women prescribed HRT, 20–30% may never fill their prescription[14]. Only a small number of women continue therapy long enough to reap maximal gains. Even in at-risk groups, continuation rates may be low. Eight months after an initial diagnosis of a low bone mineral density, nearly 40% of postmenopausal women had stopped taking their medication[82]. Wallace and colleagues assessed the acceptability of oral hormone replacement therapy in women with established osteoporosis. In the over-60 age group, only 23% agreed to take estrogen[83]. The commonest reasons for older postmenopausal women stopping estrogen treatment, as with younger patients, are side-effects of therapy (principally bleeding) and fear of developing breast cancer[84–86].

The role of the physician is of primary importance in a woman's decision to start HRT[87,88] and the majority of never users report receiving no information about the beneficial effects of estrogen. In one study involving women 65 years and older, only 4.1% of never users of estrogen reported that their physicians had ever recommended estrogen therapy[84]. Initiators of HRT in an elderly population are much more likely to be aware of the potential osteoprotective benefits of estrogen. Those patients who receive little encouragement or information from their health-care providers are a lot less likely to start treatment[85].

In the elderly, it is particularly important that there is effective patient education and encouragement, since this group will not be receiving the immediate short-term benefits such as vasomotor symptom relief that estrogen may offer to the younger postmenopausal woman.

BLEEDING PROBLEMS

Continuous combined preparations

For many women, introduction of hormone replacement therapy implies the return of menstrual bleeding. This is one of the commonest reasons for women stopping estrogen[84,86]. Continuous combined preparations have been developed whereby the administration of a daily progestogen maintains an atrophic endometrium, preventing withdrawal bleeding and endometrial hyperplasia[89]. With continuous preparations, breakthrough bleeding is less common in women with a long-standing post-menopausal state[90,91]. In early postmenopausal women, compliance has been shown to improve[92]. In elderly women, 78–86% of women were taking their continuous combined preparation after 1 year[66,93]. Significant increases in lumbar spine and proximal femoral bone density were achieved using these regimens.

Tibolone

Tibolone (Org OD14) has been developed and introduced as an alternative synthetic steroid to estrogen. It is tissue specific and exhibits different estrogenic, progestogenic or androgenic activities dependent on the target end-organ[40]. It has no stimulatory effect on the endometrium and thus has the attraction of being a no-bleed preparation. Additionally, there is no requirement for progesterone and its associated side-effects. Tibolone exerts estrogenic activity on bone, effectively reducing bone resorption. It has been shown to increase bone mineral density up to 3 years[94,95]. Studd and colleagues evaluated the effect of tibolone and calcium 800 mg daily (treatment group) versus calcium alone (placebo group) on women with established osteoporosis. After 2 years, bone mineral density had increased by 6.9% in the former group, compared to 2.7% in the placebo group ($p < 0.01$). At the femoral neck, the increase in the treatment group was 4.5% versus 1.4% in the placebo group ($p < 0.05$)[96].

There are a few studies looking at tibolone in the older age group[97,98]. Bjarnason and co-workers evaluated 91 women who were greater than 10 years postmenopausal. Tibolone was found to significantly improve vertebral bone density by 5% over 2 years, compared with placebo. The gold standard by which all osteoporosis prevention drugs are judged is the reduction in fracture incidence. As yet, there is no data on this with tibolone, although it promises to be a useful treatment for the older postmenopausal woman.

BREAST CANCER

Compared with breast cancer, cardiovascular disease kills 12 times as many women, but most women fear breast cancer more[99]. The risk of breast cancer and the use of hormone replacement therapy has always been of concern to patients and clinicians alike. Some studies have highlighted an increased risk[100,101], which worsens with duration of use[100,102]. Others have revealed no increased risk[103,104], even for durations and latencies of 20 years or longer[105]. A recent collaborative re-analysis of data from 51 epidemiological studies concluded that the relative risk of having breast cancer diagnosed increased by a factor of 1.023 for each year of use[106] (Figure 5).

Whether or not womens' mortality from breast cancer is affected by estrogen therapy is not known. It does appear that women taking estrogen and who subsequently develop breast cancer may in fact have an improved prognosis relative to non-users of estrogen[107,108]. It is important that each patient is counselled about these potential risks and that they are

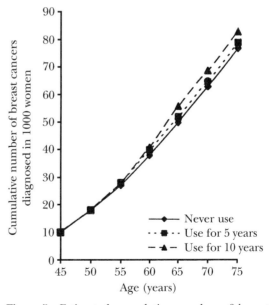

Figure 5 Estimated cumulative number of breast cancers diagnosed in 1000 never users of hormone replacement therapy (HRT), 1000 users of HRT for 5 years and 1000 users of HRT for 10 years. From reference 106)

weighed against the benefits that estrogen therapy provides against osteoporosis and cardiovascular disease. This will serve to improve compliance.

CONCLUSION

There is a great deal of uncertainty as to the optimum time to start or stop taking estrogen replacement therapy. What is certain is that bone loss continues for many years after the menopause and that estrogen is effective at combating this loss in both the younger and older postmenopausal woman. Far from estrogen therapy being useless in the elderly, they are perhaps the best beneficiaries. Debates will continue regarding the merits of deferring estrogen therapy until the later postmenopausal years, both in terms of cost-effectiveness[109,110] and reducing the morbidity of prolonged therapy. What is imperative is that estrogen is not forgotten as an important and effective treatment for the prevention of osteoporosis in the older woman.

References

1. Lindsay R, Hart DM, Forrest C, *et al*. Prevention of spinal osteoporosis in oophorectomised women. *Lancet* 1980:1151–4

2. Lufkin EG, Wahner HW, O'Fallon WM, *et al*. Treatment of postmenopausal osteoporosis with transdermal estrogen. *Ann Intern Med* 1992; 117:1–9

3. Lindsay R, Hart DM, Aitken JM, MacDonald EB, Anderson JB, Clarke AC. Long-term prevention of postmenopausal osteoporosis by oestrogen. *Lancet* 1976:1038–41

4. Munk-Jensen N, Nielsen SP, Obel EB, *et al*. Reversal of postmenopausal vertebral bone loss by oestrogen and progestogen: a double blind placebo controlled study. *Br Med J* 1988;296: 1150–2

5. Horsman A, Gallagher JC, Simpson M, *et al*. Prospective trial of oestrogen and calcium in postmenopausal women. *Br Med J* 1977;2: 789–92

6. Coope J, Thomson JM, Poller L. Effects of 'natural oestrogen' replacement therapy on menopausal symptoms and blood clotting. *Br Med J* 1975;4:139–43

7. Stampfer MJ, Colditz GA, Willett WC, *et al*. Postmenopausal estrogen therapy and cardiovascular disease. *N Engl J Med* 1991;325:756–62

8. Ross RK, Paganini-Hill A, Mack TM, *et al*. Menopausal oestrogen therapy and protection from death from ischaemic heart disease. *Lancet* 1981:858–60

9. Smith P, Heimer G, Lindskog M, *et al*. Oestradiol-releasing vaginal ring for treatment of postmenopausal urogenital atrophy. *Maturitas* 1993;16:145–54

10. Raz R, Stamm WE. A controlled trial of intravaginal estriol in postmenopausal women with recurrent urinary tract infections. *N Engl J Med* 1993;329:753–6

11. Zweifel JE, O'Brien WH. A meta-analysis of the effect of hormone replacement therapy upon depressed mood. *Psychoneuroendocrinology* 1997; 22:189–212

12. Tand MX, Jacobs D, Stern Y, *et al*. Effect of oestrogen during menopause on risk and age at onset of Alzheimer's disease. *Lancet* 1996;348: 429–32

13. Paganini-Hill A. Oestrogen replacement therapy and Alzheimer's disease. *Br J Obstet Gynaecol* 1996;103:80–6

14. Ravnikar VA. Compliance with hormone therapy. *Am J Obstet Gynecol* 1987;156:1332–4

15. Handa VL, Landerman R, Hanlon JT, *et al*. Do older women use estrogen replacement? Data from the Duke Established Populations for Epidemiologic Studies of the Elderly (EPESE). *J Am Geriatr Soc* 1996;44:1–6

16. Jensen GF, Christiansen C, Boesen J, *et al*. Epidemiology of postmenopausal spinal and long bone fractures. A unifying approach to postmenopausal osteoporosis. *Clin Orthop* 1982;166: 75–81

17. Evans JG, Prudham D, Wandless I. A prospective study of fractured proximal femur: incidence and outcome. *Public Health* 1979;93: 235–41

18. Riggs BL, Melton LJ. Involutional osteoporosis. *N Engl J Med* 1986;314:1676–86

19. Boyce WJ, Vessey MP. Rising incidence of fracture of the proximal femur. *Lancet* 1985;1: 150–1

20. Farmer ME, White LR, Brody JA, *et al.* Race and sex differences in hip fracture incidence. *Am J Public Health* 1984;74:1374–80

21. Stevenson JC, Whitehead MI. Postmenopausal osteoporosis. *Br Med J* 1982;285:585–8

22. Cummings SR, Black DM, Rubin SM. Lifetime risks of hip, Colles', or vertebral fracture and coronary heart disease among white postmenopausal women. *Arch Intern Med* 1989;149: 2445–8

23. Kanis JA. Treatment of osteoporosis in elderly women. *Am J Med* 1995;98(Suppl 2A):60S–66S

24. Kiel DP, Felson DT, Anderson JJ, *et al.* Hip fracture and the use of estrogens in postmenopausal women. *N Engl J Med* 1987;317:1169–74

25. Miller CW. Survival and ambulation following hip fracture. *J Bone Joint Surg* 1978;60A:930–3

26. Greendale GA, Barrett-Connor E, Ingles S, *et al.* Late physical and functional effects of osteoporotic fracture in women: the Rancho Bernardo Study. *J Am Geriatr Soc* 1995;43:955–61

27. Barrett-Connor E. The economic and human costs of osteoporotic fracture. *Am J Med* 1995; 98:2A3S–8S

28. Torgerson DJ, Iglesias CP. The economics and management of osteoporosis in postmenopausal women. *J Br Menopause Soc* 1999:67–71

29. Young G, Marcus R, Minkoff JR, *et al.* Age-related rise in parathyroid hormone in man: the use of intact and midmolecule antisera to distinguish hormone secretion from retention. *J Bone Miner Res* 1987;2:367–74

30. Omdahl LJ, Garry PJ, Hunsaker LA, *et al.* Nutritional status in a healthy elderly population: vitamin D. *Am J Clin Nutr* 1982;36:1225–33

31. Egsmose C, Lund B, McNair P, *et al.* Low serum levels of 25-hydroxyvitamin D and 1,25-dihydroxyvitamin D in institutionalized old people: influence of solar exposure and vitamin D supplementation. *Age Ageing* 1987;16: 35–40

32. Gallagher JC, Riggs BL, Eisman J, *et al.* Intestinal calcium absorption and serum vitamin D metabolites in normal subjects and osteoporotic patients: effect of age and dietary calcium. *J Clin Invest* 1979;64:729–36

33. Bullamore JR, Wilkinson R, Gallagher JC, *et al.* Effect of age on calcium absorption. *Lancet* 1970;2:535–7

34. Ruff CB, Hayes WC. Sex differences in age-related remodeling of the femur and tibia. *J Orthop Res* 1988;6:886–96

35. Hillard TC, Whitcroft SJ, Marsh MS, *et al.* Osteoporos Int* 1994;4:341–8

36. Hutchinson TA, Polansky SM, Feinstein AR. Post-menopausal oestrogens protect against fractures of hip and distal radius. *Lancet* 1979;705–9

37. Weiss NS, Ure CL, Ballard JH, *et al.* Decreased risk of fractures of the hip and lower forearm with postmenopausal use of estrogen. *N Engl J Med* 1980;303:1195–8

38. Ettinger B, Genant HK, Cann C. Long-term estrogen replacement therapy prevents bone loss and fractures. *Ann Intern Med* 1985;102: 319–24

39. Naessen T, Persson I, Adami H, *et al.* Hormone replacement therapy and the risk for first hip fracture. *Ann Intern Med* 1990;113:95–103

40. Ernst M, Heath JK, Rodan GA. Estradiol effects on proliferation, messenger ribonucleic acid for collagen and insulin-like growth factor-I, and parathyroid hormone-stimulated adenylate cyclase activity in osteoblastic cells from calvariae and long bones. *Endocrinology* 1989; 125:825–33

41. Keeting PE, Scott RE, Colvard DS, *et al.* Lack of a direct effect of estrogen on proliferation and differentiation of normal osteoblast-like cells. *J Bone Miner Res* 1991;6:297–304

42. Robinson JA, Riggs BL, Spelsberg TC, *et al.* Osteoclasts and transforming growth factor-β: estrogen-mediated isoform-specific regulation of production. *Endocrinology* 1996;137:615–21

43. Hughes DE, Dai A, TiHee JC, *et al.* Estrogen promotes apoptosis of murine osteoclasts mediated by TGF-β. *Nat Med* 1996;2:1132–6

44. Eastell R. Optimising the benefits of hormone replacement therapy for osteoporosis. *J Br Menopause Soc* 1999;S1:20–3

45. Steiniche T, Hasling C, Charles P, *et al.* A randomized study on the effects of estrogen/gestagen or high dose oral calcium on trabecular bone remodeling in postmenopausal osteoporosis. *Bone* 1989;10:313–20

46. Parfitt A. The physiological and clinical significances of bone histomorphometric data. In Recker RR, ed. *Bone Histomorphometry, Techniques and Interpretation*. Boca Raton, FL: CRC Press Inc., 1983:143–224

47. Garnett T, Studd J, Watson N, *et al.* A cross-sectional study of the effects of long-term percutaneous hormone replacement therapy on bone density. *Obstet Gynecol* 1991;78:1002–7

48. Naessen T, Persson I, Thor L, *et al.* Maintained bone density at advanced ages after long term treatment with low dose oestradiol implants. *Br J Obstet Gynaecol* 1993;100:454–9

49. Holland EFN, Leather AT, Studd JWW. Increase in bone mass of older postmenopausal women with low mineral bone density after one year of percutaneous oestradiol implants. *Br J Obstet Gynaecol* 1995;102:238–242

50. Khastgir G, Studd J, Holland N, *et al.* Histomorphometric evidence of an anabolic effect of oestrogen on bone in older postmenopausal women. *Br J Obstet Gynaecol* 1998;105 (Suppl 17):6

51. Quigley MET, Martin PL, Burnier AM, *et al.* Estrogen therapy arrests bone loss in elderly women. *Am J Obstet Gynecol* 1987;156:1516–23

52. Hui SL, Epstein S, Johnston CC Jr. A prospective study of bone mass in patients with type I diabetes. *J Clin Endocrinol Metab* 1985;60: 74–80

53. Riggs BL, Wahner HW, Melton LJ 3rd, *et al.* Rates of bone loss in the appendicular and axial skeletons of women. Evidence of substantial vertebral bone loss before menopause. *J Clin Invest* 1986;77:1487–91

54. Kanis JA, Adami S. Bone loss in the elderly. *Osteoporos Int* 1994;Suppl 1:S59–65

55. Resnick NM, Greenspan SL. 'Senile' osteoporosis reconsidered. *J Am Med Assoc* 1989;261: 1025–9

56. Steiger P, Cummings SR, Black DM, *et al.* Age-related decrements in bone mineral density in women over 65. *J Bone Miner Res* 1992;7:625–32

57. Looker AC, Johnston CC Jr, Wahner HW, *et al.* Prevalence of low femoral bone density in older US women from NHANES III. *J Bone Miner Res* 1995;10:796–802

58. Ensrud KE, Palermo L, Black DM, *et al.* Hip and calcaneal bone loss increase with advancing age: longitudinal results from the study of osteoporotic fractures. *J Bone Miner Res* 1995; 10:1778–87

59. Jones G, Nguyen T, Sambrook P, *et al.* Progressive loss of bone in the femoral neck in elderly people: longitudinal findings from the Dubbo osteoporosis epidemiology study. *Br Med J* 1994;309:691–5

60. Cummings SR, Black DM, Nevitt MC, *et al.* Bone density at various sites for prediction of hip fractures. *Lancet* 1993;341:72–5

61. Black DM, Cummings SR, Genant HT, *et al.* Axial and appendicular bone density predict fractures in older women. *J Bone Miner Res* 1992;7:633–8

62. Melton LJ, Atkinson EJ, O'Fallon WM, *et al.* Long-term fracture prediction by bone mineral assessed at different skeletal sites. *J Bone Miner Res* 1993;8:1227–33

63. Nevitt MC, Johnell O, Black DM, *et al.* Bone mineral density predicts non-spine fractures in very elderly women. *Osteoporos Int* 1994;4: 325–31

64. Villareal DT, Rupich RC, Pacifici R, *et al.* Effect of estrogen and calcitonin on vertebral bone density and vertebral height in osteoporotic women. *Osteoporos Int* 1992;2:70–3

65. Marx CW, Dailey GE, Cheney C, *et al.* Do estrogens improve bone mineral density in osteoporotic women over age 65? *J Bone Miner Res* 1992;7:1275–9

66. Christiansen C, Riis BJ. 17β-Estradiol and continuous norethisterone: a unique treatment for established osteoporosis in elderly women. *J Clin Endocrinol Metab* 1990;71:836–41

67. Jensen GF, Christiansen C, Transbol I. Treatment of post menopausal osteoporosis. A controlled therapeutic trial comparing oestrogen/ gestagen, 1,25-dihydroxy-vitamin D3 and calcium. *Clin Endocrinol* 1982;16:515–24

68. Ettinger B, Grady D. Maximizing the benefit of estrogen therapy for prevention of osteoporosis. *Menopause* 1994;1:19–24

69. Lindsay R, Tohme JF. Estrogen treatment of patients with established postmenopausal osteoporosis. *Obstet Gynecol* 1990;76:290–5

70. Felson DT, Zhang Y, Hannan MT, *et al.* The effect of postmenopausal estrogen therapy on bone density in elderly women. *N Engl J Med* 1993;329:1141–6

71. Orwoll ES, Bauer DC, Vogt TM, *et al.* Axial bone mass in older women. *Ann Intern Med* 1996;124: 187–96

72. Paganini-Hill A, Ross RK, Gerkins VR, *et al.* Menopausal estrogen therapy and hip fractures. *Ann Intern Med* 1981;95:28–31

73. Kanis JA, Johnell O, Gullberg B, *et al.* Evidence for efficacy of drugs affecting bone metabolism in preventing hip fracture. *Br Med J* 1992;305: 1124–8

74. Cauley JA, Seeley DG, Ensrud K, *et al.* Estrogen replacement therapy and fractures in older women. *Ann Intern Med* 1995;122:9–16

75. Schneider DL, Barrett-Connor EL, Morton DJ. Timing of postmenopausal estrogen for optimal bone mineral density. The Rancho Bernardo Study. *J Am Med Assoc* 1997;227:543–7

76. Christiansen C, Christensen MS, Transbol I. Bone mass in postmenopausal women after withdrawal of oestrogen/gestagen replacement therapy. *Lancet* 1981;459–61

77. Lindsay R, Hart DM, MacLean A, *et al.* Bone response to termination of oestrogen treatment. *Lancet* 1978; :1325–7

78. Studd J, Savvas M, Watson N, *et al.* The relationship between plasma estradiol and the increase in bone density in postmenopausal women after treatment with subcutaneous hormone implants. *Am J Obstet Gynecol* 1990;163:1474–9

79. Studd JWW, Holland EFN, Leather AT, *et al.* The dose-response of percutaneous oestradiol implants on the skeletons of postmenopausal women. *Br J Obstet Gynaecol* 1994;101:787–91

80. Holland EFN, Chow JWM, Studd JWW, *et al.* Histomorphometric changes in the skeleton of postmenopausal women with low bone mineral

density treated with percutaneous estradiol implants. *Obstet Gynecol* 1994;83:387–91

81. Cauley JA, Cummings SR, Black DM, *et al.* Prevalence and determinants of estrogen replacement therapy in older women. *Am J Obstet Gynecol* 1990;163:1438–44

82. Ryan PJ, Harrison R, Blake GM, *et al.* Compliance with hormone replacement therapy (HRT) after screening for post menopausal osteoporosis. *Br J Obstet Gynaecol* 1992;99:325–8

83. Wallace WA, Price VH, Elliot CA, *et al.* Hormone replacement therapy acceptability to Nottingham post-menopausal women with a risk factor for osteoporosis. *J R Soc Med* 1990;83:699–701

84. Salamone LM, Pressman AR, Seeley DG, *et al.* Estrogen replacement therapy: a survey of older women's attitudes. *Arch Intern Med* 1996;156:1293–7

85. Leveille SG, LaCroix AZ, Newton KM, *et al.* Older women and hormone replacement therapy: factors influencing late life initiation. *J Am Geriatr Soc* 1997;45:1496–500

86. Newton KM, LaCroix AZ, Leveille SG, *et al.* Women's beliefs and decisions about hormone replacement therapy. *J Women's Health* 1997;6:459–65

87. Newton KM, LaCroix AZ, Leveille SG, *et al.* The physician's role in women's decision making about hormone replacement therapy. *Obstet Gynecol* 1998;92:580–4

88. Wren BG, Brown L. Compliance with hormonal replacement therapy. *Maturitas* 1991;13:17–21

89. Sporrong T, Hellgren M, Samsioe G, *et al.* Comparison of four continuously administered progestogen plus oestradiol combinations for climacteric complaints. *Br J Obstet Gynaecol* 1988;95:1042–8

90. Rozenberg S, Ylikorkala O, Arrenbrecht S. Comparison of continuous and sequential transdermal progestogen with sequential oral progestogen in postmenopausal women using continuous transdermal estrogen: vasomotor symptoms, bleeding patterns, and serum lipids. *Int J Fertil* 1997;42(Suppl 2):376–87

91. Archer DF, Pickar JH, Bottiglioni. Bleeding patterns in postmenopausal women taking continuous combined or sequential regimens of conjugated estrogens with medroxyprogesterone acetate. *Obstet Gynecol* 1994;83:686–92

92. Marslew U, Riis BJ, Christiansen C. Bleeding patterns during continuous combined estrogen–progestogen therapy. *Am J Obstet Gynecol* 1991;164:1163–8

93. Grey AB, Cundy TF, Reid IR. Continuous combined oestrogen/progestin therapy is well tolerated and increases bone density at the hip and spine in post-menopausal osteoporosis. *Clin Endocrinol* 1994;40:671–7

94. Rymer J, Chapman MG, Fogelman I. Effect of tibolone on postmenopausal bone loss. *Osteoporos Int* 1994;4:314–19

95. Prelevic GM, Bartram C, Wood J, *et al.* Comparative effects on bone mineral density of tibolone, transdermal estrogen and oral estrogen/progestogen therapy in postmenopausal women. *Gynecol Endocrinol* 1996;10:413–20

96. Studd J, Arnala I, Kicovic PM, *et al.* A randomized study of tibolone on bone mineral density in osteoporotic postmenopausal women with previous fractures. *Obstet Gynecol* 1998;92:574–9

97. Bjarnason NH, Bjarnason K, Hassager C, *et al.* The response in spinal bone mass to tibolone treatment is related to bone turnover in elderly women. *Bone* 1997;20:151–5

98. Geusens P, Dequeker J, Gielen J, *et al.* Nonlinear increase in vertebral density induced by a synthetic steroid (Org OD14) in women with established osteoporosis. *Maturitas* 1991;13:155–62

99. Langer RD, Barrett-Connor E. Extended hormone replacement: who should get it, and for how long? *Geriatrics* 1994;49:20–9

100. Colditz GA, Hankinson SE, Hunter DJ, *et al.* The use of estrogens and progestins and the risk of breast cancer in postmenopausal women. *N Engl J Med* 1995;332:1589–93

101. Ross RK, Paganini-Hill A, Gerkins VR, *et al.* A case–control study of menopausal estrogen therapy and breast cancer. *J Am Med Assoc* 1980;243:1635–9

102. Bergkvist L, Adami HO, Persson I, *et al.* The risk of breast cancer after estrogen and estrogen–progestin replacement. *N Engl J Med* 1989;321:293–7

103. Dupont WD, Page DL. Menopausal estrogen replacement therapy and breast cancer. *Arch Intern Med* 1991;151:67–72

104. Kaufman SW, Miller DR, Rosenberg L, *et al.* Noncontraceptive estrogen use and the risk of breast cancer. *J Am Med Assoc* 1984;252:63–7

105. Wingo PA, Layde PM, Lee NC, *et al.* The risk of breast cancer in postmenopausal women who have used estrogen replacement therapy. *J Am Med Assoc* 1987;257:209–15

106. Collaborative Group on Hormonal Factors in Breast Cancer. Breast cancer and hormone replacement therapy: collaborative reanalysis of data from 51 epidemiological studies of 52 705 women with breast cancer and 108 411 women without breast cancer. *Lancet* 1997;350:1047–59

107. Hunt K, Vessey M, McPherson K, *et al.* Long-term surveillance of mortality and cancer incidence in women receiving hormone replacement therapy. *Br J Obstet Gynaecol* 1987;94:620–35

108. Bergkvist L, Adami HO, Persson I, *et al.* Prognosis after breast cancer diagnosis in women exposed to estrogen and estrogen–progestogen replacement therapy. *Am J Epidemiol* 1989;130: 221–8

109. Jonsson B, Christiansen C, Johnell O, *et al.* Cost-effectiveness of fracture prevention in established osteoporosis. *Osteoporos Int* 1995;5: 136–42

110. Chrischilles E, Shireman T, Wallace R. Costs and health effects of osteoporotic fractures. *Bone* 1994;15:377–86

31

Estrogens and the cardiovascular system in the over 60s

A. Pines

INTRODUCTION

Coronary artery disease (CAD) is the primary cause of death in women after the age of 60. A 50-year-old woman has about a 50% lifetime probability of developing heart disease, and about a 30% probability of dying from it. The graph of CAD mortality by age in men and women is very similar; however, there is a lag between the sexes with a delayed rise in deaths from CAD in women. The highest numbers of death in women are recorded between the ages of 75 and 85 years, as opposed to 65–80 years in men[1]. It is important to remember that, in all age categories, CAD in women carries a worse prognosis compared to men, especially in diabetics[2]. Thus, it stands to reason that preventive measures to reduce the risk for CAD should be implemented in women just as they are in men[2,3]. In addition to the well-known recommendations to stop smoking, eat a balanced diet, lower cholesterol level, treat hypertension or diabetes mellitus, and keep physically fit, there is now a growing interest in learning and understanding the advantages of hormone replacement therapy (HRT) as a powerful cardioprotective modality for postmenopausal women. Many studies, mainly observational, have shown that the prolonged use of HRT is associated with a 30–50% decrease in CAD morbidity and mortality[4]. This multifactorial protective effect is probably the result of favorable alterations in the CAD risk factor profile through various vascular and metabolic mechanisms primarily involving estrogen receptor activation and changes in gene expression[5,6]. Estrogens have antiatherosclerosis, antiischemic and antioxidant properties. These include changes in the concentrations of high- and low-density cholesterol, lipoprotein(a), plasminogen activator inhibitor-1, fibrinogen, homocysteine and insulin. They play a role in cardiac and vascular reactivity through calcium channel blocking and inhibition of angiotensin converting enzyme as well as influencing nitric oxide synthase, prostacyclins, endothelin and other vasoactive mediators. Due to some detrimental health events, which may be related to long-term hormone use, the question arises as to who would be the best candidates for HRT and what would be the best timing for HRT to achieve maximal benefits from the treatment. This risk-to-benefit equation has become a major item, discussed in recent overviews on menopause[7,8], with a focus on the important issue of assessing this equation in the elderly.

USE OF HRT IN THE ELDERLY POPULATION

A random-digit telephone survey in the USA showed that 38% of women aged 50–75 years were current users of HRT[9]. The rates of use were inversely correlated with age: 47% for those in their 50s, 32% for those in their 60s and

23% for women aged 70–74. The overall rate in hysterectomized women was 58%, in contrast with merely 19% in women with an intact uterus. In another US telephone survey among members of a health maintenance organization in Seattle aged 65–80, 10% said they had begun taking HRT at an age of 60 years or older[10]. Sixty-two per cent of past or never users claimed that they had received no information about the benefits of HRT from their health-care providers, compared with 18% of those starting HRT beyond age 60. HRT initiation was associated with the women's belief in the prevention benefits of HRT for fractures and cardiovascular disease and with reported encouragement from their physician to use HRT.

Discussion of HRT in the aged is problematic for several practical reasons. HRT is infrequently started in this age group, and the level of adherence to HRT, which means using HRT constantly for more than 5–10 years, is poor, so there are relatively few women who continue to take HRT beyond the age of 65 or 70 years. For example, a community study in North Carolina showed that only 6% of women aged over 65 years were taking hormones, although 19% reported past use[11]. In another cohort followed from the age of 58 years to 81 years, only 7% of hormone users were still taking estrogen by the end of follow-up[12]. Compliance was also found to be poor in the multicenter Study of Osteoporotic Fractures: current use of hormones declined sharply with age from 17% at 65 years of age to 4% at ages after 85[13]. The main reasons for stopping the medications were the feeling that it was not needed (31%), undesirable side-effects (16%) and a second opinion from another physician (13%). As a result, there are still unsatisfactory cardiovascular data on the protective effects of HRT in the old, with regard to both primary and secondary prevention of CAD[14].

PRIMARY PREVENTION OF CAD BY HRT IN THE ELDERLY

The results of selected studies on primary prevention of CAD by HRT are shown in Table 1. The largest published series on primary prevention was the Nurses' Health Study in the United States, in which 60 000 postmenopausal women participated[15]. The relative risk of a major coronary event over a 16-year follow-up period was 0.6 for estrogen users and 0.4 for combined estrogen– progestogen users as compared to never users. The relative risk for stroke was not

Table 1 Selected studies on primary prevention of coronary artery disease by HRT

Source	Age characteristics	Follow-up (years)	Relative risk versus non-users
Nurses' Health Study[15]	mean 58 years; maximal age at study termination 71 years	16	0.6 for coronary event in current users
Kaiser Permanente Medical Care Group[16]	mean 78 years at study termination	17	0.4 for death due to CAD in ever users
World Leisure Study[18]	mean 73 years at beginning of study	7.5	0.6 for death due to MI in ever users
Lipid Research Clinics Program Follow-up Study[20]	study included a 70–79 year category	8.5	0.5 for cardiovascular mortality in women using HRT at baseline
Uppsala study[21]	17% above age 60 at beginning of study	5.8	0.25 for first acute MI in ever users
Turku study[22]	mean 60 years at beginning of study	7	0.21 for cardiovascular death in current users
Kaiser Permanente Medical Care Group[16]	mean 64 years	retrospective analysis in women with MI	0.96 for acute MI in current users
Group Health Cooperative of Puget Sound[17]	mean 68 years, maximum 79 years	retrospective analysis in women with MI	0.7 for acute MI in current users

MI, myocardial infarction

changed by HRT use. The mean age of users was 58 years, and the oldest woman at the end of follow-up was only 71 years old. The beneficial effects of HRT for women older than 60 years were similar to those in younger women. The highest benefit was recorded in women with several risk factors for CAD, whereas healthy persons with the lowest risk profile demonstrated a relative risk for cardiac events that was much closer to 1. Another study from the United States described the results of hormone use for a mean duration of 17 years (minimum 5 years) in women with a mean age of 78 years at study termination[16]. The relative risk for death due to CAD in ever users as compared to never users was 0.4. Interestingly, a recent retrospective case–control study from the same healthcare provider looked at women hospitalized for acute myocardial infarction[17]. There was no decrease in the odds ratio for myocardial infarction associated with current use of HRT. These results are in contrast with those of Psaty and colleagues from Seattle[18]. They conducted a case–control study on a series of women aged up to 79 years (mean 68 years) who sustained a fatal or non-fatal myocardial infarction. The risk ratio for myocardial infarction associated with current hormone use was 0.69. In the World Leisure Study[19], investigators looked at mortality in a community in southern California. The median age at the beginning of the study was 73 years, and mean follow-up period was 7.5 years. All-cause mortality was 20% lower in estrogen ever users compared to never users. The relative risk for death as a result of acute myocardial infarction in ever users was 0.6 and a treatment period of more than 15 years was associated with a relative risk of 0.5. Very similar results were obtained in the Lipid Research Clinics Program[20], where estrogen users, including a group aged 70–79 years, had half the cardiovascular mortality of non-users during 8.5 years of follow-up. The data presented above were derived from US-based studies (the prescribed estrogen mainly being the conjugated equine form), but European studies (where estradiol is the common preparation) seemed to conform with those results. Of the 23 000 women who were included in a Swedish cohort

from Uppsala, about 17% were older than 60 years. During a follow-up period of 5.8 years, the relative risk for first acute myocardial infarction was 0.25 as compared to the expected rate in the general population[21]. A recent study from Turku, Finland, on 8000 postmenopausal women with a mean age of 60 years and follow-up of 7 years, concluded that current use of estrogen was associated with a decrease in cardiovascular mortality by 79%[22]. Interestingly, women at higher risk for CAD showed the largest benefit from treatment, the same as was found earlier in the Nurses' Health Study[23]. Calculating the individual risk for CAD thus becomes a potential key point to be considered prior to starting prophylactic HRT.

A less optimistic view was expressed recently in a study by Hemminki and McPherson[24]. From the literature, they randomly chose 22 controlled trials that had examined short-term outcomes of HRT other than cardiovascular events and cancer. They analyzed the adverse events reported in those studies. The cumulative results showed that there were fewer women with cardiovascular and thromboembolic events in the groups that did not receive HRT than in those that did, but the 95% confidence interval included 1. Although the article questioned the statistical significance of its results, it concluded that the pooled data did not support the notion that postmenopausal HRT prevents cardiovascular events. Nevertheless, most of the available data on the primary cardioprotection of HRT are so far encouraging, but we still await a well-designed, prospective, double-blind, placebo-controlled, long-term study on the primary prevention of CAD. The Women's Health Initiative, sponsored by the National Institutes of Health, is planned to end in 2006. It is expected to collect valuable information on this issue: 27 500 women will be studied, the follow-up will last for 9 years, two-thirds of the cohort will be 60–80 years old, and the primary end-points are morbidity and mortality from CAD.

As mentioned earlier, determining the risk profile for CAD in older women prior to HRT is important, and the influence of HRT on the risk profile in these women has to be clarified.

Unfortunately, data are lacking in this regard. The Cardiovascular Health Study examined 3000 women over 65 years of age, looking at risk factors for CAD and stroke in present, past and never users of estrogen[25]. The results resembled those found in younger women, namely, an improvement among the hormone users for all variables: better lipid profile, lower fibrinogen, factor 7 and insulin, decreased left ventricular mass, thinner carotid artery walls, fewer carotid stenoses, etc. Stratification by age showed the same effects for women aged 65–74 years and for those older than 75 years.

SECONDARY PREVENTION OF CAD BY HRT IN THE ELDERLY

A far more important issue is the effects of hormones in already established CAD. *In vitro* and *in vivo* studies showed that estrogen is capable of restoring the arterial wall and endothelial function in atherosclerotic vessels through its effect on the nitric oxide pathway, prostacyclins, endothelin and other mediators[26]. Moreover, estrogens retard the development of arterial atherosclerotic lesions. Small-scale angiographic studies showed that, at the time of the procedure, HRT use was associated with a reduced degree of coronary artery stenosis[27,28]. Several prospective studies demonstrated a better prognosis for hormone users with established CAD. Newton and colleagues examined a cohort (mean age 66 years) that was followed over a period of at least 3 years after surviving an acute myocardial infarction[29]. The odds ratios associated with current hormone use were 0.64 for reinfarction and 0.5 for all-cause mortality. A 10-year follow-up study by Sullivan and colleagues on women with angiographically proven coronary atherosclerosis at baseline showed better survival for hormone ever users, especially in cases with more severe coronary disease[30]. Women were almost 70 years old at study termination. The odds ratio associated with death reached a low value of 0.16. The same investigators also looked at survival after coronary artery bypass grafting[31]. Again, a beneficial effect of estrogen was documented;

however, the women were only 60 years old at the end of follow-up. Another study, by O'Keefe and co-workers[32], examined the consequences of coronary angioplasty in women with a mean age of 62 years at baseline. As expected, cardiovascular events (mortality or reinfarction) occurred less frequently in women using hormones over 7 years of follow-up (relative risk 0.38).

As already mentioned earlier in association with primary prevention, definitive answers on secondary prevention by HRT should be based on double-blind, placebo-controlled studies. One such investigation recently published its data[33]: the Heart and Estrogen/Progestin Replacement Study (HERS), which started in the United States in 1993. The study enrolled 2763 postmenopausal women younger than 80 years of age (mean 67 years) who had documented CAD. Women were randomly allocated into hormone (Premarin 0.625 mg plus medroxyprogesterone acetate 2.5 mg daily) or placebo treatment for a 5-year follow-up. The results of the study were surprising: there was no overall difference between HRT and placebo groups in cardiac and total mortality, nor in the incidence of myocardial infarction and stroke, despite a decrease in low-density lipoprotein cholesterol and an increase in high-density lipoprotein cholesterol in the hormone users. However, there was a significant time trend, with more cardiac events during the first year in the HRT group, but fewer events in years 4 and 5, as compared to placebo. In addition, the HRT group suffered more venous thromboembolic events, but there was no increase in the breast cancer incidence. Methodology issues clearly have utmost importance while planning and also on the later interpretation of the results of such a complex study. Indeed, there were eventually several major differences between assumptions and actual findings: there was a lower than expected cardiac event rate (3.3%/year versus 5% anticipated), the average follow-up was 4.1 years instead of 4.8 years, and there was a high drop-out rate of 18% in the first year rather than 5% as anticipated. All these facts should be taken into consideration prior to drawing conclusions from the HERS study because of its impact on the power of calculations. Doubts were also raised as to how representative the HERS cohort was of the general population of postmenopausal women with CAD. One article that compared the cohort of the NHANES III study with that of the HERS study showed that there were significant differences between the characteristics of the two cohorts[34]. There was also a lot of discussion over the issue of the study medication, which was actually a new preparation never tested in epidemiological studies before. It was a continuous combined formulation with conjugated equine estrogen and medroxyprogesterone acetate, the popular types of estrogen and progesterone used in the USA. However, medroxyprogesterone acetate is considered to have a relatively 'unfriendly' metabolic and cardiovascular profile, which also might have had an impact on event rate and prognosis. These data from the HERS study have opened a debate over the issue of whether or not long-term hormone replacement – as a prophylactic treatment for heart disease – is really advisable in the more elderly population with CAD. Should one be more cautious now in recommending HRT, or just attribute the 'bad' results to methodological flaws already detected in the HERS study? Or perhaps the specific continuous combined hormonal regimen is to be blamed and should be abandoned? So unfortunately, although we have at hand the results of a good quality secondary prevention trial in elderly women, we cannot be satisfied with what we have. Interestingly, in the 1999 annual meeting of the American College of Cardiology, researchers from Duke University looked at the incidence of post-myocardial infarction cardiac events in relation to use of HRT[35]. Thirty-seven per cent of 126 women who started HRT after the heart attack were re-hospitalized within 1 year for unstable angina (RR = 1.96), in contrast with only 17% of 1316 women never using hormones, or 21% among 411 women using HRT prior to and after their heart attack. However, mortality rates in the three groups were 0%, 4% and 1%, respectively.

CONCLUSIONS

Data so far encourage the use of HRT for primary prevention of CAD in postmenopausal women. As for secondary prevention, there might be some ill effects of HRT during the initial phase of therapy in women with established CAD. This stresses the need for implementing all other preventive measures, such as aspirin, beta-blockers, vitamin E and folic acid. A change in lifestyle is also mandatory, with cessation of smoking, watching the diet and keeping a desirable level of physical activity. A recent consensus panel statement on preventive cardiology for women, endorsed by the American Medical Women's Association, the American College of Nurse Practitioners, the American College of Obstetricians and Gynecologists and the Canadian Cardiovascular Society, addressed the issue of cardioprotection by HRT in the 'post-HERS study' era[36]. The panel's recommendations were that all women should be counselled about the potential benefits and risks of HRT, taking into consideration the individual cardiovascular risk parameters, as well as the risk of osteoporosis, breast cancer and thromboembolic disease. Indeed, it seems that individualization of treatment, based on past history and current medical status, will become the Millennium key words for hormone therapy. Therefore, suitable algorithms must be developed for the assessment of the risk–benefit equation prior to deciding on long-term HRT. Old age should not be considered an obstacle: HRT may be started at any age, and could be taken continuously for life. Low-dose estrogen (0.375 mg conjugated equine or 0.5–1 mg estradiol) may be appropriate beyond the age of 60 years since it probably provides adequate cardio- and osteo-protection on the one hand[15,37], but could be associated with fewer adverse effects and cancer risks on the other hand. Since the benefit of HRT for healthy, early postmenopausal women might be relatively small, we suggest that asymptomatic women without risk factors for CAD or osteoporosis could start HRT not at the beginning of menopause, but rather beyond the age of

60, to achieve maximal protective effects when CAD is most prevalent and possibly circumvent some of the risks associated with long-term HRT.

References

1. Tunstall-Pedoe H. Myth and paradox of coronary risk and the menopause. *Lancet* 1998;351:1425–7
2. Mosca L, Manson JE, Sutherland SE, Langer RD, Manolio T, Barrett-Connor E. Cardiovascular disease in women. A statement for healthcare professionals from the American Heart Association. *Circulation* 1997;96:2468–82
3. Rich-Edwards JW, Manson JE, Hennekens CH, Buring JE. The primary prevention of coronary heart disease in women. *N Engl J Med* 1995;332:1758–66
4. Grodstein F, Stampfer M. The epidemiology of coronary heart disease and estrogen replacement in postmenopausal women. *Prog Cardiovasc Dis* 1995;38:199–210
5. Pines A, Mijatovic V, van der Mooren MJ, Kenemans P. Hormone replacement therapy and cardioprotection: basic concepts and clinical considerations. *Eur J Obstet Gynecol Rep Biol* 1997;71:193–7
6. Mendelsohn ME, Karas RH. Mechanisms of disease: the protective effects of estrogen on the cardiovascular system. *N Engl J Med* 1999;340:1801–11
7. Greendale GA, Lee NP, Arriola ER. The menopause. *Lancet* 1999;353:571–80
8. Barrett-Connor E. Hormone replacement therapy. *Br Med J* 1998;317:457–61
9. Keating NL, Cleary PD, Rossi AS, Zaslavsky AM, Ayanian JZ. Use of hormone replacement therapy by postmenopausal women in the United States. *Ann Intern Med* 1999;130:545–53
10. Leveille SG, LaCroix AZ, Newton KM, Keenan NL. Older women and hormone replacement therapy: factors influencing late life initiation. *J Am Geriatr Soc* 1997;45:1496–500
11. Handa VL, Landerman RL, Hanlon JT, Harris T, Cohen HJ. Do older women use estrogen replacement? Data from the Duke Established Populations for Epidemiologic Studies of the Elderly (EPESE). *J Am Geriatr Soc* 1996;44:1–6
12. Ettinger B, Quesenberry C, Schroeder DA, Friedman G. Long-term postmenopausal estrogen therapy may be associated with increased risk of breast cancer: a cohort study. *Menopause* 1997;4:125–9
13. Salamone LM, Pressman AR, Seeley DG, Cauley JA. Estrogen replacement therapy. A survey of older women's attitudes. *Arch Intern Med* 1996;156:1293–7
14. Miller KL. Hormone replacement therapy in the elderly. *Clin Obstet Gynecol* 1996;39:912–32
15. Grodstein F, Stampfer MJ, Manson JE, *et al.* Postmenopausal estrogen and progestin use and the risk of cardiovascular disease. *N Engl J Med* 1996;335:453–61
16. Ettinger B, Friedman GD, Bush T, Quesenberry CP Jr. Decreased mortality associated with long-term postmenopausal estrogen therapy. *Obstet Gynecol* 1996;87:6–12
17. Sidney S, Petitti DB, Quesenberry CP Jr. Myocardial infarction and the use of estrogen and estrogen–progestogen in postmenopausal women. *Ann Intern Med* 1997;127:501–8
18. Psaty BM, Heckbert SR, Atkins D, *et al.* The risk of myocardial infarction associated with the combined use of estrogens and progestins in postmenopausal women. *Arch Intern Med* 1994;154:1333–9
19. Henderson BE, Paganini-Hill A, Ross RK. Reduced mortality in users of estrogen replacement therapy. *Arch Intern Med* 1991;151:75–8
20. Bush TL, Barrett-Connor E, Cowan LD, *et al.* Cardiovascular mortality and noncontraceptive use of estrogen in women. Results from the Lipid Research Clinics Program Follow Up Study. *Circulation* 1987;75:1102–9
21. Falkeborne M, Persson I, Adami H-O, *et al.* The risk of acute myocardial infarction after oestrogen and oestrogen–progestogen replacement. *Br J Obstet Gynecol* 1992;99:821–8
22. Sourander L, Rajala T, Raiha I, Makinen J, Erkkola R, Helenius H. Cardiovascular and cancer morbidity and mortality and sudden cardiac death in postmenopausal women on oestrogen replacement therapy (ERT). *Lancet* 1998;352:1965–9
23. Grodstein F, Stampfer MJ, Colditz GA, *et al.* Postmenopausal hormone therapy and mortality. *N Engl J Med* 1997;336:1769–75
24. Hemminki E, McPherson K. Impact of postmenopausal hormone therapy on cardiovas-

cular events and cancer: pooled data from clinical trials. *Br Med J* 1997;315:149–53

25. Manolio TA, Furberg CD, Shemanski L, *et al.* Association of postmenopausal estrogen use with cardiovascular disease and its risk factors in older women. *Circulation* 1993;88:2163–71

26. White MM, Zamudio S, Stevens T, *et al.* Estrogen, progesterone, and vascular reactivity: potential cellular mechanisms. *Endocr Rev* 1995; 6:739–51

27. Gruchow HW, Anderson AJ, Barboriak JJ, Sobocinsky KA. Postmenopausal use of estrogen and occlusion of coronary arteries. *Am Heart J* 1988;115:954–63

28. Hong MK, Romm PA, Reagen K, Green CE, Rackley CE. Effects of estrogen replacement therapy on serum lipid values and angiographically defined coronary artery disease in postmenopausal women. *Am J Cardiol* 1992;69:176–8

29. Newton KM, LaCroix AZ, McKnight B, *et al.* Estrogen replacement therapy and prognosis after first myocardial infarction. *Am J Epidemiol* 1997;145:269–77

30. Sullivan JM, Vander Zwaag R, Hughes JP, *et al.* Estrogen replacement and coronary artery disease: effect in survival in postmenopausal women. *Arch Intern Med* 1990;150:2557–62

31. Sullivan JM, El-Zeky F, Vander Zwaag R, Ramanathan KB. Effect on survival of estrogen replacement therapy after coronary artery bypass grafting. *Am J Cardiol* 1997;79:847–50

32. O'Keefe JH, Kim SC, Hall RR, Cochran VC, Lawhorn SL, McCallister BD. Estrogen replacement therapy after coronary angioplasty in women. *J Am Coll Cardiol* 1997;29:1–5

33. Hulley S, Grady D, Bush T, *et al.* Randomized trial of estrogen plus progestin for secondary prevention of coronary heart disease in postmenopausal women. *J Am Med Assoc* 1998;280: 605–13

34. Herrington DM, Fong J, Sempos CT, *et al.* Comparison of the Heart and Estrogen/Progestin Replacement Study (HERS) cohort with women with coronary disease from the National Health and Nutrition Examination Survey III (NHANES III). *Am Heart J* 1998;136:115–24

35. Alexander KP, Newby K, Harrington A, *et al.* Initiation of hormone replacement therapy after acute myocardial infarction is associated with more angina but less death/MI during follow-up. *J Am Coll Cardiol* 1999;33(Suppl A):315A

36. Mosca L, Grundy SM, Judelson D, *et al.* Guide to preventive cardiology for women. *Circulation* 1999;99:2480–4

37. Ettinger B, Genant HK, Stieger P, Madvig P. Low-dose micronized 17-β-estradiol prevents bone loss in postmenopausal women. *Am J Obstet Gynecol* 1992;166:479–88

Index